Gerontology for the Health Care Professional

Second Edition

Edited by

REGULA H. ROBNETT, PhD, OTR/L
Director and Associate Professor
Department of Occupational Therapy
University of New England

WALTER C. CHOP, MS, RRT
Chair and Professor
Respiratory Therapy Department
Southern Maine Community College

JONES AND BARTLETT PUBLISHERS
Sudbury, Massachusetts
BOSTON   TORONTO   LONDON   SINGAPORE

World Headquarters
Jones and Bartlett Publishers
40 Tall Pine Drive
Sudbury, MA 01776
978-443-5000
info@jbpub.com
www.jbpub.com

Jones and Bartlett Publishers
Canada
6339 Ormindale Way
Mississauga, Ontario L5V 1J2
Canada

Jones and Bartlett Publishers
International
Barb House, Barb Mews
London W6 7PA
United Kingdom

Jones and Bartlett's books and products are available through most bookstores and online booksellers. To contact Jones and Bartlett Publishers directly, call 800-832-0034, fax 978-443-8000, or visit our website www.jbpub.com.

Substantial discounts on bulk quantities of Jones and Bartlett's publications are available to corporations, professional associations, and other qualified organizations. For details and specific discount information, contact the special sales department at Jones and Bartlett via the above contact information or send an email to specialsales@jbpub.com.

The authors, editor, and publisher have made every effort to provide accurate information. However, they are not responsible for errors, omissions, or for any outcomes related to the use of the contents of this book and take no responsibility for the use of the products and procedures described. Treatments and side effects described in this book may not be applicable to all people; likewise, some people may require a dose or experience a side effect that is not described herein. Drugs and medical devices are discussed that may have limited availability controlled by the Food and Drug Administration (FDA) for use only in a research study or clinical trial. Research, clinical practice, and government regulations often change the accepted standard in this field. When consideration is being given to use of any drug in the clinical setting, the health care provider or reader is responsible for determining FDA status of the drug, reading the package insert, and reviewing prescribing information for the most up-to-date recommendations on dose, precautions, and contraindications, and determining the appropriate usage for the product. This is especially important in the case of drugs that are new or seldom used.

Production Credits
Publisher: David Cella
Associate Editor: Maro Gartside
Production Manager: Julie Champagne Bolduc
Production Assistant: Jessica Steele Newfell
Senior Marketing Manager: Sophie Fleck
Manufacturing and Inventory Control Supervisor:
  Amy Bacus
Composition: SNP Best-set Typesetter Ltd., Hong Kong
Cover Design: Scott Moden
Photo Research and Permissions Manager: Kimberly Potvin
Cover Image: © Halina Yakushevich/ShutterStock, Inc.
Printing and Binding: Malloy, Inc.
Cover Printing: Malloy, Inc.

Library of Congress Cataloging-in-Publication Data
Gerontology for the health care professional / [edited by] Regula H. Robnett, Walter C. Chop. — 2nd ed.
  p. ; cm.
  Includes bibliographical references and index.
  ISBN 978-0-7637-5605-5 (pbk. : alk. paper)
  1. Older people—Health and hygiene. 2. Gerontology. 3. Aging. I. Robnett, Regula H. II. Chop, Walter C.
  [DNLM: 1. Geriatrics. 2. Aged. 3. Aging—physiology. WT 100 G3753 2010]
  RA564.8.G468 2010
  618.97—dc22
                              2009008728
6048
Printed in the United States of America
13 12 11 10 09   10 9 8 7 6 5 4 3 2 1

RA
564.8
.G468
2010

DEDICATION

To our parents and grandparents, who made it to later life and taught us that "old age is not for sissies." Also, to those not pictured, but still in our hearts: Fritz, Robert, Evelyn, Alexander, Anna, Agnes, and John.

— Bette Davis

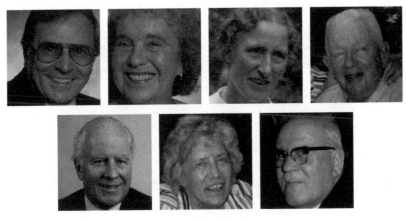

(Courtesy of the authors)

BRIEF CONTENTS

CONTENTS

INTRODUCTION

"The Times They Are a-Changin'," written by Bob Dylan in 1964,[1] seems like an appropriate introduction—more than a half century later—for a textbook related to working with older people because the times are changing: The world is getting older as the average age of human beings is increasing. The average German is already 40 years old whereas the average American is just over 35. By 2050, the average German will be nearly 52, and their American counterpart will be nearly 42.[2] The fastest growing segment of the population is composed of those older than age 85, which affects the overall population average. Also, the older population—especially if we include everyone of retirement age—is becoming more diverse. Therefore, it is increasingly more difficult to describe older people in simplistic stereotypical terms. As time goes by, each member of the older cohort becomes more distinct from the average or expected norm. We must come to realize that although some octogenarians are living well on their own, others in their 60s are already dependent and living with multiple chronic conditions.

Recently, a student reported on a case study in rehabilitation of a 94-year-old who came in following orthopedic surgery and made quick progress to return home to live independently. As a member of the audience, I asked her whether the case was surprising to her, given the patient's age. As I had anticipated, she immediately stated that yes, she was very surprised. My comment to her was that next time she works with someone that old or even older she would not be surprised but rather be open to the possibility that such progress is a pleasant and expected outcome. Hope for the future—no matter the age!

This *Second Edition* of *Gerontology for the Health Care Professional* presents an overview of the life changes associated with older age as well as the pertinent issues involved in caring for older people. Again, we present basic information often intended as a springboard for further inquiry. We hope that the chapters incentivize you to explore issues further to deepen your understanding of late life with its many convolutions and intricacies.

The text starts with a demographic overview and a review of the social aspects of aging, focusing additional information on global aging as well. An in-depth chapter on the physiologic and pathologic aspects of aging provides an excellent reference to which you can return to for valuable information time and again. In Chapters 4 and 5, we explore the cognitive and functional changes of aging and provide specific helpful hints to use when working with older adults who may have functional deficits. These are not intended to be recipes for intervention but rather offered as suggestions that may be useful and may lead to more individualized care. We added a section on sleep disturbances because individuals are more prone to developing sleep disorders with advancing age.

The text continues with Chapter 6, which provides essential content related to pharmacology; this is especially important given the fact that older adults consume more medications than other age groups. Chapter 7 provides nutritional information specifically related to late life. Those older than 65 consume approximately 30% of prescribed and 40% of over-the-counter medications.[3] Chapter 8 covers important information related to sexuality and aging, and Chapter 9 explores the continuum of care from independent to dependent living; one's environment can have a profound effect on one's performance in life. Chapter 10 explores legal issues related to aging while encouraging those needing more in-depth legal advice to contact an attorney. A compilation of information about pertinent health care providers can be found in Chapter 11, and Chapter 12 speculates about the future of aging in our society. The accelerated rate of change in our world today will likely affect the next generation of older people in unprecedented ways, just as the baby boomer generation will change the face of aging in ways about which we can only speculate. In the final chapter, Chapter 13, health literacy is the focus, specifically communicating with older people in clear and concise ways.

By providing key terms, behavioral objectives, review questions, and learning activities, each chapter is intended to be an invaluable resource for the reader interested in gerontology. The addition of a glossary to this fully updated *Second Edition* should make it easier to access the meaning of key words or phrases. We hope that the text proves to be a timely, useful, and worthwhile addition to the library of each health care professional and health care student. Thank you for picking it up. Enjoy your reading experience.

—*Regula H. Robnett, PhD, OTR/L, and Walter C. Chop, MS, RRT*
Editors

REFERENCES

1. Dylan, B. The Times They Are a-Changin'. *The Times They Are a-Changin'* [album]. New York: Columbia Records; 1964.
2. International Institute for Applied Systems Analysis. 2005. Nature: Average Remaining Lifetimes Can Increase as Human Populations Age. Retrieved January 5, 2009, from http://www.iiasa.ac.at/Admin/INF/PR/pdf-files/2005/Nature_2005_pop_pressbackground.pdf
3. National Institute of Aging. 2003. Medications and Older People. Retrieved January 7, 2009, from http://www.fda.gov/FDAC/features/1997/697_old.html

ACKNOWLEDGMENTS

Many individuals have contributed to the successful completion of this text. We would like to thank those who have helped our endeavors with compiling, writing, and reviewing the *Second Edition* of *Gerontology for the Health Care Professional*.

Our heartfelt thanks to the following people:

- Our colleagues at Southern Maine Community College and the University of New England, including Nancy Smith, Sally Doe, Bob Hawkes, Nancy MacRae, David Sandmire, Sue Stableford, and Betsey Gray. Also, particular thanks to reference librarians Bobbie Gray, Susan Nestor, and Bryan Strniste.
- All of our contributing authors, who are as devoted to this topic as we are.
- Jones and Bartlett Publishers, especially David Cella for encouraging us to proceed with a *Second Edition*, Barb Bartoszek for her assistance with marketing the text, and Maro Gartside and Jess Newell for their gentle prodding, as well as expert guiding, along the way.
- Our dear families, whose patience and understanding keep us going.

If we inadvertently let anyone out, please forgive us.

— *Regi and Walter*

CONTRIBUTING AUTHORS

Shefali Ajmera, MS, RD, LD
Chief Registered Dietitian
Dallas, Texas

Kimberly Hillman Bassett, MS
Director of Operations, Medical and
    Academic Affairs
Maine Medical Center

Nancy Brossoie, PhD
Senior Research Associate
Center for Gerontology
Virginia Polytechnic Institute

Sally Doe, MS, RTR
Chair, Radiography Department
Southern Maine Community College

Paul D. Ewald, PhD
Academic Dean of Regis College
Regis University

Betsey Gray, MSW
Director of Field Education, School of
    Social Work
University of New England

**Robert M. Hawkes, MS, PA-C,
    NREMT-P**
Chair, Emergency Medical Services
    Department
Southern Maine Community College

Nancy MacRae, MS, OTR/L, FAOTA
Associate Professor and Graduate
    Coordinator, Occupational Therapy
    Department
University of New England

John Murray, BS, RPSGT, RRT
Chair, Cardiopulmonary Sciences
    Department
Program Director, Sleep Technology
Northern Essex Community College

Thomas D. Nolin, PharmD, PhD
Assistant Professor, School of Pharmacy
University of Pittsburgh

Ann O'Sullivan, OTR/L, LSW
Family Caregiver Specialist
Southern Maine Agency on Aging

David M. Sandmire, MD
Professor, Biology Department
University of New England

Linda Simonsen, BS
Interdisciplinary Team Leader and
    Coordinator of Clinical Education
Division of Rehabilitation Medicine
Maine Medical Center

Nancy E. Smith, MS, RN
Professor and Chair, Health Science
    Division and Nursing Department
Southern Maine Community College

Sue Stableford, MPH, MSB
Director, Health Literacy Institute
University of New England

Timothy M. Vogel, Esq.
Attorney at Law
Vogel & Dubois

Lisa A. Wendler, PharmD
Clinical Pharmacy Specialist
Division of Family Medicine/Geriatrics
Maine Medical Center

Louise D. Whitney, MS, RD
Registered Dietitian

<table>
<tr><td>Chapter</td><td>1</td></tr>
</table>

DEMOGRAPHIC TRENDS OF AN AGING SOCIETY

WALTER C. CHOP, MS, RRT

I refuse to take seriously society's idea that at the arbitrary age of 65 I am suddenly a lamp going out.
—*Roger S. Mills, quoting an elder in* History of Elder Hostel, *1993*

Chapter Outline

America: An Aging Society
Global Aging
Gender and Age
Race and Aging
Geographic Distribution: Where U.S.
    Older Adults Live

Marital Status
Economic Status
Health Care
Long-Term Care

Behavioral Objectives

Upon completion of this chapter, the reader will be able to:

1. Describe why the "graying of America" is occurring.
2. Identify the fastest growing segment of the population.
3. Discuss life expectancy in terms of gender.
4. Contrast aging by races in the United States.
5. Identify the states where the largest number of individuals older than 65 years live.
6. Discuss older adults in context of their lifestyles (married or living alone).
7. Contrast the economic status of those older than 65 years in terms of race and marital status.
8. List disease conditions older adults are most likely to experience.

I

9. Discuss health care expenditures for those older than 65 years and the demand placed on the health care system by them.
10. Describe pertinent issues involving the long-term care of older adults.

Key Terms

Age cohort

Baby boom generation

Demographics of aging

Elderly, elders

Long-term care

Medicaid

Medicare

Old-old

Social Security

Third-agers

Young-old

AMERICA: AN AGING SOCIETY

The graying of America continues to accelerate as the first of the **baby boom generation** (those Americans born between 1946 and 1964) turned 60 years of age in 2006. From that time on, approximately one American will turn 60 years of age every 7.5 seconds for the next 18 years. This will have dramatic consequences on our entire society, especially our health care system.

In 1900, only 4%, or 1 in 25, of Americans were older than 65 years of age. The population of those older than 65 numbered 3.1 million in 1900. (See **Figure 1-1**.) As of July 2003, this same **age cohort** numbered 35.9 million, representing 12.7% of the total population. To put this in perspective, the population of those older than 65 years has increased by more than 2 million people (7% of the population) since 1990, while the younger-than-65 age group increased by only 4% (**Table 1-1**).

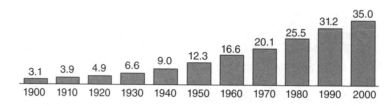

FIGURE 1-1   Population aged 65 and over: 1900 to 2000 (in millions).

Note: The reference population for these data is the resident population.

Source: 1900 to 1940, 1970, and 1980, U.S. Bureau of the Census, 1983, Table 42; 1950, U.S. Bureau of the Census, 1953, Table 38; 1960, U.S. Bureau of the Census, 1964, Table 15.5; 1990, U.S. Bureau of the Census, 1991, Table QT-P1; 2000, U.S. Census Bureau, 2001, Table PCT12.

TABLE 1-1 Total Population and Older Population by Age in the United States: 1900 to 2000 (in thousands).

Year and Census Date[1]	Total Population	65 and over						
		Total		65 to 74		75 to 84		85 and over	
		Number	Percent	Number	Percent	Number	Percent	Number	Percent
1900 (June 1)	75,995	3,080	4.1	2,187	2.9	771	1.0	122	0.2
1910 (April 15)	91,972	3,950	4.3	2,793	3.0	989	1.1	167	0.2
1920 (January 1)	105,711	4,933	4.7	3,464	3.3	1,259	1.2	210	0.2
1930 (April 1)	122,775	6,634	5.4	4,721	3.8	1,641	1.3	272	0.2
1940 (April 1)	131,669	9,019	6.8	6,376	4.8	2,278	1.7	365	0.3
1950 (April 1)	150,697	12,270	8.1	8,415	5.6	3,278	2.2	577	0.4
1960 (April 1)	179,323	16,560	9.2	10,997	6.1	4,633	2.6	929	0.5
1970 (April 1)	203,212	20,066	9.9	12,435	6.1	6,119	3.0	1,511	0.7
1980 (April 1)	226,546	25,549	11.3	15,581	6.9	7,729	3.4	2,240	1.0
1990 (April 1)	248,710	31,242	12.6	18,107	7.3	10,055	4.0	3,080	1.2
2000 (April 1)	281,422	34,992	12.4	18,391	6.5	12,361	4.4	4,240	1.5

[1]Data for 1900 to 1950 exclude Alaska and Hawaii.

Note: The reference population for these data is the resident population.

Sources: 1900 to 1940, 1970, and 1980, U.S. Bureau of the Census, 1983, Table 42; 1950, U.S. Bureau of the Census, 1953, Table 38; 1960, U.S. Bureau of the Census, 1964, Table 46; 1990, U.S. Bureau of the Census, 1991, Table 46; 1990, U.S. Bureau of the Census, 1991, Table QT-P1; 2000, U.S. Census Bureau, 2001, Table PCT12.

Growth of the older-than-65 cohort will continue to increase as baby boomers begin turning 65 in 2010. This will cause yet another rise in the **elderly** segment of the population.

Projections for the year 2030 estimate that 22%, or 70.2 million, of Americans will be older than the age of 65. To get a true feel for the changing demography of America, note the baby boom bulge on the population chart in **Figure 1-2**. You can easily envision the top-heavy appearance of this same chart 25 years from today.

An even more dramatic aging trend exists among those older than 85 years of age, often referred to as the old-old. This age cohort is expected to double—from 4.7 million in 2003 to 9.6 million in 2030—and double again to 20.9 million in 2050.[1] The number of those elderly exceeding 100 years of age reached 50,000 in 2000.[1]

Looking beyond the **demographics of aging**, let us now consider what the term *old age* implies. *Old age* is a difficult and complex concept to grasp because our idea of aging is constantly changing. What we thought of as old in the 19th century is considered middle age now. Policymakers have used the age of 65 as a marker in establishing policies affecting older adults. Some biologists, however, tell us that a person's biological age is more important than the person's chronological age when determining an individual's health status.[2] Bernice Neugarten was the first to coin the term **young-old**, which denotes relatively healthy and financially independent elders of any age, although usually those between 55 and 74 years of age.[2] The so-called **old-old** usually refers to those older than age 75 whose activities are often limited by functional disabilities. The French have a similar method of categorizing older adults. They use the terms **third-agers**, or *elder,* when referring to those persons 65 to 85 years of age. Their term *old-old* refers only to those individuals older than age 85.

Whatever classification of aging you choose to use is a matter of preference as long as you realize the limitations and variations implied by the term *old age.* The salient point to note is that there is a great amount of variability among *old-agers.* Whereas many individuals moving into the "third age" and beyond are of sound mind and body as well as financially secure, others in this same age cohort are experiencing functional declines as well as health care or financial needs.

GLOBAL AGING

In 2000, around the world, the number of persons age 60 years and older was 605 million. By 2050, that number is projected to reach 2 billion. This will make the over-60 population larger than the population of children (0–14 years) for the first time in human history.[2]

Approximately 60% of the world's older population now live in developing nations—an estimated 279 million people. This number is projected to increase to 690 million (71%) by 2030. A number of these less developed nations are also experiencing a downturn in natural population increase (births minus deaths). A similar decline has already occurred in the industrialized nations. As this rate of downturn in natural population

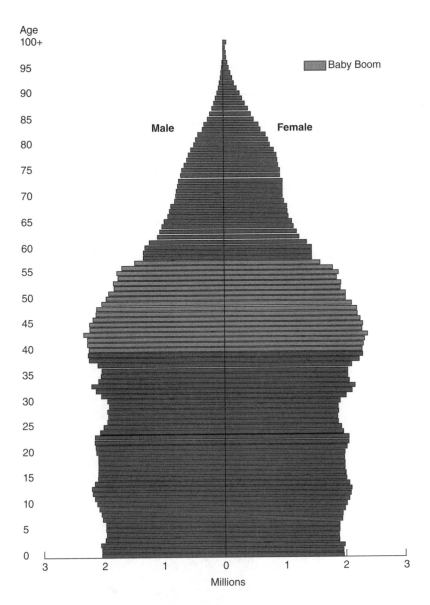

FIGURE 1-2   Population by age and sex: 2003.
Note: The reference population for these data is the resident population.
Source: U.S. Census Bureau, 2004.

continues to accelerate, elders will make up an ever greater proportion of each nation's total population.[3]

The world's oldest country is Italy, currently with 19.1% of its population over the age of 65. The world's 20 oldest countries are all in Europe (see **Figure 1-3**) except Japan, which is the second oldest with 19% of its population over 65.[3]

GENDER AND AGE

Women make up the majority of elderly people in almost every country in the world. Today in the United States, and throughout most countries, women can expect to live, on average, 7 years longer than men (Figure 1-2). As of 2003, life expectancy was 80 years for women and 74 years for men.[3] Life expectancy projections for 2020 are 81.8 years for women and 74.9 years for men.[4] This gender difference in life expectancy persists throughout the aging process.[1] In fact, among those 85 and older, there are only 46 men for every 100 women (**Figure 1-4**). This greater longevity in women is because heart

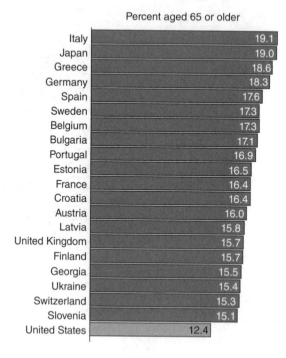

Percent aged 65 or older

Italy	19.1
Japan	19.0
Greece	18.6
Germany	18.3
Spain	17.6
Sweden	17.3
Belgium	17.3
Bulgaria	17.1
Portugal	16.9
Estonia	16.5
France	16.4
Croatia	16.4
Austria	16.0
Latvia	15.8
United Kingdom	15.7
Finland	15.7
Georgia	15.5
Ukraine	15.4
Switzerland	15.3
Slovenia	15.1
United States	12.4

FIGURE I-3 The world's 20 oldest countries and the United States: 2004.
Note: The United States ranks 38th.
Source: U.S. Census Bureau, International Data Base. Retrieved January 30, 2009, from http://www.census.gov/ipc/www/idbnew.html.

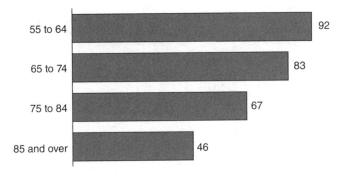

FIGURE 1-4   Sex ratio of people 55 years and over by age: 2002 (men per 100 women).
Source: U.S. Census Bureau, Annual Demographic Supplement to the March 2002 Current Population Survey.

attacks, cancer, and stroke—the major killer diseases—are or have been more common in men. Other factors influencing female longevity may have to do with women's greater sensitivity to changes in their body condition, which make them more likely to seek out earlier medical intervention. Women may also handle stress better and have better social support systems than their male counterparts do.

RACE AND AGING

The aging baby boomer generation will contain a far greater racial and ethnic mix than did any generation that preceded it. This results from both increasing immigration from primarily nonwhite countries and a lower fertility rate among the white population.[3] The U.S. Census Bureau predicts that nonwhite populations will account for approximately half (39%) of the U.S. population by 2050 (see **Figure 1-5**).[1]

Life expectancy for nonwhite Americans is less than it is for whites. African American men and women currently live on average 6 and 5 years less, respectively, than their white counterparts.[5] However, if a black person of either gender lives to age 65, his or her life expectancy is much closer to whites than it was at birth.[1] Other ethnic minorities in the United States, including Mexican Americans and Native Americans, have life expectancies lower than African Americans.[5] Even with their relatively low percentages, the population of minority older adults is growing at a faster rate than their white counterparts. The U.S. Census Bureau projects that minority populations will represent 25% of all the elderly people by 2030, up from 14% in 1990.[6] Examining this trend further, we see individuals older than 65 in specific ethnic groups increasing between 1990 and 2030 by the following percentages: Caucasians, 93%; Hispanics, 555%; African Americans, 160%; Native Americans, 231%; and Asians and Pacific Islanders, 693%.[3] Of these groups, Native Americans have the shortest life expectancy of any minority group (45–50 years of age) and also the lowest standard of living.

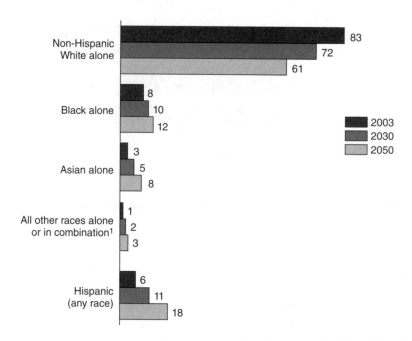

FIGURE I-5   Population aged 65 and over by race and Hispanic origin: 2003, 2030, and 2050 (percentage of total population aged 65 and over).
[1]The race group "All other races alone or in combination" includes American Indian and Alaska Native alone, Native Hawaiian and Other Pacific Islander alone, and all people who reported two or more races.
Note: The reference population for these data is the resident population.
Source: U.S. Census Bureau, 2004.

As noted previously, besides an overall increase in the number of older Americans, there will also be a more heterogeneous mix of ethnic and cultural backgrounds. This will require health care providers to become even more culturally sensitive, acquiring new knowledge and skills to better recognize and respect cultural differences. Health care professionals will also need to understand the diseases, disorders, and concerns more common not only to specific age groups but to particular ethnic groups as well (**Table 1-2**).

In some elderly minority groups, social factors may play a role in reinforcing negative health patterns and behaviors. These factors may contribute to shorter life spans of certain minorities, as in the case of African Americans. Yet this same minority can expect to outlive their white counterparts if they live to age 80. At this point a racial mortality crossover phenomenon occurs in which life expectancy for blacks exceeds that of whites.

GEOGRAPHIC DISTRIBUTION: WHERE U.S. OLDER ADULTS LIVE

As of 2000, nine states had more than 1 million people aged 65 and over—California, New York, Florida, Pennsylvania, Texas, Illinois, Ohio, Michigan, and New Jersey. Cali-

TABLE 1-2 Prevalence of Selected Chronic Conditions by Race/Ethnicity in the United States: 1997–2006.

Condition	All (%)	Hispanic (%)	Non-Hispanic White (%)	Non-Hispanic Black (%)
All types of heart disease	31	22.5	32	26.9
Coronary heart disease	21.8	17.5	22.4	19.6
Hypertension	53.3	54.1	51.2	70
Stroke	9.3	6.4	8.8	16.4
Emphysema	5.7		6.3	
Asthma	10.6	8.5	10.6	12.6
Hay fever	7.5	10.8	7	6.5
Sinusitis	13.8	9.9	14.1	15.5
Chronic bronchitis	6.1	5.1	6.4	4.4
Any cancer	21.2	12.6	23.3	11.4
Breast cancer	3.4		3.7	1.5
Cervical cancer	1		1	
Prostate cancer	10.2		10.3	11.1
Colon/rectal cancer	2.4		2.7	
Uterine cancer	1.6		1.6	
Lung cancer	1.1		1.1	
Melanoma	1.6		2	
Skin cancer	6.1		7.3	
Diabetes	18.1	24.2	16.1	27.9
Ulcer	10.8	8.4	11.1	8.7
Kidney disease	3.4		3.4	4
Liver disease	1.5		1.4	
Arthritic symptoms	—	—	—	—
Chronic joint symptoms	43.4	40.8	43.5	49.6
Doctor's diagnosis of arthritis	49.6	38.7	50.4	56.2

Source: Centers for Disease Control and Prevention, National Health Interview Survey. Prevalence of Selected Conditions by Age, Sex, and Race/Ethnicity, 1997–2006.

fornia had more than 3.5 million elder Americans, and there were more than 2.8 and 2.4 million elders living in Florida and New York, respectively (**Figure 1-6**).

In 2000, Florida registered 17.6% of its population as older than the age of 65. On a percentage basis, other states with large elderly populations include Pennsylvania

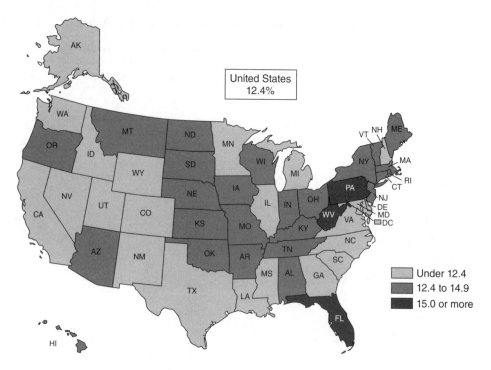

FIGURE 1-6   Percentage aged 65 and over of state population: 2000.
Note: The reference population for these data is the resident population.
Source: U.S. Census Bureau, 2001, Table P12.

(15.6%), West Virginia (15.3%), Iowa (14.9%), North Dakota (14.7%), Rhode Island (14.5%), Maine (14.4%), South Dakota (14.3%), and Arkansas (14.0%).

States experiencing a dramatic increase in their older-than-65 populations between 1994 and 2000 include Nevada (71.5%), Alaska (59.6%), Arizona (39.5%), New Mexico (30.1%), Hawaii (28.5%), Utah (29.9%), Colorado (26.3%), and Wyoming (22.2%).[1] (See **Table 1-3** for other locations.) This trend seems to indicate, for the most part, a continued movement toward warmer states, with the exception of Alaska and the Rocky Mountain states of Utah, Wyoming, and Colorado. It also points out the apparent appeal of living in less densely populated states, some of which also have lower costs of living. Older individuals moving to these states are generally affluent and well educated. They may also have existing ties to these new areas such as family, friends, or previously purchased retirement property. Many are also seeking escape from metropolitan life to the relative safety and comfort of rural or small-town USA.

In general, older Americans have a tendency to change residences less frequently than their younger counterparts do. The result of this has led to an increased "graying" of certain communities. A number of counties have elderly populations exceeding 20% of

TABLE 1-3 Population Aged 65 and Over and Percent Change for Regions, Divisions, and States: 1990 to 2000.

Region, Division, and State	65 and over		Change, 1990 to 2000	
	1990	2000	Number	Percent
West South Central	2,959,838	3,419,430	459,592	15.5
Arkansas	350,058	374,019	23,961	6.8
Louisiana	468,991	516,929	47,938	10.2
Oklahoma	424,213	455,950	31,737	7.5
Texas	1,716,576	2,072,532	355,956	20.7
Mountain	1,523,825	2,029,846	506,021	33.2
Montana	106,497	120,949	14,452	13.6
Idaho	121,265	145,916	24,651	20.3
Wyoming	47,195	57,693	10,498	22.2
Colorado	329,443	416,073	86,630	26.3
New Mexico	163,062	212,225	49,163	30.1
Arizona	478,774	667,839	189,065	39.5
Utah	149,958	190,222	40,264	26.9
Nevada	127,631	218,929	91,298	71.5
Pacific	4,249,538	4,892,283	642,745	15.1
Washington	575,288	662,148	86,860	15.1
Oregon	391,324	438,177	46,853	12.0
California	3,135,662	3,595,658	460,106	14.7
Alaska	22,369	35,699	13,330	59.6
Hawaii	125,005	160,601	35,596	28.5

Note: The reference population for these data is the resident population.
Sources: 1990, U.S. Bureau of the Census, 1991, Table P011; 2000, U.S. Census Bureau, 2001, Table P12.

the whole population. Many of these counties are located in the nation's predominantly agricultural heartland, where older persons have stayed on while the youth have moved on.

MARITAL STATUS

In 2003, 71% of elderly men were married, compared with only 41% of women.[7] What accounts for this, in large part, is the fact that women outlive men, thus increasing the ratio of widows to widowers. As of 2002, 41% of women aged 65 to 84 were widowed as compared to 11% of men in this same age group.[6] Worldwide divorce rates of older persons is relatively low. In the United States, divorce in the over-65 population has remained relatively low (9% in 2003), but it is expected that this will increase dramatically.[3] To date, worldwide divorce rates of older people are relatively low because divorce is considered less socially acceptable by this earlier generation. However, in the United States and worldwide, the number and percentage of divorcing elders are likely to increase as younger generations, who tend to find divorce a more acceptable option, reach old age.

ECONOMIC STATUS

The economic status of elderly Americans is more varied than any other age group. Looking solely at income, on average persons 65 and older, receive less income than those younger than 65. In 2004, the median income of males older than 65 was $21,102 as compared to $12,080 for females.[7] These figures may be somewhat misleading, however, because older adults have greater tax advantages, often have their home mortgages paid off, and are covered by **Medicare** insurance.[8]

Sources of income for those 65 and older in 2003 were as follows: **Social Security** (39%), asset income (14%), public and private pensions (19%), earnings (25%), and all other sources (3%).[7]

As of 2005, poverty levels for older adults were 9.8%. In terms of race, poverty figures for those older than 65 show 7.5% of whites at the poverty level, compared with 23.9% of African Americans and 18.7% of Hispanics. Older women had almost twice the poverty rate of older men (12% to 7%). Because 62% of those older than 85 years of age are women, many of whom are widows, the economic hardships of this age group are likely to intensify. The highest poverty rate among the elderly (39.9%) was experienced by African American women who lived alone.[7]

HEALTH CARE

In a 2004 assessment of general health, 36.7% of noninstitutionalized persons age 65 and older claimed their health was good to excellent. This compares with individuals younger than 65, 66% of whom considered their health to be good to excellent.[7] There was not a significant difference between the genders. However, only 25.1% of elderly African Americans rated their health as good to excellent.

The majority (80%) of elderly persons have at least one chronic condition. In 2002–2003, the most frequently occurring conditions among older adults were hypertension (51%), diagnosed arthritis (48%), heart disease (31%), cancer of any type (21%), diabetes (16%), and sinusitis (14%).[7] Heart disease, cancer, and stroke account for 6 of every 10 deaths among those older than 65 years. Other diseases that rank high as causes of death in older adults include chronic obstructive pulmonary disease (COPD), pneumonia, influenza, and diabetes. According to the 2000 U.S. Census, 14 million noninstitutionalized elderly people have some kind of disability. The good news is that studies have shown, over the past two decades, a decline in the rate of disability and functional limitation in older persons.[1] Alzheimer's disease, confirmed on autopsy, is the leading cause of cognitive impairment in older adults.

Those 65 and older visit a physician, on average, 6.8 times per year as compared with 3.8 visits per year in the younger-than-65 cohort. In 2003, approximately 1 person in 3 (13.2 million total) older than the age of 65 had a hospital stay. This is three times the comparable rate for persons of any age. Average length of stay in the hospital was 5.8 days for those over 65 as compared to 4.8 days for persons of all ages.[7] By 2030, with an estimated 71 million Americans older than the age of 65, health care spending is projected to increase by 25%.[9]

Health care expenditures are unbalanced. Most health care dollars are spent near the end of a person's life. Health care spending per person for those over age 65 was $14,797 in 2004, which was 5.6 times higher than spending per child ($2,650 in 2004) and 3.3 times higher than spending in those aged 16–64 years ($4,511 in 2004).[10] It has been estimated that by the year 2025, nearly two-thirds of the U.S. health care budget will be devoted to services for older adults.[11] This will place incredible demands on the health care system and its professionals. The question remains as to whether we will be ready to handle this staggering demand for health care services, to say nothing of affording the astronomical costs!

LONG-TERM CARE

As of 1994, approximately 7.3 million persons older than the age of 65 required some form of **long-term care**, whether in a nursing home, assisted living center, or at home with some form of provider-based health care service.[12] It is estimated that by the year 2060 this number will increase to 24 million. Since 1966, when Medicare and **Medicaid** were introduced, the percentage of older adults requiring nursing home care has more than tripled from 2.5% to 9%. The average annual cost for a private room in a skilled nursing home is $76,460.[13]

In the population of those older than 85, one in four are eligible for placement in long-term care. Because this represents the fastest-growing segment of the population, the demand for nursing home beds will increase dramatically. Right now the number of nursing home beds is increasing by only half the rate at which this age cohort is increasing.

Elders who find themselves in long-term care facilities will, on average, use their life savings within 1 year. At that point they may become eligible for public assistance or Medicaid. Considering the sharp increase in need, the question that begs asking is, Where will the funds come from to continue support of this program? This presents another problem for our ever-aging society, especially considering the ongoing debates to cut health care benefits such as Medicare.

As a result of the trend to get patients out of the hospital and back home as soon as possible, home health care has seen a dramatic increase. Expenditures for home health services were $7.9 billion in 1990. This is expected to increase to $19.8 billion by the year 2020.[1] The advantage of home care is that it allows elderly persons to remain in the community, which can be more beneficial than living in a long-term care facility from both a personal as well as a financial perspective. With an ever-increasing need for efficiency as a result of runaway costs, health care providers are being asked to become ever more productive and proficient in their delivery of elder services in alternative settings.

SUMMARY

Demographics clearly indicate that the United States, as a nation, is growing older. On January 1, 2006, one American began turning 60 years of age every 7.5 seconds. This aging baby boom generation will effect massive societal changes. These changes will occur in terms of gender, race, geography, marital status, economics, and health care. The number of women will continue to surpass the number of men, with aging African Americans, Hispanics, Native Americans, Asians, and Pacific Islanders increasing by a greater percentage than whites. Some states will be harder hit by an aging boom than others. Social Security and other government entitlement programs are likely to be stretched perhaps to the breaking point, or at least to the point where they need major revamping. The health care system, perhaps most of all, will experience demands never previously encountered.

Health care professionals will be at the forefront of this aging tidal wave as it washes over and through our health care systems. Although hospital admissions and length of stays have been on the decline since 1996, this may not be the case from 2010 to 2030 as baby boomers descend upon health care institutions. Even without dramatic increases in hospital admissions, long-term care and home care are expected to experience a dramatic rise in patient volume. It is not unrealistic to expect that two out of three health care professionals will be working in either long-term care or home care in the future. The majority of the patients in these settings will be older adults. Therefore, it benefits health care professionals to have an understanding of trends and projections as they relate to the "graying of America."

Review Questions

1. As of January 1, 2006, one American will turn 60 every _____ for the next 18 years.
   A. 7.5 minutes
   B. 7.5 seconds
   C. Hour
   D. Week

2. The fastest-growing segment of the population consists of individuals who are
   A. 1–18 years of age
   B. 24–40 years of age
   C. 30–50 years of age
   D. 50–65 years of age
   E. Older than 85 years of age

3. The young-old, according to Bernice Neugarten, refers to those who are
   A. 45–55 years of age
   B. 55–74 years of age
   C. 65–75 years of age
   D. 60–80 years of age

4. Women can expect to live, on average, _____ years longer than men.
   A. 2
   B. 5
   C. 7
   D. 10

5. Which ethnic group of those older than 65 is expected to increase at the most rapid rate between 1990 and 2030?
   A. African Americans
   B. Native Americans
   C. Whites
   D. Hispanics
   E. Southeast Asians

6. As of 2000, the state that had the largest percentage of its population older than 65 was
   A. Rhode Island
   B. California
   C. North Dakota
   D. Florida
   E. Vermont

7. In 2002, widows exceeded widowers by a ratio of
   A. 1:2
   B. 1:3
   C. 1:4
   D. 1:8

8. Poverty levels for African Americans 65 or older are approximately
   A. 10%
   B. 15%
   C. 25%
   D. 50%

9. Health care spending in those older than 65 is _____ that of those ages 16–64?
   A. 2.2 times
   B. 3.3 times
   C. 5.6 times
   D. 8.0 times

10. What type of care is likely to increase dramatically in those over 85?
    A. Home care
    B. Medicare
    C. Long-term care
    D. All of the above

Learning Activities

1. List what you believe will be some trends set by the baby boomer generation as it ages.
2. Design an elder community in a United States location. What factors would you consider in the design? Where would you place this community?
3. Which health care services and/or products are likely to be required by an aging population?
4. What will be possible roles and responsibilities of future health care professionals in long-term care facilities and home care?
5. Visualize yourself and your friends as older than 65 years of age. Where will you be living? What will you be doing? What will be your hobbies/roles? What will society be like?

REFERENCES

1. He, W, Sengupta, M, Velkoff, VA, De Barros, KA. *65+ in the United States: 2005*. U.S. Census Bureau, Current Population Reports, P23-209. Washington, DC: U.S. Government Printing Office, 2005.

2. Neugarten, B. The Rise of the Young-Old. In R Gross et al. (eds.). *The New Old: Struggling for a Decent Aging*. Garden City, NY: Doubleday Anchor, 1978.

3. Kinsella, K, Phillips, D. Global aging: The challenge of success. *Population Bulletin*, March 2005;60(1):7.

4. Kinsella, K, Velkoff, VA. *An aging World: 2001*. U.S. Census Bureau, Series P95/01-1. Washington, DC: U.S. Government Printing Office, 2001.

5. Oriol, W. The demographics of an aging revolution. In *Preparing for an Aging Society: Changes*

and Challenges. Washington, DC: National Council on Aging, 1992.

6. Smith, D. *The Older Population in the United States: March 2002.* U.S. Census Bureau, Current Populaton Reports, P20-546. Washington, DC: U.S. Census Bureau, 2003.

7. Greenberg, S. *A Profile of Older Americans: 2005.* Washington, DC: Administration on Aging, U.S. Department of Health and Human Services, 2005.

8. Grad, S. *Income of the Population 55 or Older, 2000.* Washington, DC: Social Security Administration Office of Research and Statistics, January 2000.

9. Centers for Disease Control and Prevention and Merck Company Foundation. *The State of Aging Health in America 2007.* Whitehouse Station, NJ: Merck Company Foundation, 2007.

10. Hartman, M, Catlin, A, Lassman, D, Cylus, J, Heffler, S. U.S. health spending by age, selected years through 2004. *Health Affairs,* November 6, 2007.

11. Chop, W. Resources for an aging population. *RT: The Journal for Respiratory Care Practitioners,* December/January 1995;8(1):25.

12. U.S. Care, Inc. Likelihood for Long-Term Care. Retrieved on February 10, 2009, from http://www.uscare.com/whyltc.html

13. Brandon, E. Planning to Retire. Retrieved February 10, 2009, from http://usnews.com/blogs/planning-to-retire/2009/02/05/how-much-does-long-term-care-cost.html

2

SOCIAL GERONTOLOGY

NANCY BROSSOIE, PhD

Life is not a journey to the grave with the intention of arriving safely in a pretty and well-preserved body, but rather to skid in sideways, thoroughly used up, totally worn out, and loudly proclaiming, "Wow—what a ride!"

—*Author Unknown*

Chapter Outline

Behavioral Objectives

Upon completion of this chapter, the reader will be able to:

1. Define *gerontology* and how it differs from *geriatrics*.
2. Explain why taking a biopsychosocial perspective to understanding aging is important.
3. Define *ageism*.
4. Identify common myths about aging.
5. Discuss *infantilizing* and why it is harmful to the health and well-being of older adults.
6. Describe how older adults are portrayed in the media and how that influences social thinking about older adults.

7. Describe the diversity found in the lifestyles of older adults.
8. Describe some of the social roles adults might hold in later life.
9. Describe the challenges faced by grandparents raising grandchildren.
10. Identify major sources of income for older adults.
11. Describe how different ethnic groups treat older adults.
12. Identify strategies associated with a successful retirement.
13. Identify reasons why health promotion and disease prevention programs are beneficial to aging individuals.

Key Terms

AARP
Ageism
Biopsychosocial
Caregiver
Discrimination
Fictive kin
Geriatrics
Gerontology
Gray Panthers: Age and Youth in Action
Healthy People 2010
Infantilizing
Long-distance caregiver

Long-term care insurance
Myths about aging
Older adult
Older Americans Act
Polypharmacy
Retirement
Sandwich generation
Senior Service America
Senior Volunteer Corps
Social roles
Social Security
Stereotypes

GERONTOLOGY

The aging process begins the moment we are born. As we age, our bodies and minds grow, develop, and mature. During childhood, the course of our development is influenced by many factors including our personal characteristics, our family background, how we are raised, where we grow up, and who raises us. Similarly, our development throughout adulthood continues to be influenced by our health, attitude, and behaviors and our interactions with family, friends, and the environment around us. Therefore, it is shortsighted to limit discussions about aging to matters of physical health and decline. Aging is a complex process influenced by many other personal and social factors.

Gerontology is the scientific study of aging that examines the biological, psychological, and sociological (**biopsychosocial**) factors associated with old age and aging. The factors that affect how we age are broad in scope and diverse: biological factors include genetic background and physical health; psychological influences include level of cognition, mental health status, and general well-being; and sociological factors range from personal relationships to the cultures, policies, and infrastructure that organize society.

Although sometimes confused with the term *gerontology*, **geriatrics** is a medical term for the study, diagnosis, and treatment of diseases and health problems specific to older adults. Geriatricians (medical doctors who specialize in geriatrics) increasingly recognize the importance of social and psychological influences when treating patients. In this chapter, key issues in gerontology are presented to facilitate your understanding about the lifestyles of older adults and how they may influence health status.

In the field of social sciences, the term **older adults** is used to describe people age 65 years and older and is the preferred term when speaking about aged individuals. The term *patient* is medically oriented and can refer to a person of any age. The term *elderly* has the social connotation of being white haired and medically fragile. Because many people age 65 and older do not have gray hair and live vibrant healthy lifestyles, the term *older adult* has a more positive connotation and therefore is preferred and used in this chapter.

HISTORICAL PERSPECTIVES ON AGING

Throughout history, older adults have been generally valued for the experience, insight, and wisdom they can share with others. Leadership is frequently bestowed upon older adults because of a social belief that wisdom and experience are acquired over time. However, conferring respect and responsibilities to older adults has not always been consistent. It tends to occur more in preindustrial or agrarian societies where families are intergenerational and members are dependent on one another for survival and support. For example, in 2004, hours before a tsunami in the Indian Ocean reached the shore, villagers from small fishing communities followed the leadership of their village elders and fled to safety. The suggestions of the elders were followed because the elders held the respect of the others and possessed the ability to interpret environmental cues that signaled impending danger, cues that were passed down to them from village elders long ago.[1]

In industrial societies, older adults are generally less valued than they are in agrarian societies. During the 20th century, as industrialization in the United States expanded, family members became less dependent on each other for support, frequently leaving older adults to manage for themselves, many in poverty. In 1964, President Johnson launched the War on Poverty, which fought for the development of rights, opportunities, and social services for all poor Americans to help lift them out of poverty. From this initiative, the **Older Americans Act** (OAA) of 1965 was passed into legislation specifically to address the needs and rights of older adults. The OAA continues to be reauthorized and is expected to be reauthorized indefinitely. It is one piece of legislation that represents the United States' commitment to promoting the rights and welfare of older adults.

AGEISM

How we treat older adults is influenced by many social factors including our personal assumptions, expectations, and fears about growing older.[2] Fears about aging are generally based on a lack of understanding about the aging process. Unfortunately, many people believe that old age equates to physical disabilities, poor health, the inability to think clearly and quickly, and having a negative outlook on life. These inaccurate assumptions are examples of **ageism**, that is, systematic labeling and **discrimination** against people who are old.

Ageism is based on stereotypes, **myths about aging**, and language that conjures up negative images of older adults. Ageism is to old age as racism is to skin color and sexism is to gender. Ageist thinking is detrimental to society and can result in limited opportunities (e.g., employment and workplace discrimination) and reduced access to resources (e.g., health care discrimination) for older adults. In its worst form, ageism leads to elder abuse, mistreatment, and neglect.[3]

AGEIST STEREOTYPES

Ageist comments often place older adults into set roles or categories, called **stereotypes**. Older adults are sometimes viewed as senile, rigid in thought and manner, with old-fashioned morality and skills. Similarly, older adults are also portrayed as eccentric or overly happy about life, perceiving it as rosy and carefree. When members of a younger generation see ageism in their own families and communities, they are likely to engage in ageist practices and thoughts. That is, they begin to believe that older adults are different, and they may eventually cease to view them as worthy human beings.

Ageist attitudes permeate all facets of society, especially when money is involved. Negative connotations about older adults being "greedy geezers" first surfaced in a March 1988 issue of the magazine *The New Republic*. In that issue, older adults were described as wealthy with financial and social advantages, yet eager to siphon public money (i.e., **Social Security**) that should be dedicated to poor and needy children.[4]

However, over the last 50 years there has been some gradual improvement in attitudes toward older adults in the United States, thanks to greater public education and awareness, the OAA, increased media attention, and the appearance of more positive role models, especially in movies such as *Driving Miss Daisy, Young at Heart,* and *Cocoon.* This, however, has done little to reverse the deeper undercurrents that run below the surface of ageism. Some people continue to view older adults as drains on public resources.

MYTHS ABOUT AGING

Older adults are not homogenous. They do not all look, think, or act alike. Older adults are as unique as younger adults are. Therefore, making blanket assumptions and generalizations about older adults based on knowledge about a few perpetuates myths. Following are some examples of myths that continue to promote ageism. Although the statements may be accurate for some individuals, they are not true for all older adults[3,5]:

Myth 1: Older adults are either very rich or very poor.
Myth 2: Older adults are senile (have defective memory or are disoriented or demented).

Myth 3: Older adults are neither interested in nor have the capacity for sexual relations.

Myth 4: Older adults are miserable and unhappy with the state of their lives.

Myth 5: Older adults are very religious.

Myth 6: Older adults are unable to adapt to change.

Myth 7: Older adults are unable to learn new things.

Myth 8: Older adults generally want to live in nursing homes.

Myth 9: Older adults urinate on their clothing.

Myth 10: Older adults tend to be pretty much alike.

AGEIST LANGUAGE

Ageist language is also a problem for older adults. Many negative terms are commonly used to describe older adults without much thought or understanding of how these terms hurt and degrade the individual. Some ageist terms you may have heard before include the following:

Geezer	Old duffer	Biddy	Old buck
Hag	Dirty old man	Fossil	Blue hair
Little old lady	Q-tip	Old coot	Old battleax

Boroi (Japanese slang meaning old and worn)

Phrases frequently used to disparage older adults or used in general discussions about aging include these:

Over the hill	Out to pasture	Gone senile	One foot in the grave
Old school	Older than dirt	Ol' man _____ (fill in name)	

AGEIST ATTITUDES OF HEALTH PROFESSIONALS

Unfortunately, health professionals, like the rest of the society, sometimes promote ageist attitudes in the way they treat older adults.[6,7] Those who view older adult patients sympathetically as "poor old dears" who can do little to care for themselves are actually placing little value on older adults' abilities. Referring to an unfamiliar older patient as "honey" or "dear" carries a negative connotation. This **infantilizing** of older adults encourages dependency because it devalues the individual and does not foster independence. Although those are more subtle aspects of ageism, they are not person-centered and should be avoided.

Other ageist terms used by medical professionals to describe patients in conversation or noted on medical charts include the following[8]:

"The wheelchair (or the stroke or other condition) in room number _____ . . ."

MFPB (Measure for pine box)	Bed blocker	TMB (Too many birthdays)
VAC (Vultures are circling)	GOMER (Get out of my emergency room)	

Research has shown that health care professionals are significantly more negative in their attitudes toward older patients than they are toward young patients.[7] Although not appropriate, their negative attitude can arise from one or more of the following:

- A need to justify why the medical needs of the older adult were not addressed or met
- Feelings of frustration about not being able to manage the demands of the job
- Feelings of helplessness from not being able to save or cure patients' medical problems
- Increased awareness or reminder of one's own life and mortality

Awareness is the first step in overcoming an ageist attitude. To avoid making ageist comments and remarks as a health care professional, it is important to recognize and explore personal feelings and attitudes about growing older. Stopping the spread of ageism is everyone's responsibility and starts with each individual.

THE MEDIA'S ATTITUDE TOWARD OLDER ADULTS

The media regularly perpetuate the stereotypes of older adults through inaccurate and sometimes demeaning portrayals of older adults in print, advertising, and entertainment. This is puzzling considering that older adults have the ability to purchase the products supporting the media, and thus should be able to facilitate change in the industry. Yet limited efforts have been made to alter how older adults are depicted in the media. Perhaps as more members of the baby boom generation age, positive changes will emerge.

The entertainment media play a major role in perpetuating age stereotypes. Frequently, older adults are portrayed as "more comical, stubborn, eccentric and foolish than other characters." They are also often depicted as "narrow-minded, in poor health, foundering financially, sexually dissatisfied and unable to make decisions."[9] Movie scripts tend to characterize older adults only when they are reclusive (*Finding Forrester*), dying (*The Notebook*), or facing their own mortality (*The Bucket List*). It is uncommon to watch older adult characters on the big screen portraying everyday people (*Return to Me*) in a manner that does not romanticize their lives (*Cocoon*) or portray them as behaving comically (*Grumpy Old Men*).

Television show scripting is no different. Although we do see older adults on special programming, it is unusual to see a realistic portrayal of an older person on a television show. Again, this programming decision is puzzling considering that television shows are targeted for specific demographic audiences who are apt to buy the sponsors' products. Older adults watch television more than any other age group and generally have the discretionary income to buy the products advertised during commercials. Yet limited efforts have been made to accurately depict the lives of older adults on television.[9]

Print and television advertisements tend to portray older adults at their worst—when they have some kind of physical ailment or have the desire to look and feel younger.

We see older actors in commercials for laxatives, skin moisturizers, gas elimination medications, analgesics, and hair coloring products, just to name a few. This would not be as detrimental to the image of the older adult if we also saw older adults in other types of commercials advertising general-use products. In 2007, Unilever launched an international campaign for Dove pro·age products featuring women age 50 and older as models in their commercials.[10] Their customers expressed a desire to see the bodies of everyday women represented in the commercials rather than the lithe figures of younger women. Unilever agreed and launched its successful beauty product campaign with the attitude that aging is a positive experience and should not be viewed negatively or driven by fear. However, the ads do not feature women over age 65. Our society may be making steps in the right direction, but we have yet to move enough to erase the face of ageism.

SOCIAL ROLES IN LATER LIFE

Social roles are important ways of identifying and defining members of every society. Roles define an individual's position in the community and dictate basic behaviors within social groups such as families, workplaces, and communities. They also validate a person's existence in society. Some social roles remain with us throughout our lives (e.g., father, cousin, grandmother) whereas other roles change or transform as different levels of accomplishment or development are reached. For example, individuals may transition from being a student to a teacher or from a worker to a retiree. In later life, social roles are more apt to remain in place. Older adults continue to be sisters/brothers, parents, neighbors, club members, and citizens of communities. However, their participation in those roles is generally dependent on their health status, financial resources, and mobility in the community. It is important to note that older adults can and will continue to participate in many of their social roles, even when faced with diminished capacities.[11]

One change in social role frequently faced by older adults occurs with **retirement**. Adjusting to the change in social status that results from leaving the workforce can be difficult. By the time most older adults are ready to leave their position in the workplace (regardless of position held) they have reached positions that have earned them respect, provide a regular income, and offer a social network of friends, colleagues, and acquaintances. Transitioning from a position of daily recognition and involvement to one with limited recognition and possible isolation from others can be psychologically difficult.[12] Studies have outlined several strategies for transitioning to retirement, which are identified later in this chapter. Adjusting to the lifestyle changes resulting from retirement can be easier with planning and preparation.

Becoming a **caregiver** for a family member or friend is a social role most of us do not think about until we find ourselves in the midst of providing care. Caregiving responsibilities can emerge slowly or begin suddenly after an illness or accident. Sometimes the need for assistance occurs so slowly that neither the caregiver nor the care recipient recognizes the full extent of decline over time.[13] For many older adults, providing care for a spouse gradually increases with time and becomes a full-time job before other family members are aware of the situation.

One reason many people are not ready to take on the role of caregiver is that many older adults have a strong desire to remain independent and are unwilling to relinquish their roles and responsibilities to another, even when they recognize that they need help. Many are quite adamant about not accepting support until they reach a point when they cannot function without help. At that point, adult children generally intervene, although most are ill prepared to take on the role of caregiver. Although each family is different, research has found a common pattern to providing care within the United States. In general, older adults depend on their oldest daughter (or daughter-in-law) for assistance with activities of daily living and rely on their eldest son for support with financial and estate matters.[14] This does not mean that others will not be asked to help or will not offer to help. It simply means that, culturally, older adults in the United States expect assistance in particular from these offspring.

In the past few years, more attention has been placed on the phenomenon of grandparents raising grandchildren. In 2007, it was estimated that 1.4 million grandparents had full-time caregiving responsibilities rearing grandchildren under the age of 18.[15] The benefits to engaging in this role are discussed in a later section. The role of becoming a surrogate parent can be very demanding on an older adult. Being active in a child's life requires engaging in all aspects of the child's life and associating with teachers and parents who are much younger. When combined with a fixed retirement income, the social stigma of the parent's problem and inability to parent, and the development of a parental relationship between the grandparent and the child, the new social role can become quite challenging and stressful.

CULTURAL PERSPECTIVES ON CAREGIVING AND OLDER ADULTS

Most Western societies, including the United States and western Europe, stress individualism (that is, the needs of the individual are addressed before the needs of the group). Other cultures, such as those in Asia and the Pacific Islands, are collectivist societies; that is, members place the needs of the family or collective group (which may be an intergenerational family) before the needs of the individual. Differences between individual and collective perspectives naturally inform how groups perceive older adults and place responsibility for providing care and support. Understanding how groups differ can assist in the planning and provision of effective health care services, no matter where the care is provided.

In an individualistic society, older adults are generally free to remain living independently and managing life as they see fit as long as they can afford it and they are not placing themselves or others in immediate danger. In a collectivist society, the resources of the older adults are pooled with other family resources. The activities of daily life are shared rather than lived separately. As a result, living expenses are reduced because the older adult lives with other family members. Examples of collectivist responses to caring for older adults follow.

In India, when an aging parent joins a younger household, he or she is welcomed as a member of the household. Even though the household may not have planned to include the older adult, the family members willingly make accommodations for the aging family member.[16] In a Filipino household, the youngest daughter is expected to care for the older adult at home until she married, and then the older adult moves with her to her husband's home.[17]

Some ethnic groups revere elders as authority figures who reside in positions of power within the family and community. Other ethnic groups take an almost opposite view and see older adults in terms of added responsibility, if not burden, to family and society.

The social role of the older adult within the household varies according to the society's views. In Vietnamese culture, a grandparent shares household authority with the father of the household. His or her place in the family is highly regarded.[18] In contrast, in the old Athabascan Indian culture in Alaska, older adults were seen as burdens—a drain on food and resources in the harsh and demanding climate. Older adults were expected to contribute as much as possible until the day came when the chief of the tribe would leave them to die in the wilderness in an effort to preserve resources for the healthy and strong members of the tribe.[19]

Family life and a respect for the knowledge and wisdom of the elder are central to Asian culture. This has, however, decreased somewhat in the Asian American population with modernization and assimilation into American society. However, Asian cultures remain strongly collectivistic and believe family life is central to their existence.[20,21]

Whereas collectivism may appear to be an effective approach to managing family and social resources, it is not very beneficial to people with disabilities. In general, people with disabilities are viewed as an embarrassment to the family because they are not strong enough to contribute their fair share. Often the disabled are disowned, abandoned, and end up begging on the street. This increases the collectivist society's disdain for them. This mindset can be applied to people with physical problems, mental health problems, and fragile older adults. Individuals with special needs do not have strong support from within a collectivist society to lead a productive and successful life.[16]

In the United States, our strong belief in individualism has resulted in legislation that has protected the rights of people with disabilities (e.g., the Americans with Disabilities Act) and provides accommodation for people with physical and mental health needs in communities and the workplace. Coupled with legislation through the OAA, significant strides continue to be made to ensure that older adults are legally protected to lead full and productive lives.

A great deal of research has been conducted in the United States on family dynamics and the roles and responsibilities of family members. The United States has become a mobile and independent society where intergenerational households and the reliance on family for support are no longer assumed the norm. However, studies indicate that African Americans tend to maintain extensive kin networks that continue to provide help, especially to young family members and neighbors. Community institutions, including the church, are also viewed as very important sources of physical and emotional support.[22] Likewise, Mexican Americans, who make up 9% of the U.S. population,[23] maintain close family relationships that promote family solidarity. They have more contact with their children than their white counterparts do.[24] As the baby boom generation ages beyond 65 years, additional studies will need to be conducted to specifically address how different ethnic groups are coping and meeting the needs of their aging parents.

SOCIAL RELATIONSHIPS

Older adults continue to engage in social relationships throughout later life, although relationship patterns undergo change. As personal health declines, the ability and opportunity to socialize are reduced, resulting in fewer numbers and types of relationships. Studies have shown that as we age and our health declines, we deliberately let go of some of our relationships, retaining only the ones we know we can maintain.[25] We do this because we recognize that relationships should be reciprocal, and we no longer have the ability, energy, or resources to provide the other person with the support he or she needs. The people we choose to retain in our social circle are family members and friends, the people we hold very dear and have generally known for a long time.[26]

Numerous studies have also shown that socialization is important to an individual's physical and psychological well-being and does not diminish with age.[27] Older adults are no different from younger adults when it comes to wanting to engage in relationships, although the level of engagement and the type of engagement may vary. Again, opportunities to engage and the ability to meet others influence relationship development.

Social networking through use of the Internet is booming among older adults. E-mail has replaced handwritten letters and phone calls for many older adults wanting to keep in touch with family and friends. Many older adults and their families believe that e-mail has brought them closer and more in tune with each other's lives. (See **Figure 2-1**.) Chat rooms and online dating services have also emerged as technology has enabled older adults to connect with each other for companionship and love.[28] For older adults who have never used a computer, learning to operate one may be initially challenging. However, many community centers provide periodic classes on how to send e-mail, surf the Internet, play computer games, and use basic computer programs.

The following sections provide some insight into different types of social relationships held by adults in later life.

The Aging Couple   Like other adult couples, some older adults have been married or in a committed relationship for decades, whereas others have more recently become a couple later in life. (See **Figure 2-2**.) Older men who find themselves single in later life generally

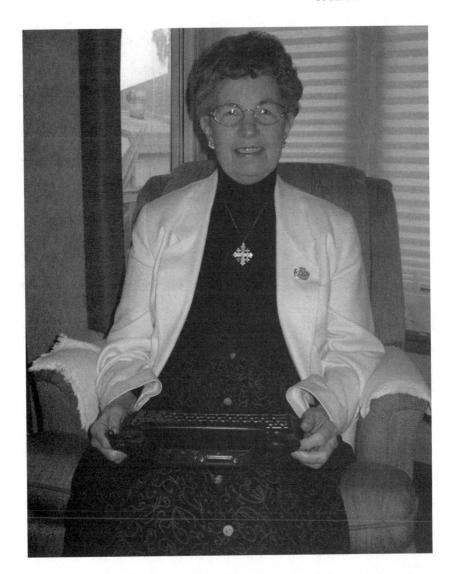

FIGURE 2-1   E-mail is any easy way for older adults to maintain communication with family and friends. (*Courtesy of C. Ernest Williams.*)

have no problem finding a female companion because, statistically, women outlive men. The U.S. Census reports that by age 85 there are 100 women for every 49 men.[29]

Relationships that have endured into old age have probably experienced and overcome many challenges and crises. Health problems aside, one of the earliest challenges faced in later life occurs around the transition into retirement. For some, it is a time of deep soul searching, redefining social roles, and wondering what the future of the relationship will

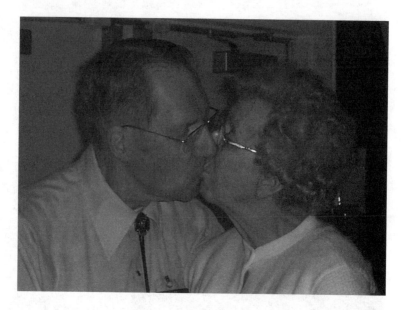

FIGURE 2-2 Expressions of love and affection. (*Courtesy of Theodore N. Brossoie.*)

be like.[30] When children leave home and people transition out of jobs, their roles change and they are faced with establishing new roles for themselves and with their partner. If a couple successfully weathers these challenges, their feelings for each other can actually become enriched and strengthened. However, problems can arise when each person experiences this internal struggle at different times. For example, if one person is ready to retire while the other one is not, or one wants to sell the family home and move to a warmer climate and the other does not, problems in the relationship often arise. In response, some couples spend considerable time reflecting on the value, purpose, and usefulness of their relationship during this stage of life. For many, this is just another one of life's challenges that they will share and work through together. Others, however, will see it as a reason and opportunity to dissolve their relationship.

Many other couples are simply not destined to grow old together. Maybe they have stayed together for the sake of the children, or perhaps they became absorbed in work or other activities over the years so that they would not have to deal with underlying relationship issues. There are also couples who are closely connected but not emotionally in touch. They may even be genuinely fond of each other but view their relationship as more of a business partnership than a marriage. A marriage of convenience is similar to this, in which each partner does "his or her own thing." Sometimes one or both partners in this type of relationship engage in extramarital affairs, which can often bring about the final unraveling of the marriage.

Although some relationships worsen or dissolve with age, others actually get better and experience a renewal or rebirth. Late life can be the most satisfying years of a marriage for the couple who has come to accept one another for who they are.[31]

Aging Parent and Adult Child   Relationships between aging parents and adult children also tend to be as varied as spousal relationships.[32] Generally, there exists a fair degree of involvement between the generations. Older parents very often provide emotional, physical, and financial support, when possible. Ideally, this is provided without strings attached and driven in part with the hope or unspoken agreement that help will be reciprocated in later years.[30]

Unfortunately, strained relations can develop between parents and a child throughout adulthood. Verbal finger pointing—unfair fighting with "you never" or "you always" statements—can upset relations, as can favoritism toward certain siblings. Sometimes parental disapproval of a lifestyle or friends also brings about disharmony. Disappointment coupled with shame may cause an older adult to place public appearances first and the son's or daughter's needs and feelings second.[30] However, if affection and communication remain open between the parent and adult child, psychological well-being will be enhanced for both.[32]

For many families, the details about daily life for older parents do not emerge until a need for help with activities of daily living arises. Until that time, many older adults do not want to live with their children, share their financial information, or include their children in their decision-making processes. Like their children, they value their independence and like to control their own lives. They do not want their children to intervene. But when the time comes when support is needed, approximately 83% of support received comes from family members.[13] One study estimated that 19% of caregivers of older adults lived with the person they were caring for, 46% lived 20 minutes away or less, and 18% lived more than 1 hour away. It is also estimated that nearly 7 million Americans are **long-distance caregivers** for an older relative.[13,33] That is, they travel a distance of 1 hour or more to the older adult to provide assistance.

We can infer from the statistics and collected stories that when the time comes to provide caregiving support, adult children may find that they have less time to spend with their own families because caregiving demands occupy more of their time. Among those caregivers, some will also be simultaneously providing care to their own children. Adults found in this position are referred to as the **sandwich generation** because they are caught between two caregiving roles. Even after the children are gown, the average American woman can expect to spend more time caring for an aging parent than she did caring for her children.[34]

One relatively recent challenge faced by many older adults has been the increased prevalence of substance abuse (alcohol and drug) and incarceration rates among their adult children. Subsequently, many older adults are forced to deal with the addictive behaviors of their adult child or grandchild, a task many are ill prepared to undertake.

Studies indicate that the problems of adult children are a significant cause of depression in older adults; the greater the child's problem, the greater the parent's depression. Older adults continue to want the best for their children, no matter what their age, and are often emotionally affected by the challenges and failures their offspring encounter.[35]

Never-Married or Childless in Late Life   In the United States, it is estimated that slightly more than 4% of the population age 65 and older have never married. That rate is almost twice the rate of never-marrieds in Europe.[36] Also notable is that nearly 19% of women older than age 44 have never given birth, contributing to a childless rate among U.S. adults that has nearly doubled since the 1980s.[36] The reasons for remaining single and for not bearing children are numerous and personal. Regardless, social roles and expectations of adults are centered around couplehood and families, leaving many people to wonder how never-marrieds and childless people receive support later in life and from whom.

Although some people may assume that never-marrieds and childless couples have been deprived of the emotional support of family in late life, research suggests otherwise. Happiness, life satisfaction, loneliness, and self-esteem appear to be unrelated to contact with adult children during late life.[37] Many never-marrieds and childless couples have adjusted by adapting their social network to include relationships generally thought to be held by partners and children. These **fictive kin** are treated as family and linked by close emotional bonds.[38] Sometimes a niece or a nephew takes on the social role of a child, or a sibling takes on some of the traditional roles of a spouse. Despite the social pressure to marry and bear children, those who do not conform to social pressure are not emotionally unstable in later life. Never marrying or remaining childless is not something to be pitied or viewed as a curiosity. It is simply another way of life.

Friendships   Friendships established early in life often continue into old age, especially if they begin during midlife. Unlike relationships with family members that are connected by blood ties and replete with social roles and expectations, friendships exist because the individuals involved share similar interests and want to maintain the relationship. Like younger adults, older adults tend to establish friendships with people similar to themselves: same gender, similar social and economic status, and from the same town or community. However, as friendships deteriorate as a result of increased distance, poor health, or death, new ones are formed if the older adult has the access and opportunity to build a new connection. The ability to form new relationships is essential because an important outcome of friendship is enhanced psychological well-being. Research indicates that friendships have an even stronger influence on well-being than do familial relationships, although the precise relationship remains unclear.[39]

Studies have also shown that women have more friends than men do because they view and engage in friendships differently.[40] Women perceive friendships to be sources of ongoing emotional and physical support and prefer to surround themselves with friends who can help them address the daily challenges they face. When a friendship ends, it is replaced with a new one. Thus, women are intentional about managing their friendships so that they maintain the desired complement of friends to help them process the events in their life. Men, however, prefer to rely on their spouse, partner, or close family members for help and emotional support rather than friends. Males' friendships are based on specific activities such as a sport or a project, rather than sharing feelings and processing a particular situation or event. As a result, men require fewer friends than women do.

Like young adults, older adults nurture their friendships and feel a sense of loss when a friendship dissolves or becomes inactive. Poor health, new living arrangements, and loss in mobility frequently change the course of friendships and make sustaining them that much more difficult. As mentioned previously, when maintaining relationships becomes too difficult to manage, older adults will break off some because they recognize they cannot reciprocate support. Instead, they choose to place their energy and resources into their most valued relationships, those with their closest family and friends.[26]

Grandparenting   Grandparenting is a social role that many adults look forward to as their children mature. Because people are living longer, it is becoming common to see great-grandparents or even great-great-grandparents within families. The U.S. Census estimated that there were approximately 70 million grandparents in the United States in 2000, with approximately 8% living with a grandchild under the age of 18.[15]

Grandparents generally welcome interactions with their grandchildren as a chance to relive their early years without balancing the stresses and responsibilities of caring for their own children the first time around. A new grandchild can be like a booster shot for some older couples, reawakening early days of marriage and the enthusiasm of early parenting.[25]

Not surprisingly, the role of grandparent is as varied as any other social role. Grandparents share multiple roles and responsibilities within families and as such can be described as one of five distinct types[41]:

- Distance figures (live far away and visit infrequently)
- Fun-seekers (provide and engage in exciting opportunities)
- Surrogate parents (take on a parenting role)
- Formal (as patriarch or matriarch of the family)
- Reservoirs of family wisdom (sources of knowledge and expertise)

Yet the role of grandparent is not static. The role of a grandparent today is generally responsive to the individual needs of the extended family. In the United States, one of the most important roles of a grandparent is that of a caregiver, in the broadest sense (**Figure 2-3**). Grandparents baby-sit, act as surrogate parents, pay educational costs, and sometimes provide the deposit for a new house. The toy industry especially likes grandparents because they purchase approximately 17% of all toys bought in the United States.[42]

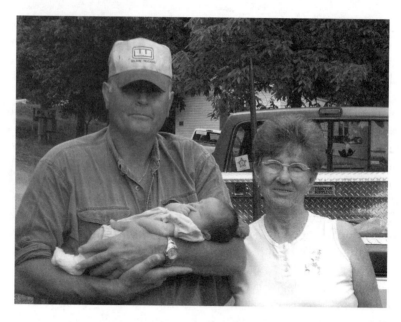

FIGURE 2-3 **Grandparents often take on a caregiving role.** (*Courtesy of Michelle Brossoie.*)

However, sometimes grandparents or adult children choose not to interact with each other and instead maintain a distance, not only physically but also emotionally. Having limited contact may be the result of personal priorities such as work or leisure or may stem from personal reasons based on unpleasant interactions in the past.[30]

The closeness felt between a grandparent and grandchild often correlates with how the grandparents saw their family members interact with their own grandparents. Healthy interactions between generations serve as positive role models for younger generations. Parents need to see grandparents spending quality time with their children to become good grandparents themselves.[30]

In addition to providing financial support, grandparents sometimes step in to take care of grandchildren when parents are abusive or addicted to drugs and are otherwise unable to parent. Grandparents also act as mediators when conflicts arise between a parent and child. Likewise, when parents divorce, grandparents can frequently offer support, comfort, consolation, and financial assistance to their child or grandchild, bringing the family closer together. Divorce, however, can also remove grandparents from their grandchild's life. In today's world of blended families and divorce, some grandparents find that they lose grandchildren as quickly as they welcome them into the family. In response, many have been fighting back for grandparent visitation rights so that they can maintain contact. Organizations that support grandparent rights include the National Coalition for Grandparenting, the Foundation for Grandparenting, and Grandparenting for Children.[43]

Arthur Kornhaber, MD, author of *The Grandparent Guide*, created the Foundation for Grandparenting to nurture and lobby for intergenerational relationships. This foundation even offers a summer camp and conference center for grandparents and grandchildren. Kornhaber's work has shown that children raised by grandparents tend to be more well rounded and have a greater respect for the past. They are more likely to speak more than one language, perform better in school, and have a good sense of family and family values.[44]

Program developers for Elderhostel[45] and other adult adventure programs have also recognized the market for offering grandparent–grandchild vacation activities. Special summer programs are being offered in which both generations can share in a cultural or environmental experience. Spending time together provides an excellent opportunity to develop the grandparent–grandchild relationship without the distractions of daily life.

Recognition of the benefits and values of grandparenting has led to the creation of Adopt a Grandparent/Grandchild programs nationwide.[46] These programs provide excellent opportunities for kids without grandparents or older adults without grandchildren to engage and learn from each other's experiences. Similar programs provide older adults with the opportunity to become "foster grandparents" through youth centers or other community organizations.[47] No matter who is the focus of the program, experiencing the grandparent–grandchild relationship is rewarding and fulfilling to everyone involved.

SOCIAL INFLUENCES ON AGING

INCOME AND FINANCIAL RESOURCES

The importance of financial security later in life cannot be overemphasized. Most older men and women have worked a good portion of their lives to establish a retirement fund or so-called nest egg from which to draw during their later years. It should, therefore, come as no surprise that older adults signal a rallying cry at every mention of reducing Social Security or Medicare benefits.

A major source of income for older adults in the United States is Social Security (SS). Ninety percent of older adults collected Social Security in 2004. The Social Security Act was signed into law by President Franklin D. Roosevelt in 1935.[48] Its original and intended purpose was and continues to be acting as a supplemental source of retirement income for older adults to help pay expenses incurred during late life when earning potential is minimal. It was never designed to be a major source of retirement income. However, nearly one-third of SS beneficiaries report that Social Security provided 89% of their income. Fifty-five percent of beneficiaries reported receiving income from assets, 41% received income from retirement plans/funds, and 24% received income from earnings.[49]

Even though growing numbers of older adults are achieving financial security, in 2006 about 3.6 million older adults in the United States lived below the federal poverty level.[50]

This group accounted for 9.4% of older adults (about the same as the rate for persons ages 18 to 64, which was 10.8%). Unlike younger adults, as older persons exhaust their resources, they are generally unable to generate the additional income necessary to improve their economic status or to leave assistance programs. Besides having diminished employment opportunities, they are also least likely to benefit from inheritance. Therefore, many are often left to fend for themselves, living off retirement savings, pension, or Social Security benefits that are marginally adjusted for inflation. Because poorer older adults have fewer resources and live off of fixed incomes, they tend to spend a much larger portion of their total income on health care and housing than do their younger low-income counterparts.[51]

For minority groups living in the United States, African American elders, the largest ethnic minority (12.4% of total population), have always lagged behind whites (81.9% of total population) in terms of social and economic status.[50] Many must continue to work into old age because they lack the resources to retire and generally receive limited Social Security benefits because of a low earnings history.

Like African Americans, Hispanic elders tend to be socioeconomically less well off than older whites and most other ethnic elders.[50] Older African American and Hispanic women who are not married or partnered have a more difficult time financially than do their white counterparts. In 2004, approximately 27% of African American women age 65 and older were living alone with household incomes at or below 100% of the federal poverty level.[50] Like most impoverished adults, their situation is the result of a lifetime of low-skill, low-paying jobs, inadequate educational opportunities, and discrimination in the labor market.

Older Asian Americans constitute a small but rapidly growing segment of the older adult population in the country. As a group, they tend to be somewhat better off, by most social indicators, than other minority groups are. This may be attributed to their collectivist lifestyle with a focus on family and emphasis on meeting the needs of the family or community before the needs of the individual. Engaging in this lifestyle is important because many immigrant elders are not covered by Social Security, never having had paid employment in this country.[52]

WORK AND RETIREMENT

Workplace Discrimination   Extensive research has been conducted on social attitudes toward older workers. Many employers and employees inaccurately perceive older workers to be rigid, inflexible, incapable of learning new skills, unproductive, and overpaid. It should, therefore, come as no surprise that the most common type of economic discrimination against older adults is work-related.[5] Research indicates that 80% of adults believe that most employers discriminate against older workers in hiring or on the job, and 61% of employers admit doing so.[53] Discrimination against older workers ignores several overall advantages to hiring them, including low absentee rates, less turnover, low accident rates, less alcohol- and drug addiction–related issues, increased job satisfaction, and company loyalty.[5] Additionally, the experiences, knowledge, and insight older workers bring to the workplace are invaluable and cannot be easily replaced by a younger person with a limited work history who is working for lower wages.

Some employers continue to believe older workers are unable to keep pace with change and learn new technologies. For example, some people believe that computers and computer software are far too difficult for older adults to learn to operate proficiently, so they will not consider them for employment. However, evidence exists that older adults can and do learn new technological skills, including computer technology. Their learning strategies and styles may be different from younger adults, but they have the ability to learn and can become quite accomplished when given the opportunity to learn and study in a way that works for them.[54]

Work discrimination against older adults is most obvious when companies attempt to reduce costs by asking older workers to take early retirement, even seducing them into it by offering a tempting retirement package, a so-called golden parachute. The offer may initially appear to be a good financial move but may short-change the worker of retirement income if not invested and managed wisely.

Retirement   Before the industrial revolution, retirement as a phase of life did not exist. Individuals worked until they became either disabled or too infirm to do otherwise. They generally died shortly afterward. If they did live a long life, they were usually supported by family or by some charitable organization such as the local church. It was only in 1889 that Chancellor Bismarck of Germany established retirement for individuals reaching age 65. He chose the age of 65 as the beginning of retirement by adding 20 years to the then normal life expectancy of 45 years. Other European countries soon followed with similar retirement systems. In 1935, the United States was the first country to establish a nationalized pension system for people age 65 and older (Social Security).[48] Since then, other countries have followed suit, and today most offer a national pension to adults age 65 and older. Variations in age of eligibility range about 5 years with most notable differences between males and females.[55]

Until 1967, retirement was compulsory for workers in the United States who reached age 65, regardless of their health status or abilities. Here again we see another myth of aging that implies there is a general loss of ability that begins occurring around age 65 or earlier. However, in adults who are aging typically, there exists no sudden or general loss of ability at age 65 or at any other age.[5] Any losses that may occur generally do so gradually over many years. Even some disorders considered inevitable as we age (such as visual and hearing impairments) are now reversible or amenable to treatment. Because of better health status, today's retirees can potentially spend 20 or more years in retirement.[55]

Older adults, like most groups of individuals, are incredibly diverse. Ken Dychtwald, president of Age Wave Inc., states, "No age group is more varied in personal background, physical abilities, personal styles, social needs, or financial capabilities than today's older population. While some older people are dreadfully sick and waiting for death, some are fit and training for marathons. Some wait in breadlines for a warm meal. Others have condos in Vail and yachts in Tahiti."[34] Additionally, many continue working in the same or some new capacity, even after reaching retirement age. In sum, retirement is a stage of life that only begins with a change in employment status.

Preparing for retirement is not a task that should be taken lightly or without preparation. Retirement requires planning, planning, and more planning. And despite what the television commercials may say, it is not all about finances. Important considerations in the retirement decision-making process include the following:

- Financial and social resources
- Spouse's/partner's retirement plans
- Desire to continue working part-time
- Need to remain active in current profession
- Desire to start a new career
- Desire to volunteer
- Desire to remain living in the same community

Prior to retirement, some older adults begin developing hobbies or spare-time occupations to engage in during retirement. Many daydream about being able to putter around their home and spend considerable time in their gardens. Although generally good ideas, hobbies and household activities are generally not intensive enough to fill the hours in a day.[56] As many older adults with a few years of retirement behind them frequently offer, you just cannot retire, you have to retire to something. Some older adults are determined to challenge themselves in pursuit of some activity that few, regardless of age, would choose to follow. Mary Harper, a 79-year-old great-grandmother (**Figure 2-4**), is one person who rose to such a challenge. In 1994, she became the oldest person to sail across the Atlantic single-handedly. Although she broke a rib in severe weather, she later said, "The whole trip was worth it just to see the waves." In answer to why she did it alone, she explained that "it was something I wanted to do . . . but didn't want to be responsible for a crew."[57] Another older adult who has refused to settle down to "quiet old age" is Corena Leslie, who completed a sky dive jump 3 days before her 90th birthday.[58]

For some older adults, engaging in lifelong learning activities helps them keep their minds active and alert. Special program topics offered at local community centers, senior centers, and colleges provide numerous opportunities for older adults to explore topics that pique their interest. Elderhostel is a not-for-profit global program that provides learning experiences for older adults on topics including history, culture, nature, music, and outdoor activities, crafts, and study cruises.[45] Participants are able to explore their interests with leading scholars and researchers in the field while sailing on cruises, walking through national parks, and visiting culturally diverse areas.

Many older adults believe that successful aging starts with mental stimulation. At the Plymouth Harbor Retirement Community in Sarasota, Florida, the longevity among

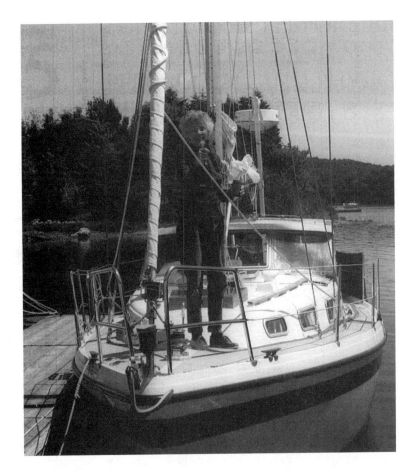

FIGURE 2-4   Mary Harper, the oldest person to sail across the Atlantic Ocean single-handedly. (*Courtesy of Mary Harper.*)

residents is greater than the national average. This unique community encourages individuals to get involved in a myriad of activities, which include electing representatives from each apartment cluster to serve on the board of residents that governs Plymouth Harbor. Residents also pool their resources in supplying volunteer lecturers on just about every topic imaginable. People at Plymouth Harbor appear more involved, interested, and perhaps *more alive* than the stereotypical portrayal of retirees.[59] As Ralph Waldo Emerson once wrote, "It is not length of life but depth of life."

Many adults take up new hobbies and activities that combine mental and physical fitness, such as tai chi or square dancing (**Figure 2-5**). Both provide retirees with the opportunity to exercise their bodies and keep a sharp mental focus. Square dance clubs travel frequently to dance with other groups, providing abundant opportunities for socializing on and off the dance floor.

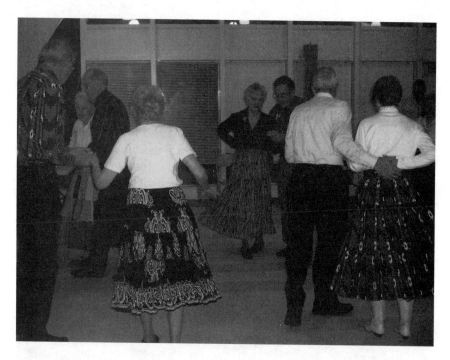

FIGURE 2-5 Square dancing helps maintain physical strength, coordination, and mental agility. *(Courtesy of Theodore N. Brossoie.)*

Many older adults have the desire to give back to their communities and devote many hours to volunteering each week, sharing their lifetime of experiences and insights. Their skills, knowledge, resources, and abilities can affect changes and make a difference in the lives of people of all ages. The **Senior Volunteer Corps** is an umbrella organization for three programs connecting adults age 55 and older to nonprofit, faith-based, and community organizations: Retired Senior Volunteer Program (RSVP), Foster Grandparents, and Senior Companions. Since the 1960s, communities have eagerly tapped into this source of people power to alleviate a number of community challenges.[60]

ADVOCACY FOR OLDER ADULTS

Advocating for the rights and needs of older adults at the local, state, and national levels can be a daunting task. However, as the baby boom generation ages and more individuals reach the age of 65, the voices of advocates are becoming louder and stronger. Several advocacy groups that help represent the needs of older adults are profiled in this section.

The most recognizable organization that has demonstrated considerable success in representing the needs of adults age 50 and older is **AARP**, a nonprofit, nonpartisan organization. It was founded in 1958 as the American Association for Retired Persons with the agenda of addressing the social needs of retirees. Today, AARP has expanded its scope of interests to include all aspects of life. In 2006, it boasted a membership of more than 37 million members. The mission of AARP is simple: "To enhance the quality of life for all of us as we age." AARP advocates for social change through information, advocacy, and service as it represents adults of all ethnicities and cultures within the United States. All of its publications (magazine, bulletins, and website) are instilled with the attitude that age is merely a number and life is what you make of it. Together with the AARP Foundation, research on topics of current interest including prescription drug costs, grandparents raising grandchildren, and civic participation is funded to generate information that can be used to promote positive social change.[61]

The Gray Panthers was founded in 1970 by Maggie Kuhn and six other women who came together to discuss and address the issue of forced retirement at age 65. However, the first issue taken on by the fledgling organization was not age discrimination, but rather opposition to the war in Vietnam. This was because the Gray Panthers did not want to be perceived as an organization that was only dedicated to fighting ageism. The Panthers believed philosophically that "gray power" should be on the cutting edge of social change by working with other organizations. Today, the Gray Panthers' mission is "work for social and economic justice and peace for all people." Armed with intergenerational support and organizational values that include honoring maturity, unifying generations, active engagement, and participatory democracy, the Gray Panthers now proudly identify themselves as **Gray Panthers: Age and Youth in Action**, to "create a humane society that puts the needs of people over profits, responsibility over power, and democracy over institutions."[62]

A third organization founded to address workplace and retirement issues is **Senior Service America** (SSA), once known as the National Council of Senior Citizens and founded by the American Federation of Labor and Congress of Industrial Organizations (AFL-CIO) in 1961. Today, the organization's fundamental purpose is broader than the scope of retirement because the group advocates for political and legislative issues that affect older adults. Legislative issues that received the organization's attention in past years have included the Older Americans Act, Medicare, Medicaid, and employment training opportunities. Today, the SSA updates members through newsletters that report on how Congress is addressing the needs of older adults. The SSA and its partner organizations also provide employment and training opportunities to more than 10,000 adults nationwide.[63]

HEALTH, WELLNESS, AND HEALTH CARE

Today, older adults are living longer and healthier thanks to improvements in health care technology and lifestyles that incorporate healthy diets and exercise. Multiple studies conducted through the National Institute on Aging have revealed that many of the health problems found in old age are not caused by age itself but rather by improper care of and use of the body over time. If the body has been subjected to overeating, exposure to toxins (such as cigarette smoke and alcohol), lack of adequate exercise, and poor nutrition, it should come as no surprise that medical problems will be greater in old age.

Teaching older adults how to manage their health conditions and educating them about their conditions requires an approach different from activities designed for patients of other ages. Older adults tend to learn more effectively in small groups that foster discussion in an informal setting. Older adults are generally more concrete learners rather than theoretical learners, and they learn best when the subject matter has direct practical application. All information presented should be developed using plain language that clearly communicates the intended message at all literacy levels. For more information about health literacy and clear health communication, see Chapter 13.

HEALTH PROMOTION AND DISEASE PREVENTION

Healthy People 2010 is a strategic plan set forth by the U.S. Department of Health and Human Services, the Healthy People Consortium, and other federal agencies to focus on preventable health threats (including disability and death) that affect citizens of all ages. The initiative challenges individuals, communities, and professionals to join together to improve the health of all citizens.[64] Healthy People 2010 is also the United States' contribution to the World Health Organization's Health for All strategy. The objectives in Healthy People 2010 fall under two overarching goals:

- Increase quality and years of healthy life
- Eliminate health disparities

The two goals include 28 focal areas that also contain concise goal statements and objectives. Healthy People 2010 emphasizes the need for vitality and independence with aging and uses a health-oriented rather than disease-oriented approach. Objectives take a true gerontological approach, accounting for socioeconomic, lifestyle, and other non-medical-related influences on personal health.

Common complaints frequently associated with old age include joint stiffness, weight gain, fatigue, loss of bone mass, and loneliness. These conditions can be slowed, prevented, or eliminated by health promotion and disease prevention activities[65] such as exercise, stress management, nutrition, and substance abuse control.

Exercise   The old adage "use it or lose it" is very applicable when it comes to making a case for exercise in the older person. Abundant studies have demonstrated the benefits of exercise throughout the life span. Exercise helps maintain fitness, stimulates and quickens the mind, helps establish social contacts, prevents and/or slows progression of some diseases, and generally improves quality of life. Inactivity leads to muscle wasting and weakening of the bones. A number of chronic conditions such as heart disease, arthritis, osteoporosis, diabetes, obesity, and depression show improvement, or at least a slowing of progression, with regular physical activity.[65]

The ideal exercise program for individuals older than age 60 should emphasize exercises that increase strength, flexibility, and endurance and should be initiated only after consultation with a medical specialist.[66] Low-impact activities such as walking, swimming, or bike riding are ideally suited for most older adults. Exercise should be preceded by stretching and should be increased in gradual increments. An exercise "prescription" from a physician is a good way to begin, especially for those who have been away from exercise for any length of time. Additionally, older participants in fitness programs need to be reminded not to exceed their ability level and to respect pain. Exercise programs specifically tailored for older adults and staffed by fitness professionals are frequently offered through hospitals, colleges, and community organizations.

Stress Management   Much has been written on the relationship between stress and disease. Stress can increase the risk of, or worsen, heart disease, cancer, or other chronic conditions. It can also dampen the immune response. Stress tends to originate from three sources: the environment, our bodies, and our minds.[4] Environmental stressors such as the weather, crime, and crowds are usually beyond one's control, whereas physical and mental stressors, although sometimes seemingly insurmountable, can often be controlled by changing behaviors. There are numerous stress management techniques such as exercise, diet, muscle relaxation, meditation, deep breathing, visualization, desensitization, and biofeedback.[65] Any individual interested in finding a stress reduction technique needs to select one that is well suited to his or her lifestyle and temperament.

Nutrition   Although we purport to be a nation of plenty, 25% of persons older than age 65 suffer from some form of malnutrition.[67] Poverty—although the major cause of malnutrition—is not the only factor. It is estimated that one-third of all nursing home patients are malnourished.[68] This, in large measure, is because few doctors are trained to recognize malnutrition in older adults. In addition to poverty, additional reasons for malnutrition in older adults include depression, limited access to buy food, unbalanced diet, problems with chewing or swallowing, chronic illness, and medications that suppress appetite or interact with nutrients. The resulting lack of physical ability and energy to cook and eat naturally compounds the problem. Poor nutrition also contributes to the progressive decline of several body functions that manifest later in life, including bone density loss, atherosclerotic lesions, opacification of eye lenses, and a blunted immune system.[69]

Substance Abuse Control   Substance abuse can become a major source of problems for older adults. Because older adults generally have less lean body mass and a lower volume of body water, substances such as alcohol, recreational drugs, and medications are absorbed at higher levels into the body and retained for longer periods of time than experienced at a younger age. The presence of alcohol and drugs increases the risk for injuries and/or accidents. Additionally, alcohol and other drugs can have an adverse effect on sleep and can sometimes mask the symptoms of underlying diseases.

Once substance abuse has been identified in an older individual, a management plan should be established. This first involves an initial screening to assess the impact of alcohol or drug abuse both physically and psychologically. Then, a treatment plan, which includes education and promotes self-responsibility, must be established. Drug use and abuse are covered in depth in Chapter 6.

Sometimes substance abuse problems develop as a result of **polypharmacy**.[70] That is, the interactions of multiple medications prescribed for multiple conditions create new disabling medical conditions in the older adult, including adverse drug reactions and addictions. Polypharmacy problems generally occur when more than one medical provider is involved in the care of an older adult. To avoid problems, the older adult should make certain that each provider is aware of what the other is prescribing. Likewise, to stem problems arising from polypharmacy issues, providers and family members should attempt to identify the source of new health problems as they arise and work together with health providers to make sure unnecessary medications are not prescribed.

HEALTH CARE FINANCES

The increased cost of health care and the aging population go hand and hand and have assumed a position on the central stage of the national policy debate. The cost of public health care programs has risen to staggering levels. The proportion of the U.S. gross domestic product for national health programs (i.e., Medicare, Medicaid, veterans' medical care) has increased from 0.4% in 1962 to approximately 5.4% in 2008.[71]

Not surprisingly, older adults with declining health spend more money on long-term institutionalized care than on any other type of health care. Most elders, however, cannot meet these overwhelming costs on their own, and Medicare coverage is limited. At an average daily cost of $183, or $66,795 annually, for a semiprivate room, many older adults in nursing homes watch their lifetime savings evaporate within a few years.[72] By 2030, the cost of institutional care is projected to increase to $190,600 per year, a sum few will be able to afford.[73]

Long-term care insurance is one method of affording nursing home care, at least for those who can afford to buy the insurance. This form of insurance has become the fastest-growing type of health insurance sold in recent years, and it promises to continue its growth in the coming years. By 2003, 13% of full-time workers in all private industry were offered long-term care insurance, while 19% of full-time workers in large private establishments (100 or more workers) were offered this benefit.[73] Although still not routinely offered or included in regular health benefit plans, some health policy analysts believe that availability will increase as the aging population grows in numbers.

SUMMARY

The aging process begins the moment we are born. Over the years our bodies and mind grow, develop, and mature. Gerontology is the scientific study of aging that examines the biological, psychological, and sociological (biopsychosocial) factors associated with old age and aging.

Ageism, a systematic stereotyping of and discrimination against people who are old, fosters the notion that older adults are not useful or valued. Ageism is fueled by numerous myths regarding aging and older adults as well as by language that conjures negative images of old persons. Ageism limits opportunities (employment and workplace discrimination), access to health care, and in its worse form can lead to elder abuse, mistreatment, and neglect.

Research has shown that health care professionals are significantly more negative in their attitudes toward older patients than they are toward younger patients.[5] To avoid making ageist comments and remarks, it is important to recognize and explore your own feelings and attitudes as a health care professional. Stopping the spread of ageism is everyone's responsibility and starts at the individual level.

The media regularly perpetuate the stereotypes of older adults through inaccurate and sometimes demeaning portrayals of older adults in print, advertising, and entertainment. This is puzzling considering that older adults have the ability to purchase the advertisers' products that sponsor media activities. Yet limited efforts continue to be made to accurately depict the daily lives of older adults through the media.

Social roles continue to be important in later life. However, relationships are often dissolved as a result of poor health, limited mobility, and the inability to reciprocate support. Relationships with close family and friends are maintained before others because they are the source of most support. Some couples find later life to be a time of closeness, after weathering life's storms together. Some choose to separate and go their own ways, while others remain single and seek support from fictive kin. Relationships between aging parents and adult children tend to be as varied and challenging as spousal relationships, yet can generally be counted on to provide support. Maintaining friendships continues to promote psychological well-being well into old age. Grandparenting has been, and remains, a rewarding and fulfilling experience in later life.

Attitudes toward retirement vary greatly, as do lifestyles of older adults. For some, retirement heralds the chance to pursue a special interest or hobby they never had time to do while working. Others see it as an opportunity to travel or return to school to pursue a second career. Others view it with a bit of disappointment, especially if they previously held an influential position. For most people, however, retirement is a time of relaxation to be spent with spouse, children, grandchildren, and/or friends.

Financial security is extremely important to older adults. Social Security was a source of income for 90% of older adults in 2004 with one-third counting it as 89% of their entire income. Unfortunately, in 2006, 3.6 million adults lived below the federal poverty level. A great many impoverished individuals include single women who are African American or Hispanic.

Several organizations advocate for the rights and needs of older adults at the local, state, and national levels: AARP, Gray Panthers: Age and Youth in Action, and the SSA. All three organizations were founded more than 40 years ago with the mission of bringing about social change for older adults.

As a result of improvements in health care, better diet, and more emphasis on exercise, Americans are entering later life healthier than ever before. Healthy People 2010 is a strategic plan focusing on health prevention efforts. It emphasizes the need for vitality and independence among older adults and uses a health-oriented rather than a disease-oriented approach. The plan addresses topics such as exercise, stress management, nutrition, and substance abuse.

One of the greatest problems facing our aging society is health care finances. The costs of financing the federal health programs including Medicare and Medicaid continue to rise. In response to rising costs, many older adults are buying long-term health care insurance.

It is important for everyone working with older adults to understand that social factors affect our aging society. By developing appreciation for the diverse backgrounds of older adults, health care professionals can better serve their needs. Additionally, this should help us in our own personal approach to coping with aging family members and our own aging processes.

Review Questions

1. Gerontologists take into account the _____ forces that influence the aging process.
   A. Organic, synthetic, and supernatural
   B. Biennial, perennial, and annual
   C. Biological, psychological, and sociological
   D. Infantile, adolescent, and middle-aged

2. Ageism is
   A. The systematic stereotyping of and discrimination against people who are old
   B. Pretending to be older than you really are
   C. Pretending to be younger than you really are
   D. Another term for racism

3. Which of the following explains some of the negative comments made by health care workers about older adults?
   A. A need to justify why the medical needs of the older adult were not addressed
   B. Provides a feeling of satisfaction for managing the demands of the job
   C. Contributes to their ability to save or cure a patient's medical problems
   D. Explains a general unawareness of their own life and mortality

4. Work discrimination against older adults is a form of
   A. Bigotry
   B. Ageism
   C. Socialism
   D. None of the above

5. Social roles are important ways of _____ members of every society.
   A. Selecting and eliminating
   B. Categorizing and sorting
   C. Identifying and defining
   D. Discovering and isolating

6. When a grandparent raises a grandchild, which of the following poses a significant challenge to the role?
   A. Limited income and resources
   B. The social stigma of the parent's problem
   C. Personal health problems
   D. All of the above

7. In collectivist societies, which role is a grandparent most likely to hold?
   A. Surrogate parent
   B. Fictive kin
   C. Reservoir of family wisdom
   D. Dowager

8. Studies have also shown that as we age and our health declines, we deliberately let go of some of our social relationships, retaining only the ones we know we can maintain. We do this because we
   A. Recognize relationships are expendable
   B. No longer have interest in the lives of other people
   C. No longer have the resources and energy to engage
   D. Realize our friends don't really need us

9. The average retirement age in most Western countries is
   A. 55
   B. 65
   C. 70
   D. 75

10. _____ is a source of income for 90% of older adults in the United States.
    A. Social Security
    B. Personal investments
    C. Retirement plans
    D. Earnings from work

11. Healthy People 2010 emphasizes the need for vitality and independence with aging and uses a _____-oriented rather than a _____-oriented approach.
    A. Health; disease
    B. Person; society
    C. Fitness; diet
    D. None of the above

12. _____ issues sometimes result when older adults take multiple medications and supplements. Interactions between the substances can create additional health problems, including addiction to prescribed medications.
    A. Polygamy
    B. Polymorphism
    C. Peer pressure
    D. Polypharmacy

13. Total nursing home costs during the last year of life are rarely covered by
    A. Medicare
    B. Medicaid
    C. Long-term care insurance
    D. None of the above

14. Which organization does not have a primary advocacy focus on older adults?
    A. Gray Panthers: Age and Youth in Action
    B. Senior Service America
    C. AAA
    D. AARP

Learning Activities

1. Role-play with a partner examples of ageism found in the workplace, in a health care setting, in social situations, and in the family.
2. Videotape television commercials or shows featuring older adults. Review the tape for how the older adults are represented. Play it for your classmates and generate a discussion.
3. Establish a "mock" advocacy group representing older adults. Develop a mission, vision statement, goals, and objectives. Describe how you might use the group to effect changes to improve the lives of older adults.
4. Role-play with a partner some of the issues and concerns of an older caregiver faced with providing care for an ailing spouse.
5. Create a retirement plan for a fictitious couple that takes into account their financial resources, their family relationships, their personal interests, and their desire to work.
6. Design a health promotion/disease prevention course or workshop for older adults.

REFERENCES

1. Associated Press. Elders' knowledge of the oceans spares Thai "sea gypsies" from tsunami disaster. December 31, 2004. Bangkok, Thailand. Retrieved April 25, 2008, from http://www.ap.org/

2. Butler, RM. Ageism: Another form of bigotry. *Gerontologist*, 1969;9:243–246.

3. Butler, RM. *The Longevity Revolution*. New York: Public Affairs, 2008.

4. Tagliareni, E, Waters, V. The aging experience. In MA Anderson, JV Braun (eds.). *Caring for the Elderly Client*. Philadelphia: F. A. Davis, 1995.

5. Palmore, EB. *Ageism: Negative and Positive*. New York: Springer, 1990.

6. Alliance for Aging Research. *Ageism: How Healthcare Fails the Elderly*. New York: Alliance for Aging Research, March 2003.

7. Simkins, CL. Ageism's influence on health care delivery and nursing practice. *Journal of Student Nursing*, 2007;1:24–28.

8. Anti-Ageing Task Force. What is ageism? In *Ageism in America*. New York: International Longevity Center-US, 2006. Retrieved April 25, 2008, from http://www.ilcusa.org/media/pdfs/Ageism%20in%20America%20-%20The%20ILC%20Report.pdf

9. Kleyman, P. Media Ageism: The Link Between Newsrooms and Advertising Suites. Retrieved April 25, 2008, from http://www.asaging.org/at/at-218/Media.html

10. Dove. Dove Is Pro-Age. Retrieved April 25, 2008, from http://www.doveproage.com/

11. Ferraro, KF. Aging and role transitions. In RH Binstock, LK George (eds.). *Handbook of Aging and the Social Sciences*. 5th ed. San Diego: Academic Press, 2001.

12. Wang, M. Profiling retirees in the retirement transition and adjustment process: Examining the longitudinal change patterns of retirees' psychological well-being. *Journal of Applied Psychology*, 2007;92:455–474.

13. Mature Market Institute. Miles Away: The MetLife Study of Long-Distance Caregiving. 2004. Retrieved on April 25, 2008, from http://www.caregiving.org/data/milesaway.pdf

14. Suitor, JJ, Pillmer, K, Keeton, S, Robison, J. Aged parents and aging children: Determinants of relationship quality. In R Blieszner, VH Bedford (eds.). *Aging and the Family*. Westport, CT: Praeger, 1996.

15. U.S. Census Bureau. Facts for Features: Grandparent's Day, 2007. July 9, 2007. Retrieved April 25, 2008, from http://www.census.gov/Press-Release/www/2007/cb07ff-12.pdf

16. Shapiro, ME. *Asian Culture Brief: India*. Vol. 2(4). Honolulu: National Technical Assistance Center, n.d.

17. Shapiro, ME. *Asian Culture Brief: Philippines*. Vol. 2(3). Honolulu: National Technical Assistance Center, n.d.

18. Shapiro, ME. *Asian Culture Brief: Vietnam*. Vol. 2(5). Honolulu: National Technical Assistance Center, n.d.

19. Wallis, V. *Two Old Women: An Alaska Legend of Betrayal, Courage and Survival*. Seattle, WA: Epicenter Press, 1993.

20. Kim-Rupnow, WS. *Asian Culture Brief: Korea*. Vol. 2(1). Honolulu: National Technical Assistance Center, n.d.

21. Brightman, J, Subedi, LA. *AAPI Culture Brief: Hawai'i*. Vol. 2(7). Honolulu: National Technical Assistance Center, 2007.

22. Charness, N, Czaja, SJ. Older worker training: What we know and don't know. *AARP*, October 2006.

23. U.S. Census, Bureau. Facts for Features: Cinco de Mayo. March 7, 2007. Retrieved April 25, 2008, from http://www.census.gov/Press-Release/www/releases/archives/facts_for_features_special_editions/009726.html

24. Garcia, EC. Parenting in Mexican American families. In NB Webb (ed.), *Culturally Diverse Parent–Child and Family Relationships: A Guide for Social Workers and Other Practitioners*. New York: Columbia University Press, 2001.

25. Carstensen, LL. Evidence for a life-span theory of socioemotional selectivity. *Current Directions in Psychological Science*, 1995;4:151–156.

26. Kahn, R, Antonucci, T. Convoys over the life course: Attachment, roles, and social support. In

P Baltes, OG Brim (eds.). *Life-Span Development and Behavior*. New York: Academic Press, 1980.

27. Berkman, L, Breslow, L. *Health and Ways of Living: The Alameda County Study*. New York: Oxford University Press, 1983.

28. Bargh, JA, McKenna, KYA. The Internet and social life. *Annual Review of Psychology*, 2004;55: 573–590.

29. Spraggins, RE. Women in the United States: A Profile March 2000. Retrieved April 25, 2008, from http://www.census.gov/prod/2000pubs/cenbr001.pdf

30. Silverstone, B, Hyman, H. *Growing Older Together*. New York: Pantheon Books, 1992.

31. Tournier, P. *Learn to Grow Old*. New York: Harper and Row, 1972.

32. Mancini, JA (ed.). *Aging Parents and Adult Children*. Washington, DC: Lexington Books, 1989.

33. MetLife and National Alliance for Caregiving. Since You Care: Long Distance Caregiving. 2005. Retrieved on April 25, 2008, from http://www.metlife.com/WPSAssets/20778401118179212V1FLong%20Dist%20Caregiving.pdf

34. Dychtwald, K. *Age Wave*. New York: Bantam Books, 1990.

35. Dunham, CC. A link between generations: Intergenerational relations and depression in aging parents. *Journal of Family Issues*, 1995;16: 450–465.

36. U.S. Census Bureau. Retrieved February 6, 2009, from http://www.census.gov/press-release/www/releases/archives/families_households/00684.html

37. Connidis, IA, McMullin, JA. To have or not to have: Parent status and the subjective well-being of older men and women. *Gerontologist*, 1993;33: 630–636.

38. Jordan-Marsh, M, Harden, JT. Fictive kin: Friends as family supporting older adults as they age. *Journal of Gerontological Nursing*, 2005; 31:2.

39. Blieszner, R, Adams, RG. *Adult Friendship*. Newbury Park, CA: Sage Publications, 1992.

40. Antonucci, TC. Social relations: An examination of social networks, social support, and sense of control. In JE Birren, KW Schaie (eds.). *Handbook of the Psychology of Aging*. San Diego, CA: Academic Press, 2001.

41. Neugarten, BL, Weinstein, KK. The changing American grandparent. *Journal of Marriage and the Family*, 1964;26:199–204.

42. Dhjama, T. Grandparents offer an expanding market niche. *TD Monthly*, 2003. Retrieved April 25, 2008, from http://www.toydirectory.com/monthly/Aug2003/Special_Grandparents.asp

43. Grandparents. Links. Retrieved April 25, 2008, from http://info.ag.uidaho.edu/grandparents/links.htm

44. Grandparenting. Home page. Retrieved April 25, 2008, from http://www.grandparenting.org

45. Elderhostel. Programs for grandparents page. Retrieved April 25, 2008, from http://www.elderhostel.org/programs/search_res.asp?keyword=grandparent

46. Adopt a Grandparent Program. Home page. Retrieved April 25, 2008, from http://www.adoptagrandparent.org

47. Foster Grandparent Program. Retrieved April 25, 2008, from http://www.fostergrandparentprogram.org/history.html

48. Social Security Administration. Traditional Sources of Economic Security. Retrieved April 25, 2008, from http://www.ssa.gov/history/briefhistory3.html

49. Social Security Administration. *Income of the Aged Chartbook, 2004*. Washington, DC: Office of Research, Evaluation, and Statistics, 2006.

50. U.S. Census Bureau. Historical Poverty Tables. Retrieved April 25, 2008, from http://www.census.gov/hhes/www/poverty/histpov/hstpov3.html

51. Koellin, K, et al. Vulnerable elderly households: Expenditures on necessities by older americans. *Social Science Quarterly*, 1995;76:619–632.

52. Maddox, G (ed.). *Encyclopedia of Aging*. New York: Springer, 1987.

53. U.S. Senate Special Committee on Aging, American Association of Retired Persons, Federal Council on the Aging, and U.S. Administration on Aging. *Aging America, Trends and Projections*. 1991 ed. Washington, DC: U.S. Department of Health and Human Services, 1991.

54. Zemke, R, Zemke, S. 30 things we know for sure about adult learning. *Innovation Abstracts*, March 9, 1984;6:8.

55. AARP International. Global Aging. Retrieved April 25, 2008, from http://www.aarpinternational.org/map/

56. Allison, R. Easy steps to tone up retirement. *Advertising Age*, November 1996;67(45):32.

57. Bennett, D. Great grandmother goes solo. *Cruising World*, December 1994;19(12):8–9.

58. Clements, M. What we say about aging. *Parade Magazine*, December 12, 1993:4–5.

59. Plymouth Harbor at Sarasota Bay. About Us. Retrieved April 25, 2008, from http://www.plymouthharbor.org/about/index.asp

60. Seniorcorp. Home page. Retrieved April 25, 2008, from http://www.seniorcorps.com

61. AARP. Home page. Retrieved April 25, 2008, from http://www.aarp.org

62. Gray Panthers: Age and Youth in Action. Home page. Retrieved April 25, 2008, from http://www.graypanthers.org

63. Senior Service America. Home page. Retrieved April 25, 2008, from http://www.seniorserviceamerica.org

64. Healthy People 2010. Home page. Retrieved April 25, 2008, from http://www.healthypeople.gov/

65. Haber, D. *Health Promotion and Aging: Practical Applications for Health Professionals.* 4th ed. New York: Springer, 2007.

66. Anderson, M, Braun, J. *Caring for the Elderly Client.* Philadelphia: FA Davis, 1995.

67. Burrell, C. Malnutrition is common among older Americans. *Maine Sunday Telegram, Health Resources Guide*, October 13, 1996.

68. Burger, SG, Kayser-Jones, J, Prince, J. *Malnutrition and Dehydration in Nursing Homes: Key Issues in Prevention and Treatment.* National Citizens' Coalition for Nursing Home Reform, The Commonwealth Fund. Washington, DC: July 2000.

69. Ahmed, F. Effect of nutrition on the health of the elderly. *Journal of American Dietetic Association*, 1992;92:1102–1108.

70. Wick, JY. Avoiding polypharmacy pitfalls: It's all in your approach. *Pharmacy Times*, 2006. Retrieved April 25, 2008, from http://www.pharmacytimes.com/issues/articles/2006-01_2981.asp

71. Outlays for Health Programs: 1962–2010. Retrieved April 25, 2008, from http://www.gpoaccess.gov/usbudget/fy06/sheets/hist16z1.xls

72. MetLife Mature Market Institute and LifePlans, Inc. *The MetLife Market Survey of Nursing Home and Home Care Costs.* Westport, CT: MetLife Market Institute, 2006.

73. Pfuntner, J, Dietz, F. Long-Term Care Insurance Gains Prominence. Retrieved April 25, 2008, from http://www.bls.gov/opub/cwc/cm20040123ar01p1.htm

Chapter 3

THE PHYSIOLOGY AND PATHOLOGY OF AGING

DAVID A. SANDMIRE, MD

It is frustrating that in a time when humans have gone into and returned from outer space and can manipulate DNA, they have not conquered death. Death, indeed, remains the last "sacred" enemy.
— *Paola S. Timiras,* Physiological Basis of Aging and Geriatrics[1]

Much of the continuing massive destruction of this planet and the consequent ills that this destruction produces for humans can be traced to overpopulation, a phenomenon that appears to show no sign of abating. Extending the life of a population that already strains global resources is, in the view of many, unconscionable.

— *L. Hayflick,* Myths of Aging[2]

Chapter Outline

Behavioral Objectives

Upon completion of this chapter, the reader will be able to:

1. Compare and contrast the concepts of aging as a "disease" and aging as a "process."
2. Compare and contrast preventive medicine and curative medicine.

3. Explain the difference between average life expectancy and maximum life span potential and describe the determinants of each.
4. Describe both molecular and evolutionary theories of aging.
5. Describe the cellular theories of aging and explain the possible role of free radical formation in the aging process.
6. Describe the cross-linking and glycosylation theories of aging.
7. Explain the effects of aging on the various organ systems of the body.
8. Understand the concept of homeostasis, or the maintenance of a stable internal environment in the body in the face of an ever-changing external environment.
9. Appreciate the interdependence among the body's organ systems and the ways in which these systems compensate for disturbances in homeostasis.
10. Describe how the compensatory capabilities of the body change with advancing age.
11. Understand the concept of *illness* as an inability of the body to adequately compensate for disturbances in homeostasis.

Key Terms

Alveoli	Gastritis
Anemia	Heat stroke
Aneurysm	Hyposmia
Atherosclerosis	Hypothalamus
Autoimmune disease	Lipofuscin
Average life expectancy	Maximum life span potential
Benign prostatic hypertrophy	Myocardial infarction
Cataract	Osteoarthritis
Chronic bronchitis	Osteoporosis
Chronic obstructive pulmonary disease	Peptic ulcer
Dementia	Pituitary gland
Diabetes mellitus	Postural (orthostatic) hypotension
Diaphragm	Presbycusis
Diverticulosis	Presbyopia
Dysphagia	Senescence
Embolism	Stroke
Emphysema	Thrombus
Fecal incontinence	Urinary incontinence
Free radical	Xerostomia

If death is our last sacred enemy, how can efforts to extend our life span be considered unconscionable? Perhaps the view of death as an enemy to be conquered emanates from one's personal perspective, whereas considering a timely death as a necessity to conserve our earth's resources reflects a more global perspective. Indeed, it is entirely possible for an individual to share both sentiments. What is certain is that death remains one of the great mysteries of our existence. Thus, how one deals with death, and the aging process that leads to it, is in large part dictated by religious, cultural, and philosophical beliefs as well as by the structure of one's national health care system. Italy's universal health care coverage is modeled after that of Great Britain, but it does not include nursing home coverage, so the care of older adults is "almost exclusively the concern of families." Thus, in a small Italian village, one finds three generations of a family living under one roof, the younger generations taking to heart a sense of obligation to the older members of the family. Contrast this with the fast-paced, highly mobile society that is the United States, where 6.5% of those 65 years and older live in institutional settings.[3,4]

Culture not only influences personal perspectives and family living arrangements but also the way that scientists approach aging (often called **senescence**) and death. Scientific enterprise is a mirror of culture, and vice versa. If society views the physiologic changes associated with aging as "diseases," researchers will do likewise. Indeed, Western medicine, with its greater emphasis on curative rather than preventive medicine, seems to favor the disease model of aging. We expend more time and resources curing cancer and treating heart attack victims than we do promoting healthful living. According to a report by the Centers for Disease Control and Prevention, only 5% of all U.S. health care dollars in 1988 were spent on preventative medicine.[5] Although that percentage may have increased in recent years, curative medicine continues to dominate our health care landscape. Curative medicine and the disease model of aging, in turn, help us rationalize the placement of older adults in nursing homes and other extended-care settings. If, instead, we accept senescence as a process that can be attenuated, we are likely to focus more on healthful living and preventive medicine throughout life than on a costly quick fix at the end of life.

From a strictly scientific standpoint, however, the distinction between aging and disease is, at best, a blurry one. Consider atherosclerosis, a pervasive affliction of older adults that predisposes them to hypertension, heart attacks, and strokes. Do the fatty plaques that develop in arteries result from degenerative changes that are inevitable with the passage of time or from specific injuries to the blood vessels, perhaps caused by turbulent blood flow or microbial infection? Do low-fat diets and exercise regimens merely slow down this unavoidable "phenomenon of aging"? Or is it more accurate to view healthy lifestyle habits as measures that prevent the "disease" atherosclerosis? Paola S. Timiras suggests the following distinctions be made between aging and disease[6]:

- Aging is a universal process, shared by all living organisms, whereas disease is a selective process, varying with species, tissue, organ, cell, and molecule.
- Aging is intrinsic, dependent on genetic factors, whereas disease is intrinsic and extrinsic, dependent on both genetic and environmental factors.
- Aging is always progressive, whereas disease may be discontinuous and may progress, regress, or be arrested entirely.

- Aging is always deleterious and likely to reduce functional competence, whereas disease is occasionally deleterious, often causing damage that is reversible.
- Aging is irreversible, whereas disease may be treatable and often has a known cause.

Whether you agree with these descriptors or not, there is good reason to continue refining definitions and conceptions of aging. Consider the following statistic: the **average life expectancy** in the United States has risen from about 45 years in 1900 to 78 years in 2004, an increase largely attributed to improvements in sanitation, food, and water supply and to the advent of antibiotics and vaccinations.[4,7,8] But during this period there has been no change in the **maximum life span potential** (MLP, that is, the oldest age reached by an individual in a population) of Americans, estimated to be about 115 (**Figure 3-1**).[9,10] Thus, although improvements in our standard of living have helped spare us from several causes of premature death, such as cholera, tuberculosis, and influenza, they have done nothing to slow down the inherent aging process. In fact, any medical intervention that claims to slow down human aging must be shown to increase the maximum life span potential, and, to date, none have done so.

Our unchanging maximum life span potential in the face of an ever-increasing life expectancy suggests two things to those who ponder growing old. First, it supports the

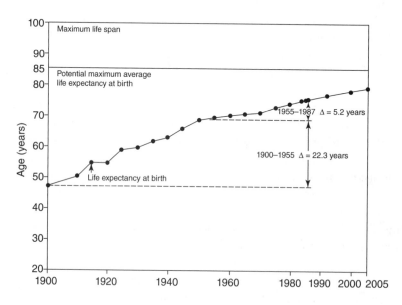

FIGURE 3-1 Life expectancy at birth and estimated maximum life span potential in the United States since 1990.

Adapted from: Harman, D. The aging process: major risk factors for disease and death. *The Proceedings of the National Academy of Sciences,* 1991;88:5362. And U.S. Department of Health and Human Services. Health: United States, 2007, Table 27, p. 192. Retrieved March 2, 2009, from http://www.cdc.gov/nchs/data/hus/hus07.pdf#027.

notion of distinguishing disease from aging. One of the most important chapters in the history of medicine has been the eradication of smallpox from the face of the earth by using vaccines. But although the child who is immunized to smallpox has been spared a devastating infectious disease, he or she is not likely to age more slowly than a nonimmunized child will. Second, a maximum life span potential that probably has not changed in centuries suggests that there exists some "biological clock" that predetermines our length of life. No such clock has been discovered, and it is perhaps an oversimplification of human physiology to suggest that one single mechanism in the body is responsible for aging. Nonetheless, it certainly appears that there are relatively fixed limits on how long the human body lasts.

A fixed life span, however, does not necessarily sentence us to pain and suffering in our twilight years. Many of the physiologic changes associated with aging can be slowed to some extent with a healthy diet and consistent regimen of moderate exercise, and many of the chronic diseases prevalent in older adults are either preventable or modifiable with healthy lifestyle habits (**Table 3-1**). Reduction of dietary fat (especially saturated fats and cholesterol) lowers one's risk of coronary artery disease and stroke[11] as well as breast and colon cancer.[12,13] A program of increased physical activity increases one's resting and maximum cardiac output (the amount of blood pumped out of the heart per minute) while decreasing one's chance of developing hypertension.[6,14] To the extent that exercise helps prevent obesity, it also decreases the likelihood that one will develop osteoarthritis and non-insulin-dependent diabetes mellitus or suffer from a heart attack.[12] Regular exercise, coupled with sufficient dietary calcium intake, lowers one's risk of osteoporosis and its complications, such as broken hips and slipped intervertebral disks.[4] Along with these physical benefits, exercise appears to have psychological benefits as well, lifting one's spirits and alleviating loneliness and depression.[15] On the other hand, sedentary lifestyles and, in particular, extended bed rest increase the chance of thromboembolic disease, respiratory infection, and decubitus ulcers (bed sores). Perhaps the most important lifestyle choice one can make is to not smoke cigarettes. Indeed, cigarette smoking is the most common preventable cause of disease and death in the United States. It leads to chronic obstructive pulmonary disease (e.g., emphysema, chronic bronchitis) and lung cancer and is a major cause of other cancers of the upper respiratory and digestive tracts.[12,16] In addition, cigarette smoking enhances one's chance of developing atherosclerosis and its complications—heart attacks and strokes. In all, cigarette smoking decreases one's life expectancy by 7 years and one's disease-free years by 14.[17]

Clearly, there are many ways to enhance our health as we age, but such modifications to lifestyle, activity level, and diet must occur in early or middle life to have the maximum effect. One of the difficulties in convincing young people to adopt these measures is that, generally speaking, they already feel healthy. Persuading a teenager to quit smoking or a 40-year-old business executive to take her blood pressure medication is difficult when doing so offers them no immediate reward—delayed gratification is not something our society seems to value highly. But the tide appears to be turning, at least on some fronts,

TABLE 3-1   Common Chronic Diseases of Aging Potentially Modifiable in Middle Age Through Personal Changes in Lifestyle.

Disorder	Preventive Strategy
Hypertension	Reduction of dietary sodium
	Reduction of body weight
Atherosclerotic cardiovascular disease	Treatment of hypertension
	Cessation of cigarette smoking
	Reduction of excess body weight
	Reduction of dietary saturated fat and cholesterol
	Increased aerobic exercise
Cancers	Cessation of cigarette smoking
	Reduction of dietary fat
	Reduction of salt- or smoke-cured food intake
	Minimization of radiation exposure
	Minimization of sun exposure
Chronic obstructive pulmonary disease	Cessation of cigarette smoking
Diabetes mellitus (type 2)	Reduction of excess body weight
	Diet consistent with atherosclerosis prevention
Osteoporosis	Maintenance of dietary calcium
	Regular exercise
	Cessation of cigarette smoking
	Avoidance of alcohol excess
Osteoarthritis	Reduction of body weight
Cholelithiasis (i.e., gallstones)	Reduction of body weight

Source: Bierman, EL, Hazzard, WP. Preventive Gerontology: Strategies for attentuation of the chronic diseases of aging. In Hazzard, WR, et al. (eds.), *Principles of Geriatric Medicine and Gerontology*, ed 3. McGraw-Hill, New York, p 188. Reprinted with permission.

as evidenced by the growing popularity of aerobic exercise over the past three decades and the legislative effort to limit the public areas where smoking is allowed. Perhaps these societal changes will accomplish what gerontologists call the compression of morbidity— that is, decreasing the period and severity of illness experienced toward the end of life.

Human aging, in its pure form, is a process that runs a fairly predictable course from infancy to senescence. Superimposed on that developmental sequence, however, are life-style choices and environmental insults that influence how far we are able to travel along life's course and how well we feel along the journey. In fact, genetic makeup may account for only 25% of the variation in human longevity, with much of our health and well-being

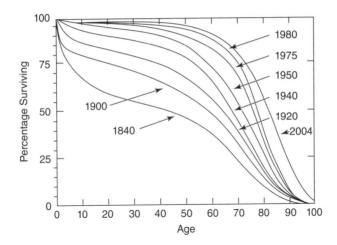

FIGURE 3-2 Specific mortality survival curve, illustrating the "rectangularization" that has taken place over the past 150 years as a growing percentage of the population approaches the maximum life span potential. (*Adapted from: Cassel, CK, Brody, JA. Demography, epidemiology, and aging. In CK Cassel (eds.). Geriatric Medicine. 2nd ed. New York: Springer-Verlag, 1990, p. 17;* National Vital Statistics Reports, *2007;56(9):6.*)

determined by environmental factors.[18] Although we may not be able to extend our maximum life span potential, we can certainly reduce the morbidity associated with aging on our way to the 115th year. In addition, healthy lifestyles may help us accomplish what epidemiologists call a rectangularization of the survival curve—a condition where nearly everyone in a population reaches the maximum life span potential (**Figure 3-2**). Perhaps there is some truth to the observation by comedian George Burns that you can never live to be 100 if you stop living at 65.[4] Burns lived to enjoy his 100th birthday.

THEORIES OF BIOLOGICAL AGING

Although research on the aging process has proceeded for decades, we now seem as far away from the fountain of youth as we ever were. One of the stumbling blocks in senescence research is the lack of a true biological marker of aging (with the arguable exception of lipofuscin accumulation in cells, discussed later). There is no single identifiable molecular, cellular, tissue, or organ change in the body that correlates closely with age.[19,20] Senescence appears to be a multifactorial process whose rate depends on both genetic and environmental phenomena.[21] The following sections briefly review some theories of aging that have been proposed over the past 55 years. It is not my intent to suggest that any single theory explains the aging process, but rather to recognize that aging is a complex phenomenon orchestrated by events at several organizational levels in the body.

MOLECULAR AND EVOLUTIONARY THEORIES OF AGING

Because the stages of cellular, tissue, organ, and body development are, for the most part, controlled by our genetic machinery, many theories of aging have focused on the role of DNA (deoxyribonucleic acid), RNA (ribonucleic acid), and the proteins made from these nucleic acid "blueprints" (**Table 3-2**).

One such theory is that senescence results from the gradual accumulation of random mutations (alterations in the DNA) in somatic cells of the body.[22] According to this *somatic mutation theory*, radiation and other environmental mutagens alter the structure of the genetic code and thus change the sequence of amino acids found in enzymes and other proteins. Such minor alterations could, in turn, have damaging effects on protein

TABLE 3-2 Theories of Biological Aging.

Somatic mutation theory	Gradually accumulating random mutations of the DNA alter gene structure and function.
Error catastrophe theory	Loss of precision in the translation of the genetic code from DNA to proteins.
Gene regulation theory	Changes in the expression of certain genes orchestrate the changes of aging.
Evolutionary theory	Aging is an inevitable by-product of evolution because of less intense selection against deleterious genes in older individuals.
Antagonistic pleiotropy theory	Evolutionary selection of genes that are favorable for younger individuals despite their harmful effect in older individuals.
Disposable soma theory	Aging is an inevitable result of the compromise that a species reaches between diverting all of its energy to reproduction and diverting all of its energy to body maintenance and repair.
Wear-and-tear theory	Cells and thus individuals wear out from continued use.
Rate-of-living theory	Version of the wear-and-tear theory that suggests that a species' average life span is inversely proportional to its basal metabolic rate per gram of metabolizing tissue.
Free radical theory	Aging results from the random damage to macromolecules by highly reactive molecules called free radicals.
Cross-linking theory	Aging results from the accumulation of cross-linkages between macromolecules.
Glycosylation theory	Aging is attributed to the accumulation of cross-linkages between macromolecules as a result of the intial attachment of glucose molecules to those macromolecules.
Telomere erosion theory	Aging and cell mortality are caused by the gradual loss of the protective telomere nucleotide sequences at the ends of the DNA strands within chromosomes with each new cell division and the resultant inability of those cells to continue to divide.

function and thus on body functions. Differences in longevity among individuals might result from varying rates of mutagenesis and varying proficiencies of DNA repair. Studies have shown that longer-lived species tend to have more effective mechanisms for repairing molecular damage than do shorter-lived species.[23,24] But although the number of DNA mutations increases with age,[25,26] proving that such changes are the cause, rather than the result, of aging has been more difficult.

The *error catastrophe theory* attributes aging to problems in the transfer of information from DNA to proteins.[27] A gradual decline in the precision of DNA transcription and RNA translation would cause the accumulation of abnormal enzymes in aging cells. If such malformed enzymes themselves were unable to play proper roles in transcription or translation, their production would, in positive feedback fashion, exacerbate the errors in transcription and translation, resulting in catastrophic changes in cellular physiology.[4,28] However, if errors in fact occurred in these critical processes, you would expect all cellular enzymes to be affected equally, and studies do not bear this out.[29–32]

In contrast to the preceding concepts of aging as something that results from molecular "mistakes," the *gene regulation theory* suggests that aging occurs along an intentional timeline that is primarily determined by changes in the regulation of gene expression.[33] If earlier stages of human development are orchestrated by the precise turning on and turning off of certain genes, age-related changes might be as well. But studies designed to look specifically for such changes in gene expression have not been fruitful.[34,35] This may be because whole organisms or tissues were studied rather than individual cell types or because the changes in gene expression are undetectable by current research techniques.

If the characteristics of growing old are indeed the result of the expression of certain genes that cause age-related changes in cells, why would such preprogrammed mortality have evolved in the first place? Some intriguing answers to this question come from evolutionary biologists. The *evolutionary theory* of aging portrays senescence as a by-product, rather than a driving force, of evolution.[36] Even if a species did not age, accidental mortality occurring at a fixed rate (e.g., resulting from predation) would cause the number of individuals reaching successively older ages to decline. Therefore, any DNA mutation that selectively affected an older individual's reproductive capability or survival in an adverse way would be less detrimental to the species as a whole than a mutation that selectively altered a younger individual's reproductive ability. There would be less intense selection pressure against "bad genes" programmed to affect older members of a species than against "bad genes" that preferentially affect its younger members. Those individuals lucky enough to escape accidental death earlier in life would eventually succumb to the effects of detrimental genes that have remained in the species' genetic pool.

But if the evolutionary theory's starting conditions dictate that aging did not exist initially and was instead an end result of the course of evolution, how could certain genes initially have had age-specific effects in a species that did not age? One possibility is that although there would be little natural selection *against* genes that adversely affected aged individuals, there would be a strong selection *for* genes that benefitted younger individuals, even if such genes had adverse side effects for older members of the species.[37] These individual genes that are beneficial early in life but detrimental late in life are said to exhibit *antagonistic pleiotropy*. For example, a gene that stimulates the deposition of calcium in the bone of young individuals (a favorable effect) may also cause calcification of arteries and other soft tissues later in life (an unfavorable effect). Similarly, a gene that promotes rapid cell division during embryonic development (favorable) may predispose an elderly individual to uncontrolled cell division, or cancer (unfavorable).[38]

Another evolutionary explanation for aging, the *disposable soma theory*, proposes that a species strikes a compromise between expending all of its energy on reproduction and spending all of its energy on maintenance and repair of the body, or *soma*.[39] Members of a species that hypothetically devote all of their available energy to reproduction without providing the necessary nutrients for feeding, growth, and tissue repair will likely die before they are able to reproduce. Conversely, organisms that devote all of their resources to maintenance of the soma would still not be able to escape the accidental mortality that all species face. In this regard, it would be wasteful to allocate too much energy to a soma that will eventually die anyway. Optimal species survival would be attained by reducing the amount of energy required for perpetual maintenance of the soma (i.e., immortality) and diverting the remaining energy to more rapid growth or greater reproductive output. Said another way, the longevity of a species would represent a balance between the natural selection for a longer reproductive period and the limits placed on the life span by environmental hazards. The soma is in this sense disposable as long as a species can survive to reproduce. A species such as the tree shrew that is relatively low on the food chain and therefore subjected to high rates of accidental death does better to focus more of its resources on rapid development and increased reproductive capability than on maintaining a viable soma. Its life span is thus relatively short. In contrast, an organism with virtually no natural predators, such as the African elephant, has a much longer life span because of its proportionately greater investment in somatic maintenance and repair. As a result, it has smaller numbers of progeny and longer gestational periods. Similarly, it is perhaps not surprising that human beings, who for all practical purposes have no natural predators, are the longest lived of all mammals.

CELLULAR THEORIES OF AGING

Although the evolutionary theories of aging provide explanations for the origin of senescence, they do not predict the specific events in the process of cellular aging. In this section, theories of aging are reviewed that either directly or indirectly relate to actual changes in cell structure and function.

The *wear-and-tear theory* of aging proposes that aging is inevitable as cells, much like machines, gradually wear out from continued use. The machine analogy is not a perfect one because cells, unlike machines, have several mechanisms to repair their injuries. But with the passage of time, the intracellular damage resulting from wear and tear might accumulate to a point at which it overcomes a cell's capacity for maintenance and repair. Cells (and therefore organisms) with higher rates of metabolism might "wear out" more quickly than do those with lower metabolic rates, thus aging more quickly and dying sooner.

The inverse correlation between basal metabolic rate and longevity across a wide number of species has led some experimental gerontologists to reformulate the wear-and-tear hypothesis into a rate-of-living theory of aging, which attributes interspecies variation in life span to varying metabolic rates per gram of metabolizing tissue.[40] Every organism, then, is endowed with the ability to burn up a fixed number of calories in its lifetime, after which the accumulation of wear and tear results in the organism's death. Members of a species with a higher metabolic rate would burn up their fixed number of total calories more quickly, suffer from accumulated wear and tear more rapidly, and die sooner than those of a species with a lower metabolic rate.

The well-documented effect of *caloric restriction* (i.e., limiting food intake) to increase average life expectancy seems on the surface to support the rate-of-living theory of aging.[41-44] Furthermore, a multitude of studies has shown that caloric restriction not only increases average life expectancy but also diminishes many of the physiologic changes associated with increasing age, such as rising serum cholesterol levels,[45] decreasing bone mass,[46] and deteriorating immune system function.[47] Nonetheless, it does not appear that caloric restriction has a significant effect on an organism's specific basal metabolic rate.[48,49] The basis for its effect must therefore lie elsewhere. Furthermore, the rate-of-living theory itself has been called into question by studies that have found exceptions to the generalization that animals with lower metabolic rates live longer than those with higher metabolic rates.[50]

Although the rate-of-living theory of aging thus far has not panned out, it nonetheless has helped focus experimental gerontology on another promising theory, the free radical theory of aging.

FREE RADICAL THEORY OF AGING

The *free radical theory* of aging is a specific version of the wear-and-tear theory that attributes cellular (and therefore organismal) aging to random accumulating damage of macromolecules by the highly reactive by-products of oxidative metabolism known as **free radicals**.[51-54] Free radicals are molecules that contain at least one unpaired electron in their outer valence shells. Free radicals most notably form in the mitochondria of cells, the site of aerobic respiration (the "burning up of food" for energy), where electrons are stripped from temporary carrier molecules and passed down a chain of membrane-bound protein carriers to be accepted by oxygen.[55,56] Free radicals are relatively rare in nature because they are chemically unstable. When formed, they usually bind with other free radicals to create more stable molecules. However, when free radicals form in cells, they can initiate chain reactions that consume oxygen and randomly damage lipid molecules, enzymes, and nucleic acids.

One part of a cell's structure that is particularly vulnerable to chemical attack by free radicals is the lipid membrane, which bounds the cell and many of its internal organelles, such as the mitochondria, endoplasmic reticulum, and Golgi apparatus. The polyunsaturated fatty acids embedded in these membranes are major targets. But cells have specific defenses against this lipid peroxidation, such as *vitamin E* (alpha-tocopherol), *vitamin C* (ascorbic acid), and several enzymes that arrest free radical chain reactions.[57]

If the levels of free radical "scavengers" such as vitamins E and C are depleted, however, damage to lipid membranes may be more permanent. Repeated peroxidation of unsaturated lipids can cause inappropriate cross-linking of lipids to proteins and nucleic acids.[58] The cross-linking of lipids with proteins leads to the formation of **lipofuscin** (or "age pigment"). Granules of this yellowish-brown pigment are found in the cytoplasm of aged cells (**Figure 3-3**). Interestingly, the slow, predictable accumulation of lipofuscin is considered to be the most reliable marker of chronological age in cells, and it has been found in nearly every eukaryotic organism studied thus far.[59]

Although evidence for the age-related accumulation of lipofuscin and other types of free radical–mediated cell damage is widespread, proving that free radical damage is the

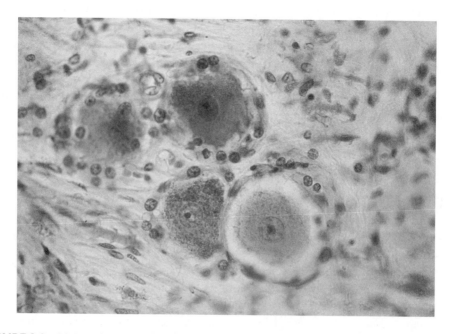

FIGURE 3-3 **Light micrograph of a dorsal root ganglion cell illustrating the accumulation of lipofuscin.** (*Courtesy of Allen Bell, University of New England.*)

primary determinant of aging has been more difficult; lipofuscin accumulation, it appears, is a result, rather than a cause, of aging.[60] Recall that any intervention that truly slows down the aging process must be shown to increase the maximum life span potential of a species. And although studies in which organisms were given supplements of vitamin E throughout life revealed that the rate of lipofuscin accumulation decreased and the average life expectancy often increased, none showed a change in the maximum life span potential.[61–66]

Nonetheless, the potential importance of free radical–mediated destruction in aging cells should not be ignored, especially when you consider its role in disease. Consider cigarette smoking, the most common preventable cause of disease and death in the United States. The smoke from cigarettes contains free radicals whose presence can alter or destroy important biological molecules such as DNA and enzymes.[67,68] Damage to DNA, in turn, may play a role in the etiology of lung cancer, whereas damage to enzymes, such as alpha-1 antitrypsin, may cause the progressive and irreversible destruction of lung tissue in patients with emphysema (see the section titled "Respiratory System" later in this chapter). Thus, smoking may accelerate the aging process by enhancing the free radical mechanism, a process that some researchers claim is at the heart of the natural aging process.[51] You can see how the distinction between disease and pure aging becomes less clear at the cellular level.

CROSS-LINKING AND GLYCOSYLATION THEORIES OF AGING

The *cross-linking theory* of aging attributes aging to the gradual accumulation of cross-linkages between organic macromolecules, particularly those that are closely packed together under normal circumstances, such as collagen and phospholipids.[69,70] Such binding together of large biological molecules might adversely alter their structure and function.

Intracellular macromolecules, such as enzymes and DNA, seem vulnerable to cross-linking as well.[71] The nonenzymatic attachment of glucose molecules to some proteins and DNA is an important preliminary step to their cross-linking. The extent of this glucose attachment increases with age, and long-term chemical modification of these glycosylated (i.e., "glucose-attached") macromolecules can lead to the formation of advanced glycosylation end products (AGEs), which are prone to further cross-linking.[72] The *glycosylation theory* of aging, really a subset of the cross-linking theory, implicates the accumulation of glycosylation-induced cross-links in the gradual aging of cells.[73]

Much of the impetus to study nonenzymatic glycosylation of proteins and DNA has come from its relevance to diabetes mellitus (DM), a disease marked by an elevated blood glucose level (hyperglycemia). Individuals with DM have glycosylated protein levels that are two to four times higher than those seen in nondiabetics.[74] Glycosylation of macromolecules might explain some of the long-term complications of DM, many of which are identical to the diseases commonly seen in aging individuals.[75] At the tissue level, long-term effects of DM include a loss of elasticity of arteries and joints, conditions that may help explain the accelerated hypertension and osteoarthritis, respectively, often suffered by diabetics.[76] In addition, excessive glycosylation and subsequent cross-linking of lens crystalline protein may contribute to the formation of **cataracts**, another diabetic complication that is also common in the nondiabetic elderly.[77,78] Finally, DM predisposes individuals to accelerated forms of atherosclerosis, emphysema, and immunosuppression—other conditions most prevalent in older individuals.[72] Although these considerations certainly do not prove that glycosylation accounts for all of the age-related changes in tissues, they are nonetheless provocative—particularly because caloric restriction in rats has been shown to decrease levels of protein glycosylation and blood glucose while at the same time increasing life expectancy.[41,74]

The proposed connections between the glycosylation process, the long-term complications of DM, and the pathologic conditions common to older adults provide but one more example of the unclear boundary between aging as a *process* and aging as a *disease*.

TELOMERES THEORY OF AGING

One of the more interesting developments in research on aging in the past decade has been in the area of *telomeres*, which are short nucleotide segments found at the ends of the DNA strands that may protect the DNA from damage. These telomere segments are of a fixed starting length in embryonic cells, but they get progressively shorter over time, most likely because of (1) oxidative stress (i.e., free radical–mediated damage), and (2) the inability of DNA polymerase enzymes to copy DNA all of the way to its ends prior to cell division. The enzyme telomerase helps maintain telomere length, but this enzyme is active only in germ cells (sperm and eggs) and certain lines of adult stem cells and cancer cells. Thus, as cells undergo repeated life cycles of cell division, the daughter cells inherit progressively shorter telomeres—a process called telomere erosion. It is believed that once these segments get too short, further cell division is not possible, thus placing a "mortality limit" on cells. Although such limits on cell division may be a protective mechanism against the development of cancers, the trade-off appears to be a fixed life span for our cells.[79–82]

As you can quickly realize from this review of the theories of aging, no one particular explanation for aging is completely satisfactory. As noted earlier, it is most likely that aging is a complex phenomenon orchestrated by events at several organizational levels in the body. Research efforts aimed at limiting the effects of aging will likely have to occur at multiple levels, from the molecular to the cellular to the organismal. Although the causes of aging remain elusive, the effects of aging on the body are more readily apparent.

The next section focuses on the actual physiologic and pathologic changes that occur in the organ systems as we grow older.

AGE-RELATED CHANGES OF THE ORGAN SYSTEMS

INTEGUMENTARY SYSTEM

The integumentary system consists of the skin and all of its accessory structures, such as hair, nails, sebaceous (oil) glands, and eccrine (sweat) glands. From outermost in, skin consists of three major layers: the epidermis, dermis, and subcutaneous layers. Because the skin covers our bodies, changes in its appearance are the most visibly noticeable of all aging phenomena. This section focuses on the particular changes that occur in the epidermis, dermis, and subcutaneous layers with age and the consequences of those changes for the structure and function of the integumentary system (**Figure 3-4**).

The *epidermis* is a multilayered sheet of epithelial cells called keratinocytes, which are named for their production of keratin, a fibrous protein that gives this layer its strength. Interspersed among the keratinocytes are smaller numbers of melanocytes, which produce

(A)

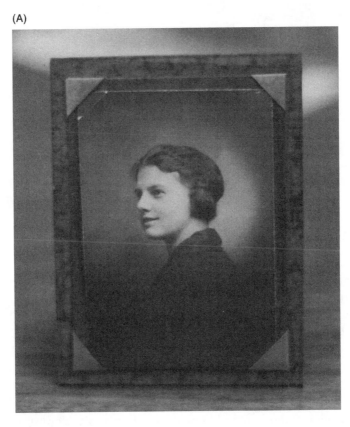

FIGURE 3-4 Change in appearance of skin with aging. The same woman is shown at (A) age 19 and (B) age 70.

(B)

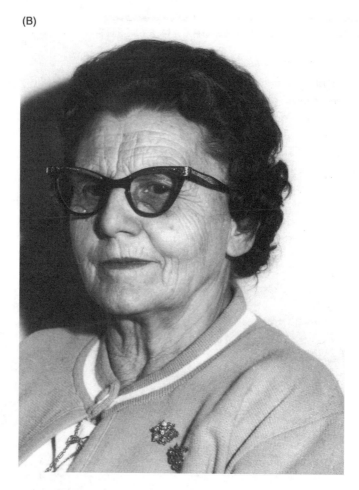

FIGURE 3-4 *continued*

the melanin pigment that browns the skin, and Langerhans cells, which play a role in the immune response, preventing the development of skin cancers, ingesting microorganisms, and in the process, stimulating white blood cells called lymphocytes.[83] The epidermal cells rest on a thin layer of tissue called the basement membrane, which separates the epidermis from the underlying dermis. This membrane is normally undulated, which helps hold the two layers together. However, with age it flattens out, making the skin more vulnerable to shearing forces, abrasion, and blister formation (**Figure 3-5**).[84] Because of the everyday wear and tear on the skin, the epidermal cells must be continuously replaced with new cells that divide by mitosis in the lowest layers. The new cells slowly get pushed up through the epidermis and ultimately are shed from the skin, a process that takes about 28 days. Thus, our epidermis is completely replaced every month. The turnover rate, however,

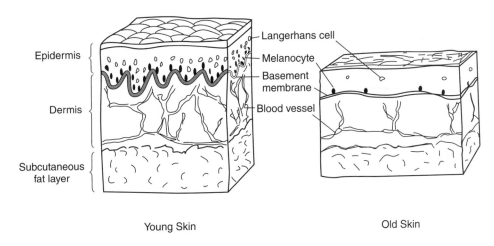

Young Skin   Old Skin

FIGURE 3-5 **Changes in the structure of skin with aging. Note that older skin has: (1) a thinner epidermis, (2) a flatter basement membrane, (3) fewer melanocytes and Langerhans cells, (4) a diminished dermal blood supply, and (5) a thinner subcutaneous fat layer.**

decreases by 30–50% between ages 20 and 70, which increases the time during which individual epidermal cells are exposed to carcinogens (i.e., cancer-causing agents) such as ultraviolet light from the sun.[85,86] Furthermore, the number of melanocytes, and therefore the amount of protective melanin pigment, decreases with age, making ultraviolet light more dangerous. Combined with the fact that the number of macrophage-like Langerhans cells also declines with age, it becomes clear why older adults are particularly prone to develop *skin cancer*.

The *dermis* is a thick layer of loose connective tissue that is well supplied with blood vessels, lymphatic vessels, nerves, and accessory organs such as sweat glands, sebaceous glands, and hair follicles. The predominant cells found in the dermis are fibroblasts, mast cells, and macrophages. Fibroblasts produce and release collagen and elastin into the extracellular matrix, which gives skin its strength and elasticity, respectively. Mast cells release substances that mediate the inflammatory response following injury to the skin. The rich supply of blood vessels in the dermis provides oxygen and nutrients as well as an efficient mechanism for regulation of body temperature. When the body is overheated, blood flow to the dermis increases so that heat can be released through the skin. This, together with the action of sweat glands, allows for the release of large amounts of heat in a short period of time.

The amount of collagen and elastin in the dermis decreases as we age, accounting for the thinning and wrinkling of the skin in older adults. Loss of collagen makes the skin more susceptible to wear and tear, while loss of elastin causes skin to lose its resilience over time. The density of the dermal blood supply also decreases with age, blunting the outward signs of inflammation in elderly skin. This is particularly important to realize because older adults often lack some of the early warning signs of tissue injury (e.g., redness and swelling) from, for example, sunburn, bacterial infection, or skin cancer. The diminished blood flow to the dermis also impairs wound healing and, together with the gradual loss of functioning sweat glands, makes older adults especially vulnerable to overheating syndromes such as **heat stroke**. The dermis contains sensory receptors called pacinian and Meissner's corpuscles, which make the skin sensitive to vibration, pressure, and light touch. The gradual loss of these receptors with age decreases the *tactile sensitivity* of the skin and probably increases the threshold for pain stimuli.

The *subcutaneous layer* of the skin is largely adipose (i.e., fat) and loose connective tissue. This fat layer provides cushioning and thus protection to the underlying tissues. It also serves to insulate the body from rapid heat loss or gain. With age comes a thinning (or atrophy) of this layer, particularly in the face, backs of the hands, and soles of the feet. Loss of this fat pad on the soles can increase the physical trauma of walking and thus exacerbate other foot conditions in older adults.

Perhaps the most striking age-related changes to the integumentary system are the graying, thinning, and loss of hair. Hair follicles are specialized epidermal cells packed into cylinders rooted in the dermis. Hair growth is made possible by mitotic cell divisions at the base of the follicle, and hair color is dependent on varying amounts of melanin pigment within the specialized cells. Blonde, brown, and black hair have successively higher concentrations of melanin. With advancing years, the number of hair follicles decreases, and those follicles that remain grow at slower rates and have lower concentrations of melanin (because of declining numbers of melanocytes at the base of the hair follicles), causing the hair to become thin and white. Such changes over the scalp hamper hair's ability to screen the skin on the scalp from the damaging effects of sunlight.

Chronic exposure to sunlight, in fact, is the biggest scourge of aging skin. It is to the skin what cigarette smoking is to the internal organs and is largely responsible for the wrinkling, yellowing, coarseness, and irregular pigmentation of the skin with advancing years. It is also implicated in the development of several benign dermatologic lesions, such as skin tags, seborrheic keratoses, and sebaceous nevi. More important, the ultraviolet component of sunlight predisposes people to the three major forms of skin cancer: *malignant melanoma*, *basal cell carcinoma*, and *squamous cell carcinoma*. The latter two comprise more than 50% of all malignancies in the United States, while malignant melanoma is the most lethal of the three and is the sixth highest in incidence among aggressive types of cancer.[87,88] Taken together, these sun-induced changes in the skin resemble an accelerated form of skin aging. Yet, despite all of the damaging effects of "photoaging," the vanity of our youth often directs us to cultivate the "great tan" rather than to protect our skin. Again, the rewards of a great tan are immediate, whereas the benefits of skin protection come decades later. Nonetheless, if you still want to look great at 80, the use of protective hats and clothing, along with sunscreens of sun protection factor 15 (SPF-15) strength or higher, is in order.

Whereas excessive exposure to sunlight has adverse effects on the skin, some exposure is still needed to stimulate the production of vitamin D in the skin. This vitamin is needed to stimulate sufficient absorption of calcium from the small intestines into the bloodstream. The ultraviolet (UV) B radiation in sunlight stimulates the conversion of 7-dehydrocholesterol to previtamin D3, which is further chemically converted to vitamin D. Approximately 5 to 30 minutes of sun exposure to the face, arms, legs, or back without sunscreen between 10 a.m. and 3 p.m. twice a week stimulates sufficient vitamin D production.[89] However, UV-B light exposure decreases the farther a person lives from the equator. Individuals living more than 42° of latitude north or south of the equator do not receive sufficient sunlight during the winter months to produce vitamin D.[90] Although vitamin D can be stored in adipose tissue, such individuals must nonetheless be sure that they have adequate dietary intake of vitamin D during those months. It is not currently known whether there is a minimal amount of sun exposure that stimulates sufficient vitamin D production without increasing the risk of skin cancer.[91]

NERVOUS SYSTEM

The nervous system is the principal regulatory system of the body. An intact nervous system, therefore, is requisite to the proper functioning of all the other systems. The central nervous system, consisting of the brain, brain stem, and spinal cord, regulates and monitors peripheral activities via the nerves, the communication networks that form the peripheral nervous system. The *neuron* is the functional unit of the nervous system, capable of transmitting electrochemical impulses (or messages) over its cell body and cell extensions (the axon and dendrites). (See **Figure 3-6**.) Neurons form functional boundaries, or *synapses*, with other neurons and with target structures such as muscles and glands. In response to electrochemical impulses, signaling chemicals called *neurotransmitters* are released from neurons at these synapses to bind with and activate (or inhibit) the next cell in the sequence. The number of neurons in the nervous system is relatively fixed early in life because most mature neurons lack the ability to divide. The continued development of the nervous system throughout life (to make possible learning and memory formation, for example) is thus not attributed to an increase in the number of cells, but most likely to an increase in the complexity of neuronal circuits (resulting from axonal sprouting) and to intracellular modifications. More than 100 billion neurons are distributed throughout the nervous system, and any single neuron can synapse with several hundred other neurons. The neurons are supported by an even larger number of *neuroglial cells* (e.g., astrocytes, microglial cells, and oligodendrocytes) that help nourish, protect, and myelinate the neurons. Given these considerations, you can understand the claim that the human nervous system is the most complex functioning system in nature.

Because of its complexity and relative inaccessibility to study, the nervous system is probably the least understood of all body systems. Thus, we know relatively little about the effects of aging on the central nervous system. Furthermore, the age-related

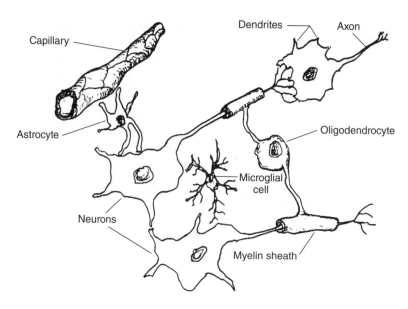

FIGURE 3-6   Neurons and related neuroglial cells.

microscopic structural alterations to this system are typically unobservable until autopsy. And even at autopsy, it is often difficult to distinguish disease-related changes from changes resulting from normal aging. Our meager progress in understanding the brain is reflected in the fact that central nervous system disorders remain one of the most common causes of disability in older adults, accounting for almost 50% of disability in those older than 65.[92] Nonetheless, some generalizations can be made concerning the appearance of the aged brain. Whereas the total number of neurons does not change much during healthy aging, certain parts of the nervous system such as the hippocampus, cerebellum, raphe nucleus, locus ceruleus, and nucleus basalis of Meynert show decreases in neuron numbers. Interestingly, Alzheimer's disease, a condition whose incidence rises as people grow older, is also marked by a loss of neurons in the locus ceruleus and nucleus basalis of Meynert, though this loss is far greater than that in the normal, aging brain. Parkinson's disease, like Alzheimer's disease, rises in incidence with age and is also marked by local loss of neurons, primarily in the substantia nigra.[93]

Important structural and functional alterations in neurons occur as people age. *Axons* in some parts of the nervous system lose moderate amounts of myelin (a lipid wrapping around the axon that increases the speed of the nerve impulse) or become swollen with age. These changes may contribute to the 10% decrease in nerve impulse conduction velocity noted with aging, a phenomenon that is partly responsible for the slowed reaction time and speed of mental processing in older adults.[94,95] The degree of branching of *dendrites* decreases with age, whereas the number of synapses between neurons remains fairly stable. There appears to be a decline in function of the neurotransmitter signaling mechanisms as well. These changes probably impair communication throughout the nervous system.

The nervous system utilizes several different neurotransmitters, some of which are excitatory and some of which are inhibitory. The more well characterized neurotransmitters include acetylcholine, dopamine, gamma-aminobutyric acid (GABA), serotonin, and glycine. Individual neurons may store and release more than one type of neurotransmitter. The smooth functioning of the nervous system appears to rely on the appropriate balance in activity among the various neurotransmitters. The neurotransmitter dysfunction that occurs with aging has more to do with a loss of this balance than with an absolute loss of any one particular neurotransmitter.

Like any other organ system, the nervous system is vulnerable to the effects of atherosclerosis with advancing age. As fatty plaques narrow cerebral arteries, blood flow to the brain diminishes. Blood clots (thrombi) developing in these narrowed arteries can block off the blood supply completely. Within minutes, brain tissue deprived of oxygen can be irreversibly damaged, resulting in infarction of tissue. The symptoms of this particular type of stroke depend on which area of the brain has been damaged. Repeated episodes of cerebral infarction can lead to multi-infarct dementia, which accounts for 8–29% of all cases of dementia in older adults, surpassed in frequency only by Alzheimer's disease, which accounts for about 50–80% of the total.[96,97] Interestingly, the risk for developing this vascular dementia appears to be 100 times greater than normal in individuals with prematurely shortened telomeres, those protective end segments of DNA whose length appears to dictate the number of times that a cell will be able to divide.[98] **Dementia** should be distinguished from the memory loss that occurs normally with age. Although most mental functions do not decline with age, mild loss of memory for recent events is quite common, whereas long-term memory remains intact in most cases. Dementia, on the other hand, is less common. See Chapter 4 for more details on this common disease of old age.

Aspects of one's intelligence appear to change with aging. *Crystallized intelligence* refers to transfer-of-learning skills, or one's ability to apply previously learned concepts to new tasks, whereas *fluid intelligence* is the ability to organize information in new ways and generate novel ideas or hypotheses about phenomena. Although our overall intelligence quotient (IQ) remains fairly stable throughout adult life, the subcomponents of intelligence do change as we age. Crystallized intelligence increases with age, perhaps because a lifetime of experiences and the cumulative exposure to ideas gives older adults a broader knowledge base to apply to problems. In contrast, fluid intelligence decreases with age, and older adults frequently score lower on timed tests of cognitive performance because they require more decision-making time and favor a slow, deliberate approach to tasks.[99]

Gradual impairment of *locomotor function* is an important contributor to disability in older adults. Chief among these symptoms are a slowing of fine motor tasks, diminished postural reflexes, and alteration of the gait, or pattern of walking. The confident, long stride of youth changes to a more hesitant, broad-based gait as people age. Such deficiencies in motor skills have been attributed primarily to an overall decrease in function of motor control centers in the brain, such as the basal nuclei, cerebellum, and cerebral cortex. However, they result in part from diminished sensory input to these areas as well-diminished *proprioception* (sense of body position), *vestibular sensation* (sense of head movement), and *kinesthetic sensation* (sense of body movement). Interestingly, many of the characteristics of the elderly stride, such as the tentative, shuffling steps and stooped posture, are identical to those seen in individuals with Parkinson's disease. These changes in balance and movement place older adults at risk for falls.

Finally, the aging process brings about notable changes in the pattern and quality of *sleep* one gets. The total amount of time spent sleeping changes little over the course of a lifetime, but as one ages, episodes of sleep are shorter and more frequent. Thus, a single 8-hour interval of sleep at night might be replaced by 6 hours of sleep a night supplemented by two or three daily naps. In addition, the proportion of stages 3 and 4 sleep decreases with advancing years. These are the deepest levels of sleep and are thought to be, physiologically speaking, the most rejuvenating forms of slumber. Their diminished presence might account for the observation that older adults are light sleepers. Conversely, the increased period of time spent in stage 1 corresponds to the common complaint that it takes longer to fall asleep as one ages. Indeed, about one-third of the elderly population suffers from insomnia.[100] The difficulties with sleep are exacerbated by the anxiety, stress, and depression that can affect the elderly population.

SPECIAL SENSES

Vision All of the special sensory systems undergo changes with aging. The changes in vision result from alterations in the structure of a number of the components of the visual system (**Figure 3-7**). The cornea and the lens are the principal focusing structures in the eye; they refract (or bend) incoming light rays so that images can be brought into focus on the retina in the back of the eye. Both the cornea and lens undergo predictable changes. The convex *cornea* is the thin and transparent anterior border of the eye. With advancing years, it becomes thicker and more opaque. The biconvex *lens* is largely acellular and transparent, consisting of several layers of crystallin lens protein. Its attachment to the surrounding sphincter-shaped ciliary muscle allows us to regulate its curvature. To focus on near objects, the ciliary muscle contracts, causing the lens to become rounder (a process called *accommodation*). Conversely, to focus on distant objects, the lens flattens out. With age, the lens increases in anterior-posterior diameter as successive layers of crystallin protein are laid down. It also becomes more opaque as its proteins become increasingly oxidized, glycosylated, and cross-linked (see earlier theories of aging)—severe degrees of which cause cataracts. These molecular changes render the lens less elastic and more rigid, which significantly impairs accommodation and thus the ability to focus on near objects,

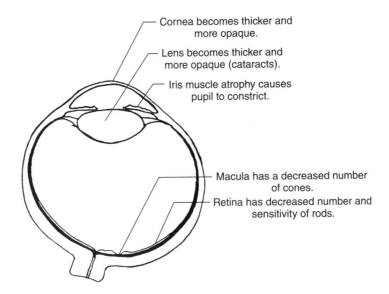

Cornea becomes thicker and more opaque.

Lens becomes thicker and more opaque (cataracts).

Iris muscle atrophy causes pupil to constrict.

Macula has a decreased number of cones.

Retina has decreased number and sensitivity of rods.

FIGURE 3-7 The structure of the eye and its age-related changes.

a condition called **presbyopia**. This change is so universal that nearly everyone older than 55 needs corrective convex lenses to read.[101]

The *iris* is a pigmented ring of tissue whose opening, or pupil, regulates the amount of light entering the eye. Two sets of smooth muscle, the dilator and constrictor muscles, regulate the diameter of the pupil. Over time, the dilator muscle atrophies to a greater extent than the constrictor muscle, causing the average diameter of the pupil to decrease. The *retina* is the photoreceptive surface in the back of the eye. It is covered with highly sensitive *rods* (which detect white light) and less sensitive *cones* (which detect colored light). With aging comes increased lipofuscin accumulation in these photoreceptive cells, a change that might cause cell death.[102] Both the number and photosensitivity of the rods decrease with age, which, coupled with the inability to completely dilate the pupils, makes night vision more difficult for the elderly. There is also a gradual loss of cones, which are normally densely packed in the *macula* of the retina. This may contribute to the decreased visual acuity common with aging. Possibly related to these changes is age-related macular degeneration, one of the most common causes of blindness among older adults in the United States.[103]

Hearing   As with vision, impairment of hearing is very common in older adults, affecting about 40% of those older than 63 years and 64% of those aged 80; it is the third most common chronic disease in the elderly.[104,105] We normally hear and interpret sounds through a multistepped process that converts sound waves (air pressure) into nerve

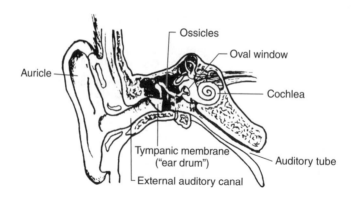

FIGURE 3-8 The auditory system.

impulses (**Figure 3-8**). The sound waves travel through the external auditory canal and set the *tympanic membrane* (eardrum) into vibration, which in turn causes the lever-like *ossicles* (middle ear bones) to vibrate, all at the same frequency as the original sound. The smallest ossicle "taps" on the oval window, which creates a fluid pressure wave that travels through the *cochlea* of the inner ear. Specialized cochlear *hair cells* sense this wave and generate nerve impulses that travel via the auditory nerve to the brain stem and brain. Hair cells at the base of the spiral-shaped cochlea are sensitive to high-pitched sounds, whereas hair cells at the apex are sensitive to low-pitched sounds. Hearing impairment related to problems of the outer ear canal (e.g., excessive wax) or middle ear (e.g., damage to the ossicles or middle ear infection) is called conductive hearing loss, whereas difficulty hearing caused by alteration of the inner ear or auditory nerve function (e.g., Meniere's disease or acoustic neuroma) is called sensorineural hearing loss.

With aging comes a gradual, progressive hearing loss called **presbycusis**. Presbycusis is the most common form of sensorineural hearing loss in adults. Men are affected more than women, and urban dwellers suffer greater losses than those living in rural areas (suggesting a role played by chronic exposure to environmental noise). The degree of loss is more severe for high-frequency sounds than for low-frequency sounds. This selectivity suggests that the origin of the problem is in the inner ear and/or the nerve pathways to and through the brain. Cochlear hair cells near the base of the cochlea, for example, accumulate lipofuscin in proportion to the degree of high-frequency loss. Other likely mechanisms for age-related damage include altered mechanical function of the basilar membrane (on which the hair cells sit), damage to the neurons in the auditory nerve, and diminished blood flow to the cochlea. The selective loss of high-frequency hearing makes it especially difficult for the elderly to hear consonants. Vowel sounds, on the other hand, are lower pitched and can still be heard fairly well. Overall, these changes cause speech to sound muffled. Many elderly compensate for this loss by lip-reading, which is easier to do for consonant sounds than for vowel sounds. Hearing conversations in a crowded room can be very difficult for an elderly person, not only because of the presbycusis, but also because older adults have a diminished ability to localize sound and to ignore those sounds that are deemed less important.

Taste There appears to be a decline in sensitivity to taste with age as well. Our ability to taste results from the activation of taste cells, which are clustered together in the taste buds on our tongue and other regions of the oral cavity. Nerves transmit this information to the brain stem and on to higher centers in the brain. Taste buds have been classically described as being of four types—sweet, sour, bitter, and salty—which are regionally distributed over the tongue. The degree of taste impairment with age seems to vary from taste to taste, being least profound for sweet and most profound for salt.[106] The decline in taste is consistent with the age-related loss in the number of taste buds on the tongue but may also be caused by the decreased production of saliva and resultant dry mouth older adults experience with aging. Older adults also have more difficulty gauging the intensities of tastes and identifying individual tastes, such as salty, in a mixture of flavors. This impairment may cause older individuals to add excessive amounts of salt to foods, which could be detrimental, particularly if they have hypertension or congestive heart failure.

Smell Another functional decline with important ramifications is the impairment of the ability to smell, a condition known as **hyposmia**. Similar to taste, the degree of impairment varies with the particular odor, and the ability to identify individual odors in a mixture is gradually lost with age. Interestingly, men are more profoundly affected than women are. Smell is made possible by the activation of sensory cells in the upper mucosal surface of the nasal cavity, which pass the sensory information through the bony roof into the *olfactory bulb* at the base of the frontal lobe. From there, the information is processed and relayed through the *olfactory tract* to higher brain centers. As you might expect, there is an age-related decline in the numbers of mucosal sensory cells and olfactory bulb relay cells, accounting for the decreased sensitivity to smell.

Because of the crucial role played by smell in distinguishing the tastes of different foods, hyposmia makes foods less desirable, causing a decreased appetite and irregular eating habits with subsequent weight loss and malnutrition in the elderly. In addition, the inability to smell can have dire consequences if a person fails to notice a poison gas leak or other toxic inhalant. Older adults, for example, have a 10 times higher threshold than younger individuals for the smell of ethyl mercaptan, an odiferous substance added to propane gas to warn individuals of gas leakage.[107] Clearly, the sense of smell has protective value.

MUSCULOSKELETAL SYSTEM

Musculoskeletal dysfunction is a major cause of disability in older adults, altering mobility, fine motor control, and the mechanics of respiration. As a result, older adults are more prone to falls (and thus fractures), respiratory infections, and the general physiologic decline that accompanies an increasingly sedentary lifestyle. One of the most significant changes in the aging skeleton is **osteoporosis**. Defined as a reduction in bone mass and bone density, this condition predisposes an individual to fractures, especially in the vertebrae, proximal femur, and distal radius. In the United States, an estimated 10 million people over the age of 50 have osteoporosis, and another 34 million have lower than normal bone mass. About 1.5 million fractures per year result from osteoporosis, the morbidity of which accounts for about $18 billion in health care costs annually.[108,109] The average lifetime cost for the care of an individual's hip fracture is about $81,000. Clearly, with the shifting demographics of the U.S. population and the aging of the baby boomer generation, these costs will rise further over the next few years.[109] Important risk factors for osteoporosis include estrogen depletion (in postmenopausal women), calcium deficiency (exacerbated in older adults because of decreased intestinal absorption of calcium), decreased bone mass at the end of development, physical inactivity, testosterone depletion (in males), alcoholism, and cigarette smoking. The loss of bone mass in the vertebrae and the thinning of the intervertebral disks account for a gradual decrease in height of about 2 inches between ages 20 and 70.[110] Collapse or severe wedging of the vertebrae cause the characteristic appearance of kyphosis, an exaggerated convex curvature of the upper spine leading to a "hunch-backed" posture. Concomitant deformity of the rib cage can alter the normal mechanics of breathing. At about age 40, the rate of bone resorption surpasses the rate of new bone formation, with a subsequent loss of about 40% of total bone mass in women and 30% in men over the course of the life span.[111] Bone resorption is most extreme in the inner spongy bone at the enlarged ends (epiphyses) and along the inside rim of long bones, making older bones more vulnerable to fractures from both compression and lateral impact.

Osteoarthritis, also called degenerative joint disease, is the second most common cause of disability in this country, affecting more than 27 million Americans.[112,113] Its incidence increases with age, affecting about 50% of those older than 65 and 85% of those older than 75 years.[114] It is estimated that 9.6% of men and 18% of women aged 60 and older worldwide have symptoms related to osteoarthritis.[115] So common is this disease in older adults that, for many years, it was believed to be a normal aspect of aging. More recent histological studies, however, have revealed clear differences in joint and cartilage structure between the healthy aged and those with osteoarthritis. Osteoarthritis is marked by ulceration and destruction of joint cartilage, leading eventually to exposure and destruction of underlying bone. The normal cushioning effect of cartilage is lost, causing bone to rub on bone. As you might guess, the weight-bearing joints are the most commonly affected (e.g., knee and hip joints), and obesity is a major risk factor. Osteoarthritis is the most common cause of total knee and hip replacements,[116] but other highly used, freely movable joints, such as the proximal and distal interphalangeal joints of the fingers, are also commonly affected. Inflamed joints are marked by pain, swelling, and decreased range of motion. Other less common forms of arthritis that increase in incidence with age include rheumatoid arthritis, gout, pseudogout, and polymyalgia rheumatica.

Skeletal muscle undergoes changes with aging as well. Overall, the number of skeletal muscle fibers (cells) decreases with age,[117] although the rate of decline varies from muscle to muscle. For example, little change is noted in the diaphragm, the primary breathing muscle that never relaxes for more than a few seconds; muscles used less frequently, such as those of the extremities, exhibit greater rates of muscle cell loss. Other microscopic changes in aging skeletal muscle include a variable decrease in muscle fiber size (atrophy) and capillary supply, an increase in deposition of lipofuscin and adipose (fat) cells, and a spotty loss of the motor neuron innervation. These microscopic changes result in a gradual decline in muscle strength and efficiency over time, although this too varies from one muscle group to the next. It cannot be overemphasized, however, that regular physical training can improve muscle strength and endurance, even in the very old.[118] This fact, coupled with the benefits of exercise in maintaining bone strength and cardiovascular fitness, argues for a cautioned exercise regimen for almost everyone.

CARDIOVASCULAR SYSTEM

The cardiovascular system consists of the *heart* and *blood vessels*. It is responsible for the circulation of the blood that allows for the delivery of oxygen and nutrients to and removal of waste products from all parts of the body. Damage to this system, therefore, can have negative implications for the entire body. The *ventricles* of the heart generate the pressure that propels the blood through the arteries, arterioles, capillaries (the site of nutrient and waste exchange), venules, and finally the veins, the blood vessels that return the blood to the *atria* of the heart. The left ventricle has the thickest muscular wall and pumps blood out to the systems of the body (via the higher pressure *systemic circulation*) while the right ventricle pumps blood to the lungs (via the lower pressure *pulmonic circulation*). (See **Figure 3-9.**)

The significance of cardiovascular disease in middle-aged and elderly adults cannot be overemphasized. It is the most common cause of death worldwide. Although mortality resulting from cardiovascular disease has been decreasing in the United States since the late 1960s, probably as a result of healthier diets, increased exercise, less smoking, and better control of hypertension (high blood pressure), it is nonetheless still a major killer.

Although the heart may increase in size considerably as a result of chronic congestive heart failure, its size and weight change very little with age in healthy individuals. Nevertheless, the heart exhibits several structural alterations with advancing years. Lipofuscin is deposited at a regular rate and mitochondrial DNA is damaged in cardiac muscle cells. Adipose tissue accumulates in and around the heart. The inner lining, or endocardium, undergoes fibrosis (i.e., scarring), and there is a gradual loss of the specialized conduction cells (autorhythmic cells) that coordinate the events of the cardiac contraction cycle.

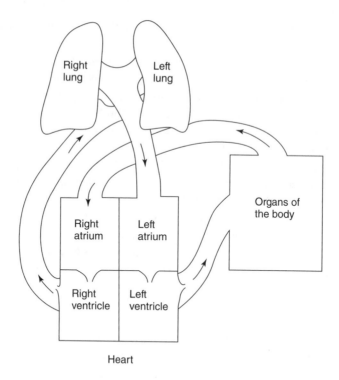

FIGURE 3-9 The cardiovascular system.
Note: The arrows indicate the direction of blood.

Coinciding with these changes are important functional alterations. The resting *cardiac output*, defined as the total volume of blood pumped out of the heart in 1 minute while at rest, decreases by 1% per year after age 30.[110] To understand the reasons for this, you must be familiar with the determinants of cardiac output, which is computed by multiplying the *heart rate* (in beats per minute) by the *stroke volume* (the volume of blood pumped out of the ventricle in one contraction). A decline in the resting cardiac output with age is primarily caused by a decrease in stroke volume, which in turn is caused in part by a decreased efficiency of cardiac muscle as well as a decreased responsiveness of the heart to the sympathetic nervous system, the branch of the nervous system whose effect is normally to increase the strength of the heart's contraction, or *contractility*.

Other factors influencing stroke volume, and therefore the cardiac output, are the preload and afterload work requirements placed on the heart. *Preload* is a measure of the amount of blood filling the ventricles just prior to contraction. When the volume of blood filling the ventricles increases, the heart responds by contracting more strongly, pumping out more blood to keep pace. Conversely, a decreased preload causes a weaker contraction. This phenomenon, known as *Starling's law of the heart*, ensures that blood does not get "backed up" in the venous circulation. However, with aging comes changes in the elasticity and smooth muscle of the venous walls and subsequent dilations, or varicosities, of the veins. This increases the capacity of the veins to hold blood and decreases the rate of venous return to the heart, ultimately causing a decreased preload and cardiac output. Afterload is a measure of the pressure against which the ventricles must pump to force blood out into the arteries. All other things being equal, the greater the afterload, the smaller the stroke volume, and therefore cardiac output. Systemic hypertension is defined as a resting blood pressure greater than 140 mmHg/90 mmHg on three separate occasions or the condition of being treated with antihypertensive medications. Hypertension is more prevalent in the aged population. In the United States, more than 70% of men and women aged 75 and older have hypertension.[119]

Hypertension increases afterload and thus reduces cardiac output. Successful treatment of high blood pressure, therefore, reduces the workload placed on the heart and thus the severity of heart disease. It has become clear in the past 15 years that for those people in their 50s and older, an elevated systolic blood pressure (i.e., the higher number in the blood pressure measurement) is an even more significant risk factor for strokes and other hypertension-related complications than is an elevated diastolic blood pressure (i.e., the lower number).[120] Thus, much emphasis has been placed in the health care arena on the treatment of isolated systolic hypertension in older adults.

Despite the cardiovascular changes associated with aging, cardiac output generally remains sufficient for the body's resting needs well into old age. It is during physical exertion that the decreased work capacity of the heart becomes more evident. During exercise, heart rate and stroke volume normally rise to meet the body's increased metabolic needs. These changes, which are part of the so-called fight-or-flight response to stress, occur largely under the direction of the sympathetic nervous system. At the same time that the heart is working harder, the sympathetic nervous system preferentially redirects blood flow to skeletal muscles, the brain, and heart muscle while limiting blood flow to the "less vital" organs of the digestive, reproductive, and urinary systems. But these normal responses to exercise are dampened as we age, largely because of decreased sympathetic nervous system activity. The maximum heart rate during exercise, calculated roughly as 220 minus one's age, decreases with advancing years. Thus, older adults become short of breath (*dyspnea*) and tire more quickly than younger individuals do during exercise. A related problem, probably also caused in part by insufficient sympathetic nervous system activity, is **postural**, or **orthostatic**, **hypotension**, which is a fall in systemic blood pressure upon rising from a supine to a standing position (usually too quickly). It can cause lightheadedness when a person stands up and can thus increase the risk of falling.

These age-related changes in heart structure and function may result from aging per se or from an increasingly sedentary lifestyle or a combination of both. Because regular exercise improves cardiac functioning in the young and middle-aged, it is likely to have similar benefits in older adults, provided the regimen is safe and commensurate with the abilities of the individual. In fact, one study found that healthy 60- to 71-year-old subjects improved their maximal oxygen consumption (a measure of physical fitness) in response to regular exercise to the same relative extent as younger individuals did, independent of initial level of fitness.[121] In another study, a meta-analysis of 13 studies, individuals older than age 60 experienced an 8.4% decline in resting heart rate following an endurance training regimen.[122]

The predominant change that occurs in the blood vessels with age is **atherosclerosis**, defined as the development of fatty plaques and the proliferation of connective tissue in the walls of arteries. The slow destruction of the arterial wall can lead to blockage of the artery, particularly when a blood clot develops on its damaged surface. So prevalent is this condition that one may argue that it is an inevitable phenomenon of aging. And although the clinical consequences of atherosclerosis are often sudden and life-threatening (e.g., heart attacks and strokes) and come toward the end of life, it has become clear in recent years that the earliest evidence of fatty accumulation is detectable in the first decade of life, and that the lesions progress throughout life.

Knowledge of the normal structure of the artery wall is necessary to understand the changes of atherosclerosis. The three major layers of arteries, from the innermost out, are the intima, media, and adventitia (**Figure 3-10A**). The *intima* is a thin layer of connective tissue covered on the inner surface by endothelial cells. The *media* is primarily smooth

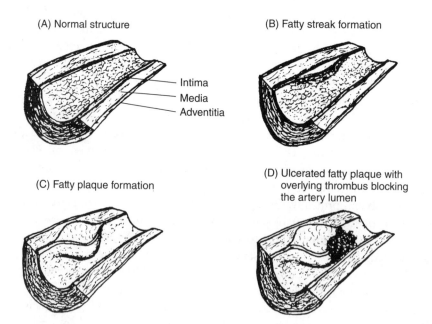

(A) Normal structure

(B) Fatty streak formation

Intima
Media
Adventitia

(C) Fatty plaque formation

(D) Ulcerated fatty plaque with overlying thrombus blocking the artery lumen

FIGURE 3-10   The progressive changes in arteries resulting from atherosclerosis.

muscle, bounded on its inner and outer surfaces by elastic connective tissue. The *adventitia* is a connective tissue layer that contains the tiny blood vessels (vasa vasorum) that nourish the outer half of the arterial wall. The inner half of the artery wall receives its nutrients by direct diffusion from the blood in the lumen of the artery.

According to one widely held theory of atherogenesis (fatty plaque formation), white blood cells called monocytes adhere to the surface of the intima in areas where microscopic damage has occurred (e.g., because of turbulent blood flow). These cells transform into macrophages and begin to ingest lipids from the bloodstream. Lipids and proteins from the blood begin to accumulate in the intra- and extracellular spaces of the intima and media as endothelial, smooth muscle, and macrophage cells begin to proliferate. As the lipid deposits enlarge, they become visible as *fatty streaks*, which form as early as the first decade of life (**Figure 3-10B**). As the fatty deposits grow and the arterial wall thickens, cells of the intima and media are forced farther away from their nutrient supplies and ultimately die and disintegrate, leaving behind a fatty paste, or *atheroma*. In an effort to contain the damage, fibroblasts form a fibrous connective tissue capsule around the atheroma. The encapsulated lesion, referred to as a *fibrous* (or *fatty*) *plaque*, appears as early as the second decade of life (**Figure 3-10C**).

Fatty plaques create several problems for us as we age. First, enlargement of the fatty deposits may partially or completely block blood flow through the artery. Second, the thickening of artery walls makes them more rigid, which in turn can raise systolic blood pressure and increase the afterload work requirement of the heart. Third, destruction of the inner layers of the artery wall can weaken it and cause it to balloon out under the force of the blood pressure. These dilations, called **aneurysms**, are prone to rupturing and causing severe internal bleeding. Finally, breaks in the fibrous capsule of fatty plaques can cause ulcerations, leaving the underlying fat deposits exposed to the bloodstream. This is ominous because such ulcerations attract platelets from the bloodstream, which clump and release substances that stimulate the formation of a blood clot, or **thrombus (Figure 3-10D)**. Enlarging thrombi can very quickly occlude arteries, or break off and travel farther down the bloodstream to lodge in a smaller vessel, a phenomenon known as **embolism**.

The complications of atherosclerosis begin as early as the fourth decade of life and increase in frequency with each succeeding decade. The particular consequences of the disease depend on the artery or arteries involved. Blockage of the coronary arteries can cause **myocardial infarction** (heart attack), whereas occlusion or rupture of a cerebral artery can result in a **stroke**. The development of fatty plaques in the renal arteries can cause hypertension and kidney failure, whereas blockage of an artery in the leg can cause peripheral vascular disease marked by severe pain (called claudication) and ulcerations of the skin. Although nearly everyone is prone to some degree of atherosclerosis, there are several risk factors that seem to accelerate the disease process. They include age, genetic predisposition, hypertension, diabetes mellitus, high blood cholesterol level, cigarette smoking, obesity, poor physical fitness, and "type A" personality. The confluence of many of these risk factors in older adults makes the complications of atherosclerosis more prevalent in this age group. Heart attacks are more common in individuals older than age 50, and the coronary artery disease that causes heart attacks is the number one killer of Americans.[123] Worldwide, cardiovascular disease accounts for about 29% of all deaths.[124] Unfortunately, the warning signs of an impending heart attack are not always as obvious in the elderly population and those with diabetes mellitus, making immediate treatment less likely. Peripheral vascular disease, by some estimates, affects more than 30% of individuals older than the age of 80.[125] And although the lifetime risk of stroke at age 65 has decreased over the past 40 years, it is still high (14.5% in men and 16.1% in women).[126] Given the increased risk of atherosclerosis in older adults, it makes good sense for everyone, young or old, to "eat right," exercise, keep trim, avoid cigarettes, and comply with any prescribed blood pressure medications. Indeed, as is true of most preventive health measures, these interventions are more effective if initiated early in life.

RESPIRATORY SYSTEM

The function of the respiratory system is to transport oxygen to and remove carbon dioxide from the bloodstream. The air breathed in is warmed, humidified, and cleansed as it passes successively through the mouth and nasal cavity, pharynx, larynx, trachea, and bronchi to reach the lungs (**Figure 3-11**). In the lungs, the inhaled air continues through smaller bronchi, bronchioles, and alveolar ducts to finally reach the **alveoli**, the tiny, thin-walled air sacs covered by capillaries that are the major site of gas exchange between the air and the bloodstream. The 300 million alveoli in the lungs account for most of the lung volume and provide about 75 square meters of surface area for gas transport to and from the blood. The lungs, located in the thoracic cavity (or thorax), are enclosed on the sides and top by the thoracic vertebrae and rib cage and from below by the **diaphragm**, a dome-shaped skeletal muscle. During inhalation, the diaphragm contracts, lowering the floor of the thorax while the external intercostal muscles between the ribs contract to swing the ribs forward and upward. Both of these actions help expand the thorax, creating a vacuum-like effect that draws air into the respiratory tract and lungs. The lungs expand passively during this process because of their adherence to the inner wall of the thorax. Exhalation is normally a passive process whereby the relaxation of the breathing muscles causes the thorax to contract down to a smaller volume, largely by elastic recoiling of the rib cage and lung tissue. The elastic recoiling (and lowering of volume) of the lungs during exhalation results from two factors (**Figure 3-12A**):

- The tendency of individual alveoli to become smaller at lower air pressures because of the surface tension generated by the watery inner alveolar lining
- The recoiling of elastic tissue around the respiratory airways that was stretched out during inhalation

The elastic tissue in the lungs is tethered between alveoli and bronchioles in such a way that actually prevents the bronchioles from completely collapsing during exhalation.

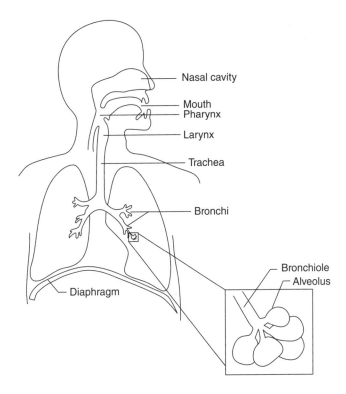

FIGURE 3-11 The respiratory system.

Elastic recoiling of the rib cage and lungs decreases the thoracic volume, thus increasing air pressure in the thorax and creating the necessary pressure gradient to force much of the air back out of the respiratory system.

A major indicator of pulmonary fitness is the *forced vital capacity* (FVC), defined as the maximal volume of air breathed out during one forced exhalation after maximal inhalation. The normal FVC in adults is 3 to 4 L in women and 4.5 to 5.5 L in men. FVC increases with growth of the body during childhood, adolescence, and early adulthood, reaching a peak at about age 25. Thereafter, FVC declines at a steady rate of about 21 mL/year, primarily because of changes in the soft tissue of the lungs.[127] As we age, the elastin fibers in the lungs are altered, probably by both excessive cross-linking between fibers and breakage of individual fibers. As a result, the lungs, as a whole, lose some of their elastic recoil, and the small bronchioles tend to partially or completely collapse during exhalation, causing obstruction of air flow and trapping of air in the alveoli (**Figure 3-12B**). Air trapping decreases the rate of oxygen delivery to and carbon dioxide delivery from the bloodstream. In addition, air trapping in the alveoli increases the *residual volume*,

(A) Normal elastic recoil of the alveoli and unobstructed bronchiolar airflow in healthy lungs.

(B) Decreased elastic recoil of alveoli and obstructed bronchiolar airflow noted with emphysema.

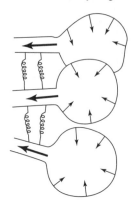 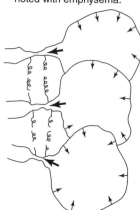

FIGURE 3-12   Elastic recoiling.

which is the volume of air remaining in the lungs after a forced exhalation. Because the *total lung capacity* (or maximum volume of air that the lungs can hold) changes very little in a healthy aging person, any increase in the residual volume comes at the expense of decreasing the FVC. Further hampering of gas exchange occurs with age as a result of a gradual loss of alveolar wall surface area, estimated to be a 4% decline per decade after age 30.[128] These changes in lung elasticity and alveolar surface area are similar to, but smaller in scale than, the changes that occur in emphysema.

Coupled with the changes in the lung tissue are changes in the mechanical properties of the wall of the thorax. As we grow older, the rib cage stiffens largely because of the calcification of the cartilage between the ribs and the vertebrae and the exaggerated curvature of the thoracic spine (kyphosis). These skeletal changes limit the mobility of the rib cage, making it difficult for the external intercostal muscles (as well as the accessory muscles of inhalation, such as the sternocleidomastoid and pectoralis major and minor) to expand the rib cage. Although a healthy elderly person might breathe adequately to meet the body's needs at rest, the previously described changes may limit his or her tolerance for exercise, especially when coupled with the age-related decrease in cardiac output described earlier in this chapter. Thus, it is not surprising that older adults, in general, experience shortness of breath (dyspnea) more quickly during exercise than do younger individuals.

Superimposed on the normal age-related changes to the respiratory system are certain diseases that increase in frequency from the fifth decade of life onward. They include emphysema, chronic bronchitis, pneumonia, and lung cancer. The first two are referred to together as **chronic obstructive pulmonary disease** (COPD), and along with lung cancer, are caused primarily by cigarette smoking or chronic exposure to unhealthy air. The steps leading to **emphysema** begin when cigarette smoke irritates the respiratory tract, stimulating proliferation of white blood cells called macrophages. These macrophages release chemicals that attract large numbers of another type of white blood cell, the neutrophil, to the inflamed area. Neutrophils, in turn, release protease enzymes, one of which called elastase can damage the elastin protein found in elastic tissue of the lungs. The effects of elastase are limited by a protective enzyme called alpha-1 antitrypsin, which inactivates elastase. However, alpha-1 antitrypsin is damaged by the free radicals produced from cigarette smoke. Thus, elastase is free to destroy lung tissue. The stage is then set for the slow, irreversible loss of functional elastic tissue in the lungs, resulting in the loss of alveolar wall surface area and the premature collapsing of small bronchioles during exhalation (hence, the "obstructive" in chronic obstructive pulmonary disease).[129–133] As more air gets "trapped" distal to the bronchiolar obstruction, the lung volume increases, creating the classic "barrel chest" appearance. In the end stages of emphysema, destruction of alveolar walls can be so extreme that large, visible air pockets form in the lungs. Collapsed bronchiolar airways are more difficult to reopen on inhalation. Thus, emphysema increases the work of breathing so that an individual must use the accessory muscles of inhalation to supplement the activity of the diaphragm and external intercostal muscles. Because of the diminished rate of gas transport and the increased work of breathing, the sufferer of emphysema is short of breath and cannot tolerate rigorous exercise well.

Chronic bronchitis, like emphysema, is more common in the elderly, especially in those with a long history of cigarette smoking. It is clinically defined as a chronic cough ("smoker's cough") productive of sputum, occurring on most days for at least 3 months duration over at least 2 consecutive years. Whereas emphysema primarily affects the smallest airways, chronic bronchitis is inflammation of the larger bronchi, brought about by the irritating effects of cigarette smoke or other environmental inhalants. The inflammatory process causes excessive mucus production, which is difficult to clear from the lungs not only because of its abundance but also because the tiny, beating cilia covering the bronchi that normally help move the mucus upward are damaged by smoking. The pooling of excessive mucus can block the bronchi (hence, the "obstructive" in chronic obstructive pulmonary disease) and provide a nutrient-rich environment for bacterial infection. When you consider that the elderly immune system is not as efficient, and neither does the cough reflex that helps clear excess mucus and aspirated food from the respiratory tract work as well, you can easily understand why an older smoker with chronic bronchitis is at increased risk for the spreading of the inflammation and infection to the bronchioles and alveoli—the development of *pneumonia*. Collectively, the number of people who die each year of respiratory illnesses is considerable. COPD and other chronic lower respiratory tract diseases (e.g., asthma) represent the fourth leading cause of death in the United States, while pneumonia and influenza collectively rank seventh on the list.[134] The World Health Organization estimates that 300 million people worldwide suffer from asthma and an additional 210 million have chronic obstructive pulmonary disease.[135]

HEMATOLOGIC SYSTEM

The hematologic system consists of those organs and tissues in the body that contribute red blood cells (RBCs), white blood cells (WBCs), and platelets to the bloodstream. Production of these cells from precursor stem cells, a process called *hematopoiesis*, occurs primarily in the bone marrow. The WBCs, or *leukocytes*, protect the body from infectious organisms and cancer cells, coordinate the events of the inflammatory and allergic responses, and participate in tissue and organ transplant rejection. Following their production in the bone marrow, WBCs travel through blood and lymphatic vessels to "seed" other organs, such as the spleen, tonsils, and lymph nodes, where they provide a continuous supply for life. Their role in aging is discussed in the next section. Platelets, or *thrombocytes*, are really cell fragments produced by the disintegration of large megakaryocyte cells in the bone marrow. They play a role in hemostasis (i.e., the stoppage of bleeding) by clumping together and releasing chemicals that stimulate blood clot formation in damaged blood vessels.

This section focuses on RBCs, called *erythrocytes*, which are flexible, disk-shaped cells filled with hemoglobin, an iron-containing protein that reversibly binds to and helps transport oxygen and carbon dioxide through the bloodstream. The life span of a RBC is relatively short, lasting only about 120 days. This is because RBCs undergo significant wear and tear as they are repeatedly squeezed through the small capillaries of the circulation. In addition, mature RBCs lack a nucleus (it is extruded from the RBCs during their final stage of development) and thus cannot repair themselves when damaged. For these reasons, RBCs must be produced at the astonishing rate of more than 2 million per second in healthy bone marrow (a process called *erythropoiesis*). They are broken down by macrophages at the same rate in the spleen. When the rate of erythropoiesis is equal to the rate of RBC destruction, there is no net change in the oxygen-carrying capacity of the blood over time. This capacity is often gauged by measuring the *hematocrit*, defined as the percentage of total blood volume taken up by red blood cells. The normal range for hematocrit is 42–54% and 37–47% in healthy men and women, respectively.[136]

A major hematologic concern in geriatric medicine is the high prevalence of **anemia** (defined as a lower than normal oxygen-carrying capacity of the blood) in older adults, particularly those older individuals in acute and long-term care settings. Anemia, however, is not a single disease, but rather a syndrome that has several different causes. Individuals with anemia often have pale skin, shortness of breath, and fatigue as a result of the subnormal hematocrit. The majority of the blood's oxygen is carried in RBCs, and anemias are caused by inadequate production or premature destruction of these RBCs. It has become clear in recent years that the high incidence of anemia in the elderly is not caused by aging per se, but rather to the high frequency of other age-related illnesses that can cause anemia. In healthy elderly individuals, there is no significant decline in the rate of erythropoiesis under normal conditions. However, when the body is stressed in ways that require an increase in erythropoiesis (e.g., chronic bleeding), aged bone marrow has a more difficult time "keeping up" than does young bone marrow.

The most common category of anemia diagnosed in older adults is *hypoproliferative anemia*, anemia resulting from a lower rate of RBC production than would be expected for the degree of hematocrit decline. The most common cause of hypoproliferative anemia in older adults is an inadequate supply of iron to make the hemoglobin in RBCs. However, the problem in most cases is not insufficient iron in the diet, but rather excessive loss of iron and/or the inability to recycle the iron that collects in macrophages from broken-down RBCs. Excessive loss of iron is caused by acute or chronic bleeding, which in older adults occurs most frequently in the digestive tract (e.g., from ulcers, diverticulitis, or colon cancer). Another type of hypoproliferative anemia, the anemia of inflammation, affects those individuals undergoing inflammatory responses as a result of conditions such as infection, tissue damage, or cancer. Extensive inflammation hampers the recycling of iron from macrophages in the spleen and liver. Thus, as older RBCs are continuously broken down, the supply of iron available for erythropoiesis in the bone marrow is inadequate. Chronic diseases such as rheumatoid arthritis and inflammatory bowel disease (e.g., ulcerative colitis and Crohn's disease) have a similar effect. These anemias can be exacerbated by protein and caloric malnutrition, which appears to decrease levels of the protein erythropoietin, a hormone produced by the kidneys, whose normal effect is to stimulate erythropoiesis in the bone marrow.

Other types of anemia that can afflict older adults fall under the category of *ineffective erythropoiesis*, defined as a group of anemias that result from destruction of developing RBCs while they are still in the bone marrow or immediately after they are released into the circulation. Anemia resulting from vitamin B_{12} deficiency is an example of ineffective erythropoiesis often diagnosed in older adults. Vitamin B_{12} is a coenzyme required for DNA production. When levels of this vitamin are deficient, RBCs develop abnormally in the bone marrow. Specifically, the cells cannot divide efficiently, and maturation of the cell nucleus lags behind maturation of the cytoplasm. The large, nucleated RBC precursors called megaloblasts (hence, the disease's alternative name, megaloblastic anemia) that form are often destroyed in the bone marrow before they can be released into the bloodstream. The cause of the vitamin B_{12} deficiency may be any of the following:

- Insufficient dietary intake (particularly in those who suffer from alcoholism)
- Inflammation or destruction of the ileum, the terminal portion of the small intestine, where vitamin B_{12} is absorbed
- Inflammation or destruction of the stomach lining (e.g., because of an autoimmune disorder called pernicious anemia) and thus the cells that produce intrinsic factor, a glycoprotein required for successful vitamin B_{12} absorption in the ileum

Having just reviewed the cardiovascular, respiratory, and hematologic systems, it becomes clear that all three of these systems are required to ensure adequate delivery of oxygen to the tissues. An age-related decline in the function of one or two of these systems will exacerbate any physiologic dysfunction present in the others. The presence of anemia in someone with congestive heart failure would be much more detrimental than it would be in an otherwise healthy individual. If that person with anemia and congestive heart failure also had emphysema, the disruption to the body would be still more extreme. It is this interdependence of our organ systems that, on the one hand, allows for appropriate compensatory adjustments to homeostatic disturbances in younger, healthy individuals but, on the other hand, can create a "chain reaction" of dysfunction in older, less healthy persons with decreased physiologic functional reserve.

IMMUNE SYSTEM

The ability of our bodies to remain free of infections and cancer requires that the WBCs of our immune system are able to distinguish "self" cells (i.e., our own healthy cells) from "nonself" cells (i.e., invading microorganisms and parasites or structurally altered cancer cells). To appreciate the enormity of this task, think about the thousands of different types of organisms that can invade the body, each of which must be specifically recognized by the immune system as foreign and destroyed without damaging the integrity of our own tissues in the process. Similarly, imagine the countless number of precancerous cell types, each of which may differ from normal cells in only very subtle ways, that are recognized and destroyed by the immune system on a regular basis. Indeed, in its prime, the immune system is to be marveled for its fidelity. But, as is true of most systems, age takes its toll. A discussion of the most important aspects of the immune response is followed by a review of those age-related changes in immunity that have implications for our health and well-being.

To be immune to an infection implies being protected from it. The development of immunity to a particular infectious organism, however, usually requires initial exposure to it, which in turn often causes mild illness. Nonetheless, on recovery from the sickness, the individual is immune to subsequent infection and illness from that organism; the body has developed an "immunological memory" (sometimes called adaptive immunity) so that it can act more swiftly and effectively the next time it is exposed to the same invader. The development of this immunological memory occurs by one of two general processes, called the humoral-mediated and cell-mediated immune responses. The former process produces proteins called antibodies, which circulate through the blood (or "humor") and specifically bind to the foreign organism; the latter process activates white blood cells called killer T-lymphocyte cells, which directly destroy the invading organism.

In the *humoral-mediated immune response*, the invading organism, for example, a streptococcal bacterium, is initially "trapped" and ingested by scavenger *macrophage* cells "hiding out" in the lymph nodes (**Figure 3-13A**). The macrophage digests the bacterium but re-presents some of the bacterial molecules (or antigens) on its own cell surface. This

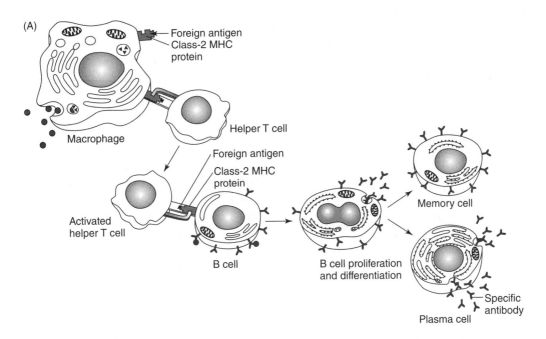

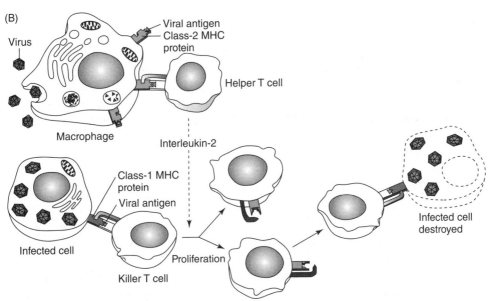

FIGURE 3-13 **(A) Humoral-mediated immune response. (B) Cell-mediated immune response.**
Adapted from: Van de Graff, KM, Fox, SI: *Human Anatomy and Physiology*, ed 4. William C Brown, Pub., Dubuque, IA, 1994, pp. 672–673. Reprinted with permission.

antigen presentation signals a helper T-lymphocyte (or *T-helper cell*) to bind to the macrophage. Several distinct populations of T-helper cells are available in our body for this purpose, but the beauty of our immune system is that only the T-helper cell with the appropriate receptor for that particular presented streptococcal antigen will bind to the macrophage. Other T-helper cells will not bind because their receptors do not make a nice hand-in-glove fit with that specific antigen. The macrophage, once bound to the appropriate T-helper cell, releases a chemical called interleukin-1, which, in turn, stimulates the T-helper cell to mature and multiply, forming a large population of clones, all bearing receptors for the streptococcal antigen. These activated T-helper cells then bind to and activate another type of white blood cell called the B lymphocyte (or *B cell*), which is specialized to make antibodies. But again, the correct population of B cells is selected (clonal selection). In other words, only that particular population that makes the antibody that binds specifically to the streptococcal antigen is selected. These activated B cells multiply, forming an entire army of fully developed, antibody-producing cells called *plasma cells*. The abundant supply of antistreptococcal antibodies released from the plasma cells binds to the streptococcal bacteria in the tissues, lymphatics, and bloodstream, tagging them for efficient destruction by other macrophages and by membrane-piercing chemicals called complement factors. In the process, some of the dividing B cells are stored away as memory B cells, primed and ready to go for the next time the same strain of streptococcus enters the body.

Although antibodies are effective in neutralizing extracellular microorganisms, another strategy must be used to destroy those microbes that hide out inside our cells, most notably viruses. This strategy, called the *cell-mediated immune response*, is similar in many respects to humoral-mediated immunity (**Figure 3-13B**). The invading virus enters the macrophage, and some of its protein coat antigen is presented on the surface of the macrophage. This signals the correct T-helper cell to bind, become activated, and subsequently activate the correct clone of killer T-lymphocytes (or *T-killer cells*). As a result, a growing population of T-killer cells is formed, each cell of which is specifically programmed to kill those of our body cells that have been infected by that particular virus. In addition, some of the primed T-killer cells are stored away as memory T cells, poised for the next invasion by that same virus. The ability to detect and destroy cancer cells in the body also involves populations of these T-killer cells, along with another population of white blood cells called *natural killer cells*. As can be concluded from the this discussion, lymphocytes play a critical role in the development of immunity to infections and cancer. Unfortunately, it is these lymphocytes whose function most noticeably diminishes with aging.[137]

The age-related decline of immune system functioning gives rise to three general categories of illness that preferentially afflict the elderly:

- Infections
- Cancer
- Autoimmune disease

The overall incidence of *infectious disease* rises in late adulthood. Particularly prevalent among the aged are influenza, pneumonia, tuberculosis, meningitis, and urinary tract infections. Deficiencies in both humoral- and cell-mediated immunity have been implicated in the increased incidence of infections as well as the decreased immune response to vaccines in older adults.[138] Utsuyama et al. (1992) studied human blood from individuals ranging from newborn to 102 years old and found that numbers of both B and T cells remain somewhat stable between the third and seventh decades of life but then decline thereafter.[139] The age-related decreases in the numbers and activities of various clones of T cells may be caused by the slow, postpubertal destruction of the thymus gland, an organ that stimulates the development of T-helper and T-killer cells by releasing various hormone-like chemicals. Another possible reason for diminished functioning of T cells is the derangement of precursor stem cell development in the bone marrow. Regardless of the cause, it is important to bear in mind that any decline in T-helper cell function will have widespread repercussions for our health because this cell is the catalyst for both humoral- and cell-mediated immunity. It is, incidentally, the destruction of these cells by the human immunodeficiency virus (HIV) that makes acquired immune deficiency syndrome (AIDS) such a devastating disease. There appears to be an age-related decline in the number and function of different B cell clones as well. Thus, there is a general decline in the body's ability to generate antibody responses to certain infections.

Cancer increases in prevalence with age as well, particularly leukemia, lung, prostate, breast, stomach, and pancreatic cancer. This rise may be caused in part by the altered immune surveillance of precancerous and cancer cells that comes with aging. Several components of the immune system play roles in cancer protection, including the previously mentioned natural killer cells. Both the number and function of natural killer cells in animals decline with aging. If this is the case in humans, it may partly explain the rising incidence of cancer in older adults.

Autoimmune diseases also are more common in older adults. These diseases are marked by the mistaken immunological destruction of the body's own cells. In such diseases, the body loses the ability to distinguish self from nonself. Prominent examples of autoimmune diseases affecting the elderly are rheumatoid arthritis, Hashimoto's thyroiditis, lupus, and chronic hepatitis. Tolerance to our own tissues develops early in life (during development of the immune system), when the thymus gland selects out and eliminates those clones of T cells programmed to destroy our own tissues—a process called *clonal deletion*. However, with the slow, age-related destruction of the thymus gland, the body may lose the ability to detect and destroy these potentially self-harming T cells. Indeed, with aging comes increased levels of autoantibodies.

DIGESTIVE SYSTEM

The primary function of the digestive system is to process incoming food so that nutrients can be absorbed into the body. The primary structural feature of this system is the

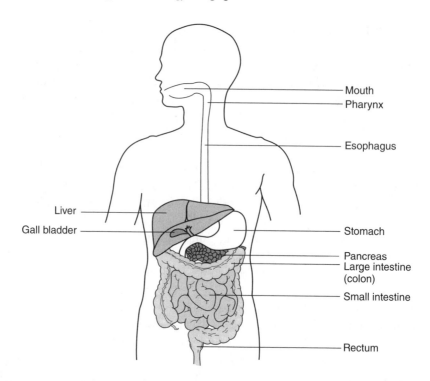

FIGURE 3-14   The digestive system.

digestive tract, made up of the mouth, pharynx, stomach, small intestine, large intestine (or colon), rectum, and anus (**Figure 3-14**). This canal works like an assembly line, with each part having a specialized function in digestion. Attached to the digestive tract along the way are exocrine glands, such as the salivary glands, pancreas, and liver, which secrete substances to aid in digestion and absorption. Although aging in an otherwise healthy individual has minimal effects on the digestive system, many specific diseases of this system increase in frequency with advancing years. The age-related alterations in structure and function are discussed in descending order, starting with the mouth and proceeding to the rectum.

Food entering the *mouth* undergoes the initial stages of mechanical digestion (via chewing) and chemical digestion (via release of salivary amylase enzyme). In the mouth, the teeth undergo perhaps the most visible changes with age, becoming yellowish-brown (because of exposure to coffee, cigarette smoke, and other staining agents) and worn on the surface (because of years of chewing, night grinding, and jaw clenching). Osteoporotic changes of the jaw bones (maxilla and mandible) can cause teeth to loosen from their sockets. This change, coupled with the recession of the gums (*periodontal disease*), can cause loss of teeth in older adults. Indeed, about half of U.S. citizens have lost the majority of their teeth by age 65.[140] Although dental caries (cavities) are not an inevitable result of aging, the diminished strength and dexterity of older adults can make teeth brushing difficult, thus increasing the likelihood of dental caries. **Xerostomia**, or dry mouth, is another problem of aging and has several causes, including decreased saliva production, cigarette smoking, and medication side effects (e.g., from certain blood pressure medications).

Once sufficiently chewed, the food is swallowed by the complex coordination of several muscles of the tongue, palate, pharynx, and esophagus. In this regard, a common problem in the elderly is **dysphagia**, or difficulty swallowing. This may be caused by weakness of the tongue muscles, improper nervous system control of the swallowing reflex, or uncoordinated muscular action of the pharynx or esophagus. Severe dysphagia can cause aspiration of food into the larynx and farther down the respiratory tract, which in turn puts one at risk for aspiration pneumonia. Treatment of more severe cases of dysphagia may require the expertise of a speech and language pathologist.

In the *stomach*, the swallowed food is chemically digested by virtue of hydrochloric acid (gastric acid) and pepsin enzyme secretion and is mechanically digested by the stomach's muscular churning action. The rate of gastric acid secretion decreases with age, while the incidence of **peptic ulcers** and **gastritis** (i.e., inflammation of the stomach lining) increases. The latter two phenomena may be a result of an increased incidence of *Helicobacter pylori* bacterial infection in older adults, drug ingestion (e.g., aspirin, caffeine, alcohol), or genetically programmed changes with age. Chronic bleeding from a peptic ulcer or gastritis can result in iron-deficiency anemia, whereas acute bleeding can place severe stress on the elderly individual's cardiovascular system. *Carcinoma* (or cancer) of the stomach is most common in the very old and carries a poor prognosis for survival.

The initial section of the *small intestine*, called the *duodenum*, receives the partially digested food (or chyme) from the stomach and continues the process of digestion with the help of secretions from the liver and gallbladder (the bile) and from the pancreas (digestive enzymes and bicarbonate-rich fluid). As the chyme is further digested, nutrient molecules become small enough to be absorbed through the wall of the small intestine, a process that occurs primarily in the more distal parts of the small intestine (the *jejunum* and *ileum*). Movement of the chyme through the small intestine by peristaltic contractions of the muscular wall is fairly slow to allow sufficient time for nutrient absorption. Aging has surprisingly little effect on the small intestine's digestive function and smooth muscle contractility. In addition, with the possible exceptions of calcium, vitamin D, and iron, most nutrients are absorbed efficiently in the small intestine in healthy older adults. The decreased calcium and vitamin D absorption may contribute to the increased incidence of osteoporosis in older adults.

The *liver* has several functions, some related to digestion and others not. It produces the bile that is stored below in the gallbladder until its release into the duodenum. Bile is required for the emulsification of fats in chyme. Without bile, fats would pass through the digestive tract without being absorbed, a condition called *steatorrhea*. The storage of

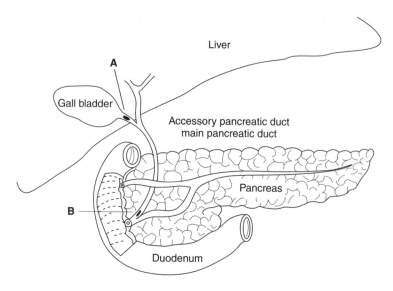

FIGURE 3-15 **Hepatobiliary tree with gallstone lodged in (A) the cystic duct and (B) the common bile duct.**

bile in the gall bladder can lead to its precipitation into solid stones, or *gallstones*, a phenomenon that is increasingly likely as we age. Gallstones, in turn, can get lodged in the ducts that normally convey the bile to the duodenum, resulting at times in obstructive jaundice, inflammation of the gallbladder (*cholecystitis*) or pancreas (*pancreatitis*), and steatorrhea (**Figure 3-15**).

The liver also detoxifies many of the foreign and potentially damaging chemicals that enter or are produced within the body. Indeed, many of the medications given for disease and illness are broken down by the liver and are either released through the bile or in the bloodstream to be eliminated by the kidneys in the urine. But with age, this detoxifying ability is diminished. This is particularly important to realize because it means that many drugs given to older adults remain in the body for longer periods of time. Thus, recommended dosages of many drugs for older adults are smaller than they would be for younger individuals. Failure to consider this leads to the dangerous overdosing of medications for older adults (see Chapter 6).

The remainder of the small intestinal contents (largely water and undigestible fiber) enters the *large intestine* (or *colon*), an area of the digestive tract that is heavily colonized by a normal flora of bacteria. The large intestine reabsorbs much of the remaining water and stores the feces until defecation. One common problem in the elderly is **diverticulosis**, which is the development of small sacs where the large intestinal lining has herniated through the intestinal muscular wall. These herniations usually result from the muscular spasms and increased intracolonic pressure associated with diets low in fiber. These pockets, or diverticuli, can become impacted with feces, resulting in ulceration and inflammation of the mucosal lining (*diverticulitis*). Also with age comes decreased motility of the smooth muscle in the large intestinal wall, prolonging the time that feces are stored in the colon and rectum. This, in turn, causes excessive water reabsorption and hardening of the feces, leading to *constipation* and, in extreme cases, intestinal obstruction. On the other end of the spectrum, older adults may suffer from **fecal incontinence** (the inability to voluntarily control defecation), largely because of the weakening of the external anal sphincter muscle. This can be exacerbated when there is a simultaneous increase in intra-rectal pressure caused by episodes of *diarrhea*.

The small and large intestines, like most other parts of the body, are vulnerable to the ravages of atherosclerosis. Blockage of the mesenteric arteries supplying the intestines can result in *ischemia* (reversible tissue damage caused by oxygen depletion) and, ulti-mately, *infarction* (tissue death and breakdown). In the latter case, perforations can develop in the intestinal wall, allowing the bacteria-laden feces to spill out into the nor-mally sterile peritoneal cavity, causing severe inflammation (*peritonitis*), a life-threatening condition. Finally, the large intestine is susceptible to cancer as well. In fact, in those people 70 and older, colon cancer is the second most common malignancy (behind lung cancer).[141]

GENITOURINARY SYSTEM

The paired *kidneys* serve two principal, and somewhat overlapping, functions:

- Excretion of certain waste products from the body
- Maintenance of homeostasis (stability) in the fluid compartments of the body, such as the plasma and the interstitial fluid

The fact that these two fairly small organs (each weighing only 5 ounces) receive about 20% of the cardiac output illustrates their importance in carrying out these tasks. Failure to perform these functions can result in the buildup of nitrogenous waste products (e.g., urea) in the bloodstream and in the imbalanced levels of water, electrolytes, or acids in the body, any of which can in turn alter normal physiologic processes. One would expect organs of such importance to have considerable functional reserve so that they could make the necessary compensations when damaged in any way. For the most part, this is true. Consider the *nephrons*, the microscopically sized functional units of the kidneys that filter the blood and then "choose" which substances of the filtered fluid to excrete and which substances to place back in the bloodstream. At age 25, there are approximately 1 million nephrons in each kidney. By age 85, 30% to 40% of them have been lost, yet an otherwise healthy 85-year-old can still maintain homeostasis under normal circumstances.[110]

Nonetheless, because of the loss of nephrons and the less efficient functioning of those that remain, the kidneys of older adults have a more difficult time responding to any added metabolic stressor on the body. Thus, as is true of the other organs discussed, older kidneys work well under normal conditions but have reduced tolerance for disease processes, whether originating from the kidneys themselves or from other organs. This is why, compared with younger individuals, older adults more commonly suffer from *acute* and *chronic renal failure*, conditions in which toxic metabolites build up in the body because of the inability of the kidneys to remove them at a sufficient rate. It is also important for the health care provider to understand that the kidneys, like the liver, help eliminate drugs and their breakdown products from the body. The decreased functional reserve capacity that comes with age makes it more difficult for the kidneys to efficiently excrete drugs. Thus, to prevent overdosing of medications, older adults typically require smaller drug dosages than do younger individuals (see Chapter 6).

One of the major roles of the kidneys is to maintain water balance in the body. Indeed, the amount of water in fluid compartments such as the blood, interstitial fluid, and intracellular fluid is a major determinant of the concentrations of all the substances dissolved in those fluid compartments. Therefore, to maintain levels of sodium, potassium, calcium, and other vital components within the appropriate narrow concentration ranges, the kidneys must regulate the rate of water removal from the body. Severe dehydration (e.g., resulting from excessive sweating or inadequate fluid intake) might increase the concentration of dissolved substances in the body to dangerously high levels, if not for the ability of the kidneys to respond by producing smaller volumes of very highly concentrated urine, thus minimizing the amount of water lost. On the other hand, when someone is overhydrated, the kidneys respond by producing large volumes of very dilute urine. But this ability to regulate the concentration according to the body's needs diminishes with age. For this reason, older adults are more likely to become dehydrated, especially when confusion, immobility, or fear of urinary incontinence (discussed later) prevents them from drinking adequate amounts of liquids. This dehydration may be exacerbated by the overdosing of diuretics, medications used for congestive heart failure and hypertension, whose effect is to increase urinary output.

Other age-related changes in the genitourinary system pertain to the structures required for urinary collection and removal—that is, the *ureters, urinary bladder,* and *urethra* (**Figure 3-16**). Normally, urine produced by the kidneys flows continuously through the ureters to be temporarily stored in the bladder. As the bladder fills with urine, its walls stretch out, initiating a reflexive contraction of the bladder wall. The expanding bladder compresses the ureteral openings, preventing the reflux of urine in the bladder back into the ureters. In addition, the smooth muscle sphincter at the urethral opening (internal urethral sphincter) prevents urine in the bladder from entering the urethra. Nonetheless, as the fluid pressure in the bladder rises, the internal urethral sphincter opens up and urine enters the proximal urethra. However, a more distal, voluntary, skeletal muscle sphincter (the external urethral sphincter, located in the pelvic floor) must relax before urine can exit through the urethra. Thus, although the release of urine, called micturition, is made possible by an involuntary reflex, we nonetheless have voluntary control over it under normal conditions.

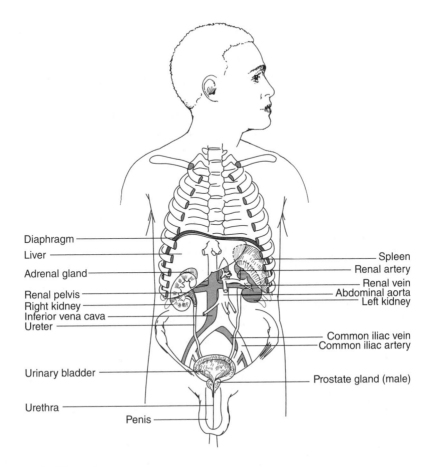

FIGURE 3-16 The urinary system.
Adapted from: Van Wynsberghe, D, et al. *Human Anatomy and Physiology*, ed 3. McGraw-Hill, New York, 1995, p. 889.
Reprinted with permission.

The loss of this voluntary control of micturition, called **urinary incontinence**, is a common problem in the elderly population. Indeed, 50–60% of those living in institutions suffer from this embarrassing and distressing condition.[142] Postmenopausal women are prone to this problem because lowered estrogen levels cause the skeletal muscles of the pelvic floor and the smooth muscle of the urethra to weaken. Women who have had multiple pregnancies are particularly susceptible and may involuntarily urinate whenever intra-abdominal pressure rises, for example, when coughing, sneezing, or laughing. This is called stress incontinence. In elderly men, urinary incontinence is often caused by an enlarged *prostate gland*. The prostate gland, which produces some components of semen, is wrapped around the beginning of the urethra. It undergoes enlargement as a man ages, which can in turn partially or completely obstruct the urethra. This enlargement is either benign (**benign prostatic hypertrophy** [BPH]) or malignant (*prostate cancer*). In either case, the bladder must contract more forcefully to eliminate the urine. Over time, the bladder can become very distended (a condition called *urinary retention*) and its muscular wall can weaken, leading to a lack of coordination of micturition and, in turn, incontinence. Urinary retention, in turn, increases the chance of *urinary tract infection* and kidney damage (caused by the buildup of fluid pressure). To avoid these complications, surgery is often performed to remove that part of the prostate gland blocking the urethra (a procedure called transurethral resection of the prostate, or TURP).

ENDOCRINE SYSTEM

Like the nervous system, the endocrine system is a principal regulatory system in the body. It helps control several aspects of our physiology, such as body temperature; basal metabolic rate; growth rate; carbohydrate, lipid, and protein metabolism; stress responses; and reproductive events. Clearly, dysfunction of this system could have widespread ramifications for one's health and well-being. Only a few of the many age-related changes to this system are highlighted here.

The endocrine system is a collection of glands that produce and secrete into the bloodstream chemical messengers called *hormones* that have physiologic effects on various *target organs* throughout the body. The cells of target organs have protein *receptors* that specifically bind to the hormone in question. This binding initiates a cascade of metabolic events within the target cell that mediate the effects of the hormone.

Although the endocrine glands are spread throughout the body, there is a hierarchical control of the release of most hormones, which begins in the central nervous system (CNS) (**Figure 3-17**). Neural activity from higher centers in the CNS is relayed to the **hypothalamus**, a small but extremely important structure that, in turn, controls the activity of the **pituitary gland** by releasing hormones that stimulate or inhibit its hormonal production and release. The pituitary gland, under the influence of these higher control centers, releases a battery of tropic hormones that have selective stimulatory effects on glands such as the thyroid, adrenal, and gonadal glands (ovaries and testes). It should be emphasized, however, that even the structures at the top of this endocrine hierarchy are influenced by "lower" events. For example, the thyroid gland is stimulated to release thyroid hormone in response to the sequential release of thyrotropin-releasing hormone (TRH) from the hypothalamus and thyroid-stimulating hormone (TSH) from the pituitary gland. But as its level in the blood increases, thyroid hormone "turns off" further production of TRH and TSH in the higher centers in a negative feedback fashion—in effect, the endocrine system operates under a system of checks and balances so that under normal conditions the appropriate levels of all hormones are maintained.

The *thyroid hormone* released from the *thyroid gland* has many physiologic effects, such as regulation of tissue growth and development (particularly of the skeletal and nervous systems), regulation of the basal metabolic rate (BMR) by promoting oxygen

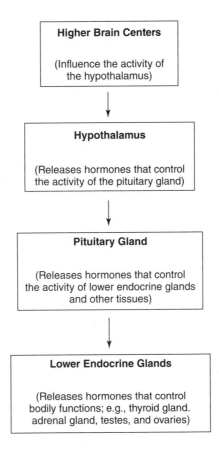

FIGURE 3-17   The hierarchy of control over the endocrine system.

consumption and heat production in most tissues (i.e., a calorigenic effect), enhancement of the effects of the sympathetic nervous system (or fight-or-flight response), increased mental alertness, and possibly regulation of cholesterol metabolism. As one ages, the level of thyroid hormone secretion declines. However, this decrease is matched by a decline in its rate of removal from the bloodstream so that, overall, levels change very little over the years. Furthermore, aging per se does not appreciably affect the increased release of TRH, TSH, or thyroid hormone required in times of greater need. However, several characteristics of older adults, such as a reduced metabolic rate, suboptimal regulation of body temperature, decreased effectiveness of the fight-or-flight response, reduced mental alertness, and increased incidence of cholesterol-related atherosclerosis, are also symptoms of reduced thyroid activity (hypothyroidism). Thus, it is possible that the age-related changes in thyroid function result from inadequate responses of target cells to thyroid hormone rather than from direct damage to the thyroid gland.

The paired *adrenal glands* consist of an outer layer called the adrenal cortex and an inner section called the adrenal medulla (which, from a functional standpoint, is more aptly considered part of the sympathetic nervous system, and thus is not discussed here). The *adrenal cortex* produces a number of corticosteroid hormones, such as cortisol, which helps the body adapt to stress; aldosterone, which helps the body conserve sodium and thus water; androgens, which have masculinizing effects; and estrogens, which have feminizing effects. The latter two hormones, whose levels decline with age, supplement the action of the testosterone and estrogen released from the testes and ovaries, respectively. The loss of estrogen production from postmenopausal ovaries appears to upset the androgen–estrogen balance in favor of the androgens produced in the adrenal gland. This might explain the mild masculinization of a woman's physique as she ages.

Aldosterone levels also fall as one ages, impairing an important component of blood pressure regulation. Normally, this hormone stimulates the reabsorption of sodium ions from the renal tubules back into the bloodstream, which osmotically draws water back in as well, thus increasing blood volume and therefore blood pressure when needed. Although the aldosterone mechanism is just one of many ways to increase blood pressure, its loss may bring the body one step closer to disruption of homeostasis.

Cortisol is the quintessential stress hormone, released into the bloodstream during prolonged periods of physical or psychological stress. It is a catabolic hormone whose function is to mobilize the body's energy reserves, increasing blood levels of glucose, fats, and amino acids during times of illness, physical injury, or emotional distress. In addition, baseline cortisol release (in conjunction with release of the hormone glucagon from the pancreas) in the absence of stress helps prevent blood glucose levels from falling dangerously low during sleep and in between meals.

As was true of thyroid hormone, cortisol levels remain normal well into old age because of a balance between the hormone's decreased production and its decreased excretion. In addition, stress-induced increases in cortisol release are not affected by aging. However, it appears to take older adults longer to reestablish normal blood cortisol levels following the stressful event, possibly as a result of a faulty negative feedback system in which the hypothalamus and pituitary gland fail to slow down the release of corticotropin-releasing hormone (CRH) and adrenocorticotropic hormone (ACTH), respectively, when cortisol levels are increased. The persistently elevated cortisol level may actually have a negative impact on the health of older adults. Some of the well-documented effects of chronically high blood cortisol levels include hyperglycemia (excessively high blood glucose level), hypertension (high blood pressure caused by the aldosterone-like effects of cortisol), and immunosuppression (increased susceptibility to infection and cancer). It is plausible then that elevated cortisol responses to stress might exacerbate concomitant diabetes mellitus, hypertension, and infectious disease in older adults.

Unlike in the thyroid gland, adrenal cortex, and gonads, control of hormone release from the endocrine cells of the *pancreas* is not primarily controlled by the hypothalamus and pituitary gland. Instead, the two major hormones produced by the pancreas, *insulin* (which decreases the blood glucose level) and *glucagon* (which increases the blood glucose level), are released at various rates based primarily on blood glucose levels. Deficient insulin action causes **diabetes mellitus** (DM), a condition marked by hyperglycemia and long-term complications such as blindness (resulting from cataracts and retinal damage), renal failure, nerve damage, atherosclerosis, and gangrenous infection often necessitating amputation of all or part of the leg. Non-insulin–dependent diabetes mellitus (NIDDM) is a type of diabetes mellitus that increases in frequency with age and accounts for about 90–95% of all cases. It appears to be caused by deficient target organ responses to the effects of insulin—the level of insulin itself is actually normal or increased. It is estimated that, in the United States, 20.8 million people (7% of the total population) suffer from diabetes, the vast majority having NIDDM.[143] Because it is so common in older adults, affecting more than 15% of those aged 65 and older, non-insulin–dependent diabetes mellitus is of great interest to geriatric medicine.[144]

SUMMARY

It is clear that our health and well-being depend on the degree to which our organ systems can successfully work together to maintain homeostasis, or internal stability, in the body. Diminished function in one organ system is minimized by appropriate compensatory mechanisms in other systems. An elderly individual with emphysema, and therefore less efficient ventilation of the lungs, often has an elevated hematocrit (i.e., a greater proportion of RBCs in the blood) to maintain adequate oxygen delivery to the bloodstream and tissues. An individual with systemic hypertension will have enlargement of the muscle in the heart's left ventricle, generating a greater force of contraction to maintain adequate cardiac output in the face of the increased afterload. A person's excessive exposure to sunlight not only stimulates increased production of the protective melanin pigment in the skin but may also heighten immune surveillance for precancerous epidermal cells.

However, also apparent is the gradual impairment of these homeostatic mechanisms with age, most likely as a result of the linear decline that seems to characterize many physiologic functions such as cardiac output, forced vital capacity, the number of functioning nephrons, bone mass, and epidermal melanocyte density. What is gradually lost with age is the functional reserve capacity of our organ systems. A physiologic disturbance that is easily correctable at age 30 may cause significant illness at age 60 or death at age 90. Perhaps it should not be surprising that coinciding with the linear decline in physiologic functioning is a logarithmic increase in mortality.[4] It is as though our bodies function well during the younger years despite the accumulation of environmental and genetic insults. However, at some stage in life, we reach a "critical mass" of impairment, a point beyond which our homeostatic correction mechanisms are no longer able to keep pace. When this point is reached, the likelihood of illness, disease, and death rises exponentially.

We may take comfort in the fact that much of the illness and suffering that tends to come with old age can be delayed or at least modified by taking care of ourselves. And it must be remembered that the hallmarks of preventive medicine, such as eating right, exercising, and avoiding cigarettes, are most effective when initiated early in life. Although there may be wisdom in the adage "live for the day," it is equally wise, from a health perspective, to "live for tomorrow."

Review Questions

1. Which of the following statements is correct?
   A. Improvements in sanitation have helped to increase the maximum life span potential of U.S. citizens over the past 100 years.
   B. Most of the increase in average life expectancy over the past 100 years can be attributed to advances in medical technology.
   C. The percentage of U.S. citizens nearing the maximum life span potential is higher today than it was 100 years ago.
   D. In the effort to increase the average life expectancy, curative medicine is more cost-effective than preventive medicine.
   E. Dietary practices such as vitamin intake and caloric restriction can prevent aging.

2. Match the following theories of aging with their most appropriate descriptions.
   _____ Rate of living theory
   _____ Free radical theory
   _____ Error catastrophe theory
   _____ Disposable soma theory
   _____ Gene regulation theory
   _____ Somatic mutation theory
   _____ Evolutionary theory
   _____ Glycosylation theory
   A. Aging results from the compromise that a species reaches between devoting all of its energy to reproduction and devoting all of its energy to body maintenance and repair.
   B. Aging results from accumulating damage to cells caused by molecules that have unpaired electrons in their outermost valence shells.
   C. Certain species live longer because they have lower metabolic rates.
   D. Aging is an inevitable result in a species that faces the possibility of accidental death (e.g., caused by predation).
   E. The random accumulation of DNA mutations and subsequent errors in protein production cause aging.
   F. Aging results from a gradual decline in the precision of DNA transcription and RNA translation.
   G. The aging process begins with the attachment of glucose to important molecules such as proteins and DNA.
   H. Aging occurs along an intentional timeline dictated by the sequential expression of particular genes in cells.

3. The skin gradually loses its brown tone with age as a result of a decrease in the number of _____ in the skin.
   A. Melanocytes
   B. Keratinocytes
   C. Fibroblasts
   D. Mast cells
   E. Langerhans cells

4. Which of the following is *not* a characteristic change in the nervous system as one ages?
   A. A decrease in the nerve conduction velocity
   B. A loss of moderate amounts of myelin around some axons
   C. A generalized and substantial decrease in the number of neurons
   D. A decrease in the number of dendrites
   E. An increase in the size of fatty plaques in the cerebral arteries

5. Which of the following is not a risk factor for osteoporosis?
   A. Cigarette smoking
   B. Sedentary lifestyle
   C. Depletion of estrogen levels following menopause
   D. High blood pressure
   E. Calcium deficiency

6. Which of the following statements regarding the cardiovascular system is false?
   A. With aging comes a gradual decline in the maximal heart rate during exercise.
   B. Insufficient activity of the sympathetic nervous system can cause postural hypotension in older adults.
   C. The cardiac output is obtained by multiplying the heart rate by the stroke volume.
   D. The walls of arteries become more rigid with age, increasing the likelihood that an older individual will develop hypertension.
   E. The first changes of atherosclerosis are not detectable in arteries until middle age.

7. Occasionally a blood clot can dislodge from its area of formation and travel farther down the bloodstream to block a more distal artery. This is called a(n)
   A. Thrombus
   B. Embolism
   C. Aneurysm
   D. Infarction
   E. Atheroma

8. Which of the following statements about chronic bronchitis is false?
   A. It is marked by excessive production of mucus in the bronchi.
   B. It is a condition that typically lasts only a week to 10 days.

   C. Cigarette smoke can play a key role in its development by irritating the respiratory lining.
   D. It is more likely to cause pneumonia in the very old because of the diminished effectiveness of their immune system.
   E. It can lead to blockage of the bronchi.

9. An elderly woman complains of bruising and bleeding easily. A deficiency of which of the following types of cells might cause these symptoms?
   A. Erythrocytes
   B. Thrombocytes
   C. Macrophages
   D. Fibroblasts
   E. Leukocytes

10. A decline in the functioning of the immune system in the elderly population may help directly explain the increased prevalence of all of the following categories of illness except
    A. Cancer
    B. Renal failure
    C. Viral infection
    D. Autoimmune disease
    E. Bacterial infection

11. Older adults are at increased risk of developing small, sac-like herniations through the wall of the large intestine. This condition is called
    A. Cholecystitis
    B. Peritonitis
    C. Fecal incontinence
    D. Steatorrhea
    E. Diverticulosis

12. Which of the following statements about non-insulin–dependent diabetes mellitus (NIDDM) is false?
    A. Poorly treated NIDDM results in elevated blood glucose levels.
    B. Individuals with NIDDM are at increased risk for cataracts.
    C. One's risk of developing NIDDM increases with age.
    D. NIDDM is caused by the inability of the pancreas to secrete insulin.
    E. Sufferers of NIDDM are more likely to develop hypertension than are healthy individuals.

13. The clouding of the lens of the eye is called
    A. Presbyopia
    B. Cataract

C. Dyspnea
D. Presbycusis
E. Hyposmia

14. Elderly individuals commonly experience an inability to focus on near objects because of the inelasticity of the lens of the eye. This is called
   A. Presbyopia
   B. Cataract
   C. Dyspnea
   D. Presbycusis
   E. Hyposmia

15. Older individuals who have lost the coordination of their tongue, palatal, and pharyngeal muscles find it difficult to swallow food. This phenomenon is called
   A. Dyspnea
   B. Dysphagia
   C. Xerostomia
   D. Emphysema
   E. Dementia

Learning Activities

1. Compare and contrast aging and disease. How do the effects of cigarette smoking on the body illustrate the difficulty of distinguishing aging from disease?
2. A 76-year-old man with a long history of peptic ulcer disease has become increasingly fatigued and short of breath over the past 3 weeks. He complains of a dull pain below his sternum that is worse following meals. On physical examination, he looks pale and has a slightly elevated heart rate.
   A. What might be this man's diagnosis?
   B. Suggest some possible explanations for his
      i. Shortness of breath
      ii. Elevated heart rate
   C. From a physiologic standpoint, why might it be more difficult for this man to compensate for his current problem than it would be for a 30-year-old man? In your answer, explore possibilities from at least three different organ systems.

REFERENCES

1. Timiras, PS. Introduction: Aging as a stage in the life cycle. In PS Timiras (ed.). *Physiological Basis of Aging and Geriatrics*. 2nd ed. Boca Raton, FL: CRC Press, 1994, p 1.

2. Hayflick, L. Myths of aging. *Scientific American*, 1997;276:110.

3. Ribbe, MW, et al. Nursing homes in 10 nations: A comparison between countries

and settings. *Age and Ageing*, 1997;26(Suppl 2):3–12.

4. Schneider, EL. Aging research: Challenge of the twenty-first century. In AD Woodhead et al. (eds.). *Molecular Biology of Aging*. New York: Plenum Press, 1985, p 1.

5. Centers for Disease Control and Prevention (CDC). Estimated national spending on prevention—United States, 1988. *Morbidity and Mortality Weekly Report*, 1992;41(29):529–531.

6. Timiras, PS. Aging and disease. In PS Timiras (ed.). *Physiological Basis of Aging and Geriatrics*. 2nd ed. Boca Raton, FL: CRC Press, 1994, p 23.

7. National Center for Health Statistics. *Vital Statistics of the United States 1985*. PHS Publication No. 88-1104, Life Tables, Vol. 2, Sect 6. Hyattsville, MD: U.S. Department of Health and Human Services, 1988, p 9.

8. National Center for Health Statistics. *National Vital Statistics Reports 2004*. United States Life Tables, Vol. 56, No. 9. Hyattsville, MD: U.S. Department of Health and Human Services, 2007, p 3.

9. Comfort, A. *The Biology of Senescence*. 3rd ed. New York: Elsevier, 1979, p 81.

10. Finch, CE. *Longevity, Senescence, and the Genome*. Chicago: University of Chicago Press, 1990.

11. Spence, JD. Stroke prevention in the high-risk patient. *Expert Opinion on Pharmacotherapy*, 2007;8(12):1851–1859.

12. Bierman, EL, Hazzard, WR. Preventive gerontology: Strategies for attenuation of the chronic diseases of aging. In WR Hazzard et al. (eds.). *Principles of Geriatric Medicine and Gerontology*. 3rd ed. New York: McGraw-Hill, 1994, p 187.

13. Committee on Diet and Health, Food, and Nutrition Board, Commission on Life Sciences, National Research Council. *Diet and Health*. Washington, DC: National Academy Press, 1989.

14. Evans, W, Rosenberg, I. *Biomarkers*. New York: Simon & Schuster, 1991.

15. Ruuskanen, JM, Ruoppila, I. Physical activity and psychological well-being among people aged 65 to 84 years. *Age and Ageing*, 1995;24:292–296.

16. Wynder, EL. Etiology of lung cancer: Reflections on two decades of research. *Cancer*, 1972;30:1332.

17. Bernhard, D, et al. Cigarette smoke: An aging accelerator? *Experimental Gerontology*, 2007;42(3):160–165.

18. Cournil, A, Kirkwood, TBL. If you would live long, choose your parents well. *Trends in Genetics*, 2001;17:233–235.

19. Timiras, PS. Demographic, comparative, and differential aging. In PS Timiras (ed.). *Physiological Basis of Aging and Geriatrics*. 2nd ed. Boca Raton, FL: CRC Press, 1994, p 7.

20. Martin, GM. Interactions of aging and environmental agents: The gerontological perspective. In SR Baker, M Rogul (eds.). *Environmental Toxicity and the Aging Process*. New York: Alan R Liss, 1987, p 25.

21. Tosato, M, et al. The aging process and potential interventions to extend life expectancy. *Clinical Interventions in Aging*, 2007;2(3):401–412.

22. Szilard, L. On the nature of the aging process. *Proceedings of the National Academy of Sciences USA*, 1959;45:30.

23. Ogburn, CE, et al. Exceptional cellular resistance to oxidative damage in long-lived birds requires active gene expression. *Journals of Gerontology. Series A, Biological Sciences and Medical Sciences*, 2001;56:B468–B474.

24. Burkle, A, et al. Poly(ADP-ribose) polymerase-1, DNA repair and mammalian longevity. *Experimental Gerontology*, 2002;37:1203–1205.

25. Martin, GM, et al. Increased chromosomal aberrations in first metaphases of cells isolated from the kidneys of aged mice. *Israel Journal of Medical Sciences*, 1985;21:296.

26. Curtis, HJ. Cellular processes involved in aging. *Federal Proceedings*, 1964;23:662.

27. Orgel, LE. The maintenance of the accuracy of protein synthesis and its relevance to aging. *Proceedings of the National Academy of Sciences USA*, 1963;49:517.

28. Medvedev, ZA. The nucleic acids in development and aging. In BL Strehler (ed.). *Advances in Gerontological Research*. Vol 1. New York: Academic Press, 1964.

29. Holliday, R, Tarrant, GM. Altered enzymes in aging human fibroblasts. *Nature*, 1972; 238:26.

30. Lamb, MJ. *Biology of Aging*. New York: John Wiley & Sons, 1977.

31. Reiss, V, Gershon, D. Comparison of cytoplasmic superoxide dismutase in liver, heart, and brain of aging rats and mice. *Biochemical and Biophysical Research Communications*, 1976;73:255.

32. Kanungo, MS, Gandhi, BS. Induction of malate dehydrogenase isoenzymes in livers of young and old rats. *Proceedings of the National Academy of Sciences USA*, 1972;69:2035.

33. Kanungo, MS. A model for ageing. *Journal of Theoretical Biology*, 1975;53:253.

34. Sierra, F, et al. T-kininogen gene expression is induced during aging. *Molecular and Cellular Biology*, 1989;9:5610.

35. Friedman, V, et al. Isolation and identification of aging-related cDNAs in the mouse. *Mechanisms of Ageing and Development*, 1990;52:27.

36. Medawar, PB. *An Unsolved Problem in Biology*. London: HK Lewis, 1952.

37. Williams, GC. Pleiotropy, natural selection and the evolution of senescence. *Evolution*, 1957;11:398.

38. Miller, RA. The biology of aging and longevity. In WR Hazzard et al. (eds.). *Principles of Geriatric Medicine and Gerontology*. 3rd ed. New York: McGraw-Hill, 1994, p 3.

39. Kirkwood, TBL. Evolution of ageing. *Nature*, 1977;270:301.

40. Pearl, R. *The Rate of Living*. London: University of London Press, 1928.

41. McCay, CM, Crowell, MF. Prolonging the life span. *Scientific Monthly*, 1934;39:405.

42. Barrows, CH, Kokkonen, GC. Relationship between nutrition and aging. *Advances in Nutritional Research*, 1977;1:253.

43. Bishop, NA, Guarente, L. Genetic links between diet and lifespan: Shared mechanisms from yeast to humans. *Nature Reviews Genetics*, 2007;8(11):835–844.

44. Dilova, I, et al. Calorie restriction and the nutrient signaling pathways. *Cellular and Molecular Life Sciences*, 2007;64(6):752–767.

45. Masoro, EJ, et al. Temporal and compositional dietary restrictions modulate age-related changes in serum lipids. *Journal of Nutrition*, 1983;113:880.

46. Kalu, DN, et al. Life-long food restriction prevents senile osteopenia and hyperparathyroidism in F344 rats. *Mechanisms of Ageing and Development*, 1984;26:103.

47. Weindruch, R, et al. Influence of controlled dietary restriction on immunologic function. *Federal Proceedings*, 1979;38:2007.

48. Masoro, EJ, et al. Action of food restriction in delaying the aging process. *Proceedings of the National Academy of Sciences USA*, 1982;79:4239.

49. McCarter, R, et al. Does food restriction retard aging by reducing the metabolic rate? *American Journal of Physiology*, 1985;248:E488.

50. Austad, SN, Fischer, KE. Mammalian aging, metabolism, and ecology: Evidence from the bats and marsupials. *Journal of Gerontology*, 1991;46:B47.

51. Harman, D. The aging process: Major risk factor for disease and death. *Proceedings of the National Academy of Sciences USA*, 1991;88:5360.

52. Harman, D. Aging: A theory based on free radical and radiation chemistry. *Journal of Gerontology*, 1956;11:298.

53. Chance, B, et al. Hydrogen peroxide metabolism in mammalian organs. *Physiological Reviews*, 1979;59:527.

54. Von Zglinicki, T, et al. Stress, DNA damage and ageing: An integrative approach. *Experimental Gerontology*, 2001;36:1049–1062.

55. Nohl, H, Hegner, D. Do mitochondria produce oxygen radicals in vivo? *European Journal of Biochemistry*, 1978;82:563.

56. Lippman, RD. The prolongation of life: A comparison of antioxidants and geroprotectors versus superoxide in human mitochondria. *Journal of Gerontology*, 1981;36:550.

57. Leibovitz, BE, Siegel, BV. Aspects of free radical reactions in biological systems: Aging. *Journal of Gerontology*, 1980;35:45.

58. Pryor, WA. The formation of free radicals and the consequences of their reactions in vivo. *Photochemistry and Photobiology*, 1978;28:787.

59. Sohal, RS (ed.). *Age Pigments*. Amsterdam: Elsevier/North-Holland, 1981.

60. Timiras, PS. Degenerative changes in cells and cell death. In PS Timiras (ed.). *Physiological Basis of Aging and Geriatrics*. 2nd ed. Boca Raton, FL: CRC Press, 1994, p 47.

61. Berg, BN. Study of vitamin E supplements in relation to muscular dystrophy and other diseases in aging rats. *Journal of Gerontology*, 1959;14:174.

62. Porta, EA, et al. Effects of the type of dietary fat at two levels of vitamin E in Wistar male rats during development and aging. I. Life span, serum biochemical parameters and pathological changes. *Mechanisms of Ageing and Development*, 1980;13:1.

63. Blackett, AD, Hall, DA. Vitamin E: Its significance in mouse ageing. *Age and Ageing*, 1981; 10:191.

64. Ledvina, M, Hodanova, M. The effect of simultaneous administration of tocopherol and sunflower oil on the life-span of female mice. *Experimental Gerontology*, 1980;15:67.

65. Tappel, AI. Lipid peroxidation damage to cell components. *Federal Proceedings*, 1973;32:1870.

66. Packer, L, Smith JR. Extension of the lifespan of cultured normal human diploid cells by vitamin E: A reevaluation. *Proceedings of the National Academy of Sciences USA*, 1977;74:1640.

67. Nakayama, T, et al. Generation of hydrogen peroxide and superoxide anion radical from cigarette smoke. *Gann*, 1984;75:95.

68. Church, DF, Pryor, WA. Free radical chemistry of cigarette smoke and its toxicological implications. *Environmental Health Perspectives*, 1985;64:111.

69. Nagy, I. Memorial lecture: Verzar's ideas on the age-dependent protein cross-linking in the light of the present knowledge. *Archives of Gerontology and Geriatrics*, 1986;5:267.

70. Bjorksten, J. The crosslinkage theory of aging. *Journal of the American Geriatrics Society*, 1968;16:408.

71. Kohn, RR. *Principles of Mammalian Aging.* 2nd ed. Englewood Cliffs, NJ: Prentice Hall, 1978.

72. Monnier, VM. Nonenzymatic glycosylation, the Maillard reaction and the aging process. *Journal of Gerontology*, 1990;45:B105.

73. Cerami, A. Hypothesis: Glucose as a mediator of aging. *Journal of the Ameircan Geriatrics Society*, 1985;33:626.

74. Masoro, EJ, et al. Evidence for the glycation hypothesis of aging from the food-restricted rodent model. *Journal of Gerontology Series A: Biological Sciences and Medical Sciences*, 1989;44:B20.

75. Cerami, A, et al. Role of nonenzymatic glycosylation in the development of the sequelae of diabetes. *Metabolism*, 1979;28:431.

76. Kohn, RR, Schneider, SL. Glycosylation of human collagen. *Diabetes*, 1981;(suppl)31:47.

77. Araki, N, et al. Immunochemical evidence for the presence of advanced glycation end products in human lens proteins and its positive correlation with aging. *Journal of Biological Chemistry*, 1992;267:10211.

78. Monnier, VM, Cerami, A. Nonenzymatic browning in vivo: Possible process for aging of long-lived proteins. *Science*, 1981;211:491.

79. Ahmed, A, Tollefsbol, T. Telomeres and telomerase: Basic science implications for aging. *Journal of the American Geriatrics Society*, 2001;49(8): 1105–1109.

80. Kim, S, et al. Telomeres, aging and cancer: In search of a happy ending. *Oncogene*, 2002;21: 503–511.

81. Von Zglinicki, T. Oxidative stress shortens telomeres. *Trends in Biochemical Sciences*, 2002;27: 339–344.

82. Kipling, D. Telomeres, replicative senescence and human ageing. *Maturitas*, 2001;38(1):25–38.

83. Romani, N, et al. Epidermal Langerhans cells—changing views on their function in vivo. *Immunology Letters*, 2006;106(2):119–125.

84. Montagna, W, Carlisle, K. Structural changes in aging human skin. *Journal of Investigative Dermatology*, 1979;73:47.

85. Grove, GL, Kligman, AM. Age-associated changes in human epidermal cell renewal. *Journal of Gerontology*, 1983;38:137.

86. Leyden, JJ, et al. Age-related differences in the rate of desquamation of skin surface cells. In RD Adelman et al. (eds.). *Pharmacological Intervention of the Aging Process.* New York: Plenum Press, 1978, p 297.

87. Kaminer, MS, Gilchrest, BA. Aging of the skin. In WR Hazzard et al. (eds.). *Principles of Geriatric Medicine and Gerontology.* 3rd ed. New York: McGraw-Hill, 1994, p 414.

88. U.S. Cancer Statistics Working Group. *United States Cancer Statistics: 1999–2004 Incidence and Mortality Web-Based Report.* Atlanta, GA: U.S. Department of Health and Human Services, Centers for Disease Control and Prevention, and National Cancer Institute, 2007.

89. Holick, MF. Vitamin D deficiency. *New England Journal of Medicine*, 2007;357(3):266–281.

90. Cranney, C, et al. Effectiveness and safety of vitamin D. Evidence Report/Technology Assessment No. 158 prepared by the University of Ottawa Evidence-Based Practice Center under Contract No. 290-02.0021. AHRQ Publication No. 07-E013. Rockville, MD. Agency for Healthcare Research and Quality, 2007.

91. Office of Dietary Supplements. *Dietary Supplement Fact Sheet: Vitamin D.* Betheseda, MD: National Institutes of Health, 2008. Retrieved January 20, 2009, from http://ods.od.nih.gov/factsheets/vitamind.asp

92. Timiras, PS. Aging of the nervous system: Functional changes. In PS Timiras (ed.). *Physiological Basis of Aging and Geriatrics.* 2nd ed. Boca Raton, FL: CRC Press, 1994, p 103.

93. Palmer, AM, DeKosky, ST: The neurochemistry of ageing. In MSJ Pathy (ed.). *Principles and Practice of Geriatric Medicine.* 3rd ed. Chichester, England: John Wiley and Sons, 1998, pp 65–76.

94. Shock, NW. The physiology of aging. *Scientific American,* 1962;206:100.

95. Ferro, JM, Madureira, S. Age-related white matter changes and cognitive impairment. *Journal of the Neurological Sciences,* 2002;15:221–225.

96. Alzheimer's Association. *2008 Alzheimer's Disease Facts and Figures.* Chicago, IL, 2008. Retrieved January 20, 2009, from http://alz.org/national/documents/report_alzfactsfigures2008.pdf

97. Jarvik, LF, et al. Dementia and delirium in old age. In JC Brocklehurst et al. (eds.). *Textbook of Geriatric Medicine and Gerontology,* 4th ed. London: Churchill Livingstone, 1992, pp 332, 338.

98. Von Zglinicki, T, et al. Short telomeres in patients with vascular dementia: An indicator of low antioxidative capacity and a possible prognostic factor? *Laboratory Investigation,* 2000;80:1739–1747.

99. Szwabo, PA. Psychological aspects of aging. In MSJ Pathy et al. (eds.). *Principles and Practice of Geriatric Medicine.* 4th ed. Chichester, England: John Wiley and Sons, 2006, pp 53–57.

100. Morgan, K. Sleep in normal and pathological aging. In JC Brocklehurst et al. (eds.). *Textbook of Geriatric Medicine and Gerontology.* 4th ed. London: Churchill Livingstone, 1992, p 122.

101. Pointer, JS. The burgeoning presbyopic population: An emerging 20th century phenomenon. *Ophthalmic and Physiological Optics,* 1998;18(4):325–334.

102. Shamsi, FA, Boulton, M. Inhibition of RPE lysosomal and antioxidant activity by the age pigment liposfuscin. *Investigative Ophthalmology and Visual Science,* 2001;42:3041–3046.

103. Kevorkian, R. Physiology of aging. In MSJ Pathy et al. (eds.). *Principles and Practice of Geriatric Medicine.* 4th ed. Chichester, England: John Wiley and Sons, 2006, p 39.

104. Gates, GA, et al. Hearing in the elderly: The Framingham cohort, 1983–1985. *Ear Hear,* 1990;11:247.

105. Lewis, TJ. Hearing impairment. In RJ Ham, PD Sloane, GA Warshaw, MA Bernard, E Flaherty (eds.). *Primary Care Geriatrics: A Case-Based Approach.* 5th ed. Philadelphia: Mosby, 2007, p 334.

106. Stalworth, M, Sloane, PD. Clinical implications of normal aging. In RJ Ham, PD Sloane, GA Warshaw, MA Bernard, E Flaherty (eds.). *Primary Care Geriatrics: A Case-Based Approach.* 5th ed. Philadelphia: Mosby, 2007, p 23.

107. Stevens, JC, et al. Aging impairs the ability to detect gas odor. *Fire Technology,* 1987;23:198.

108. Berg, RL, Cassells, JS. *The Second Fifty Years: Promoting Health and Preventing Disability.* Washington, DC: National Academy Press, 1990, p 76.

109. Office of the Surgeon General. *Bone Health and Osteoporosis: A Report of the Surgeon General.* Hyattsville, MD: U.S. Department of Health and Human Services, 2004.

110. Kallenberg, GA, Beck, JC. Care of the geriatric patient. In RE Rakel (ed.). *Textbook of Family Practice.* 3rd ed. Philadelphia: W. B. Saunders, 1984, p 249.

111. Mazess, RB. On aging bone loss. *Clinical Orthopaedics and Related Research,* 1982;165:239–252.

112. Sorensen, LB. Rheumatology. In CK Cassel et al. (eds.). *Geriatric Medicine.* 2nd ed. New York: Springer-Verlag, 1990, p 185.

113. Arthritis Foundation. Osteoarthritis: Who Is at Risk? Retrieved January 20, 2009, from http://www.arthritis.org/disease-center.php?disease_id=32&df=whos_at_risk

114. American Geriatrics Society Panel on Exercise and Osteoarthritis. Exercise prescription for older adults with osteoarthritis pain: Consensus practice recommendations. *Journal of the American Geriatrics Society*, 2001;49:808–823.

115. Murray, CJL, Lopez, AD. The Global Burden of Disease: A Comprehensive Assessment of Mortality and Disability from Diseases, Injuries, and Risk Factors in 1990 and Projected to 2020. Harvard School of Public Health, 1996. Retrieved January 20, 2009, from http://www.scielosp.org/scielo.php?script=sci_arttext&pid=S00429686 2003000900007&nrm=iso&tlng=pt

116. Felson, DT, et al. Osteoarthritis: New insights. Part 1: The disease and its risk factors. *Annals of Internal Medicine*, 2000;133:635–646.

117. Brunner, F, et al. Effects of aging on type II muscle fibers: A systematic review of the literature. *Journal of Aging and Physical Activity*, 2007;15(3):336–348.

118. Mian, OS, et al. The impact of physical training on locomotor function in older people. *Sports Medicine*, 2007;37(8):683–701.

119. Wolz, M, et al. Statement from the national high blood pressure education program: Prevalence of hypertension. *American Journal of Hypertension*, 2000;13:103–104.

120. Lewington, S, et al. Age-specific relevance of usual blood pressure to vascular mortality: A meta-analysis of individual date for one million adults in 61 prospective studies. *Lancet*, 2002;360:1903–1913.

121. Kohn, WM, et al. Effects of gender, age, and fitness level on response of val max to training in 60–71-year-olds. *Journal of Applied Physiology*, 1991;71:2004.

122. Huang, G, et al. Resting heart rate changes after endurance training in older adults: A meta-analysis. *Medicine and Science in Sports and Exercise*, 2005;37(8):1381–1386.

123. Johnson, D, Sandmire, D. *Medical Tests That Can Save Your Life: 21 Tests Your Doctor Won't Order Unless You Know to Ask*. New York: Rodale and St. Martin's Press, 2004, p 68.

124. World Health Organization. Cardiovascular Disease: Prevention and Control. World Health Organization, 2008. Retrieved January 20, 2009, from http://www.who.int/dietphysicalactivity/publications/facts/cvd/en/

125. Ness, J, et al. Risk factors for symptomatic peripheral arterial disease in older persons in an academic hospital based geriatrics practice. *Journal of the American Geriatrics Society*, 2000;48:312–314.

126. Carandang, R, et al. Trends in incidence, lifetime risk, severity, and 30-day mortality of stroke over the past 50 years. *Journal of the American Medical Association*, 2006;296(24):2939–2946.

127. Crapo, RO, et al. Reference spirometric values using techniques and equipment that meet ATS recommendations. *American Review of Respiratory Diseases*, 1981;123:659.

128. Timiras, PS. Aging of respiration: Erythrocytes, and the hematopoietic system. In PS Timiras (ed.). *Physiological Basis of Aging and Geriatrics*. 2nd ed. Boca Raton, FL: CRC Press, 1994, p 226.

129. Pryor, WA, et al. The inactivation of alpha-1-proteinase inhibitor by gas-phase cigarette smoke: Protection by antioxidants and reducing species. *Chemico-Biological Interactions*, 1986;57:271.

130. Weiss, SJ. Tissue destruction by neutrophils. *New England Journal of Medicine*, 1989;320:365.

131. Travis, J, Salvesen, JS. Human plasma protease inhibitors. *Annual Review of Biochemistry*, 1983;52:655.

132. Janoff, A. Elastase in tissue injury. *Annual Review of Medicine*, 1985;36:207.

133. Boross, M, et al. Effect of smoking on different biological parameters in aging mice. *Z Gerontol*, 1991;24:76.

134. Anderson, RN, Smith, BL. *Deaths: Leading Causes for 2002*. National Vital Statistics Report, Vol. 53, No. 17. Hyattsville, MD: U.S. Department of Health and Human Services, 2005, p 7.

135. World Health Organization. Chronic Respiratory Diseases. World Health Organization, 2008. Retrieved January 20, 2009, from http://www.who.int/respiratory/en/

136. Marieb, EN. *Human Anatomy and Physiology*. 6th ed. San Francisco, CA: Benjamin Cummings, 2004, p 1162.

137. Linton, PJ, Dorshkind, K. Age-related changes in lymphocytes development and function. *Nature Immunology*, 2004;5(2):133.

138. Kovaiou, RD, et al. Age-related changes in immunity: Implications for vaccination in the

elderly. *Expert Reviews in Molecular Medicine*, 2007;9(3):1–17.

139. Utsuyama, M, et al. Differential age-change in numbers of CD4+CD45RA+ and CD4+CD29+ T cell subsets in human peripheral blood. *Mechanisms of Ageing and Development*, 1992;63: 57–66.

140. Timiras, PS. Aging of the gastrointestinal tract and liver. In PS Timiras (ed.). *Physiological Basis of Aging and Geriatrics*. 2nd ed. Boca Raton, FL: CRC Press, 1994, p 248.

141. Nelson, JB, Castell, DO. Gastroenterology. In CK Cassel et al. (eds.). *Geriatric Medicine*. 2nd ed. New York: Springer-Verlag, 1990, p 356.

142. Herzog, AR, Fultz, NH. Prevalence and incidence of urinary incontinence in community dwelling populations. *Journal of the American Geriatrics Society*, 1990;38:273.

143. Centers for Disease Control and Prevention. *National Diabetes Fact Sheet: General Information and National Estimates on Diabetes in the United States, 2005.* Atlanta, GA: U.S. Department of Health and Human Services, Centers for Disease Control and Prevention, 2005.

144. Goldberg, AP, Coon, PJ. Diabetes mellitus and glucose metabolism in the elderly. In WR Hazzard et al. (eds.). *Principles of Geriatric Medicine and Gerontology*. 3rd ed. New York: McGraw-Hill, 1994, p 826.

THE COGNITIVE AND PSYCHOLOGICAL CHANGES ASSOCIATED WITH AGING

REGULA H. ROBNETT, PhD, OTR/L

In the central place of your heart there is a wireless station. So long as it receives messages of beauty, hope, cheer, grandeur, courage, and power from the earth, from men and from the Infinite—so long are you young. When the wires are all down and the central places of your heart are covered with the snows of pessimism and the ice of cynicism, then are you grown old, indeed!

—*Samuel Ullman (1840–1924) "Youth"*

Chapter Outline

Behavioral Objectives

Upon completion of this chapter, the reader will be able to:

1. List the three basic factors that cause cognitive impairments in older adults.
2. Describe how general (fluid and crystallized intelligence) and specific aspects of cognition (attention, orientation, memory, executive functioning, and learning) may change with the aging process.

3. Describe compensatory measures related to decreased or changed cognitive functioning.
4. Compare and contrast signs of delirium, depression, and dementia.
5. Complete a screen for depression to make a referral for assistance.
6. List general guidelines for working with people who have dementia.
7. Describe the bereavement process, and state recommendations for health care professionals who are working with bereaved individuals.
8. Differentiate aspects of personality that may tend to change over time from those that may not, based on current research.
9. Describe factors believed to contribute to a positive quality of life in elderly people.

Key Terms

Age-associated memory impairment	Learned helplessness
Alzheimer's disease	Long-term memory
Anhedonia	Malnutrition
Attention	Mild cognitive impairment
Bereavement	Orientation
Cerebrovascular accident	Personality
Cognition	Primary memory
Crystallized intelligence	Procedural memory
Delirium	Prospective memory
Dementia	Quality of life
Depression	Self-efficacy
Episodic memory	Semantic memory
Failure to thrive	Short-term memory
Fluid intelligence	Stereotypes
Gerotranscendence	Suicide
Heterogeneous	Working memory

Aging is often viewed through a distorted lens, although the truth is hard to grasp with absolute certainty. The trajectory of human performance has been determined to "develop" through young adulthood, reach a plateau through middle age, and "decline" in old age. For example, cognition from birth to maturity is seen as *development*, whereas the changes of cognition from the age of maturity onward have been viewed as part of the *decline* of aging. Development is described as a positive emerging state, whereas aging is viewed as a negative state moving toward the inevitable end of life.[1] The simple statement—cognition decreases with age—although widely accepted as hard-core fact, is suspect.

This chapter explores human development throughout life in the typical aging process and juxtaposes it with the atypical, or abnormal, aging process with which it is sometimes confused. Although change is a constant in our lives and the aging process inevitably entails change, not all changes are negative, and not every aspect of our lives or our state of humanness experiences change. Sometimes we need to question whether the negative changes that occur result from the aging process alone or from the accumulation of poor lifestyle choices, to expectations of decline, or to a combination of these forces.

Not all behaviors undergo transformation over time. In working with older people, knowledge of the typical aging processes and the importance of individuality cannot be overstated. This chapter demonstrates that chronological age is less a predictor of cognitive performance than other factors such as subjective and objective health status, personality traits, and lifestyle choices (especially as the impact of these choices accumulates over decades of time).

Levy, in conducting important research on the **stereotypes** associated with aging, concluded that aging stereotypes may become self-fulfilling prophecies actually leading to poorer performance among elders.[2] Levy researched children's views of older people and found them to be already predominantly negative. The majority of children in her study stated they would prefer not to get old. Levy proposes the idea that over the course of life negative stereotypes get reinforced repeatedly to the point where they become internalized, resulting in a situation in which older people tend to be even more negative about old age than younger people are. Levy suggests that we need to restructure our heretofore ingrained views by focusing on the positive changes of aging. By activating more affirmative stereotypes and increasing societal awareness of the strong impact of negative stereotypes (i.e., not actual changes of aging, but merely the associated expectations), we can promote a more realistic image of aging, improved health, and better performance over time.

Aging, or just living life, does entail inevitable change, but when people age well, they become more aware of, and more determined to take advantage of, the positive changes they encounter (wisdom, maturity, increased self-esteem, increased level of confidence, increased ability to appreciate ambiguity). They also take actions to counteract the negative changes (potential declines in physical and cognitive realms). Older people deserve the hope and a caring positive attitude that we, as health care professionals, can share with them to promote an optimal, individualized aging process.

Another factor promoting the current less-than-rosy outlook on the aging process is the increase in the prevalence of dementia, a condition that now touches nearly every extended family. More than 5 million people in the United States currently have Alzheimer's disease, the most common form of dementia.[3] Ironically, the disease is a gift of our scientific progress. As a greater proportion of the population lives longer, more people are getting dementia. The incidence of dementia increases with advancing age, although it never becomes an inevitable diagnosis even among the oldest-old. We are also more apt to hear about the "suffering" of old age (e.g., cancer, arthritis, stroke), not realizing that many people can still live well and happily even with health problems. A recent study of centenarians found that a significant proportion of the oldest-old has been living with chronic conditions (associated with suffering) for decades. The majority of older people do not "suffer" through life but rather learn to live well despite pain or bodily restrictions.[4]

Finally, because of the cumulative nature of lifestyle choices (i.e., in the realms of nutrition and substance use or abuse) and the impact of disabling conditions on some older people but not others, elders tend to become more and more different from each other over time—they become a more **heterogeneous** group. Yet often those of an advanced age (age 60 or 65 and older) are lumped together into a single group, as if they were all more alike than different. Older people who have inherited the right genes, make positive choices throughout life (e.g., with regard to exercise, nutrition, and managing stress), and perhaps have a little luck may be able to function as well as or even better than when they were young, whereas others succumb to disease, functional decline, or may even begin "dying by degrees" (described by an elder who felt he was experiencing this prior to his eventual death). As caring health care professionals, we can help elders to live well until they die and to "rage, rage against the dying of the light."[5]

COGNITION

Preconceived notions are the locks on the door to wisdom.

—Merry Browne

Cognition includes thinking, learning, and memory.[6] Our brains control everything we do intentionally and much of our unintentional behavior as well. A well-known assertion posits that cognition declines with older age. This premise is only partially true. Zec asserts that cognitive impairments in older adults are primarily caused by three factors[7]:

1. Disease
2. Disuse
3. Aging

Several disease processes affect cognition, and these diseases are more common in elderly than in younger people. Diseases related to cognitive performance include the most common debilitating disease of old age, **Alzheimer's disease** (AD), and other dementias, as well as Parkinson's disease, diabetes mellitus, cardiac disease, and the sequelae of acquired brain injuries such as stroke. Those with an interest in the problems of aging related to specific diseases are encouraged to investigate these on their own because detailed information about individual disease processes is beyond the scope of this chapter. Only AD is considered in more depth because of its prevalence.

Often simple old age is implicated as the cause of cognitive declines, but disuse may be as much to blame as the impact of just living a certain number of years. We have all heard the advice "use it or lose it" to keep our brains active and performing optimally. We explore optimal brain functioning later in the chapter. First, we delve into various aspects of cognition and how each aspect may change over the course of typical (i.e., healthy) aging. To simplify the presentation, cognition is divided into several sections. However, keep in mind that these cognitive components rarely have distinct boundaries;

because of vast interconnecting brain networks, each aspect of cognition influences many other aspects as we perform our daily tasks. In fact, it is rare to have an isolated cognitive deficit because the human brain tends to work in a highly integrated fashion.

Table 4-1 gives a brief overview of the cognitive changes associated with advanced age, along with a few helpful hints for health care providers. An important caveat is that these hints just briefly scratch the surface. People need individualized care, and these ideas may occasionally help. A few areas are described in more depth in the body of the chapter.

ORIENTATION

People who are aging typically are generally alert and oriented in all realms, (A&O × 3 or A&O × 4) as described in Table 4-1.* However, retirement—rather than a specific disease process—may contribute more to apparent disorientation to exact date or time of day. Without a planned schedule or daily appointments, it is easy to lose track of the exact day and time. Therefore, when determining someone's level of **orientation**, allow a little flexibility and consider the potential influence of an unstructured lifestyle. A psychiatric disturbance is indicated when a person is alert but is not oriented at least to him- or herself. This is not a common occurrence in elderly people, except for those with severe dementia, another psychiatric illness, or those who are currently delirious, perhaps under the influence of medication.

DELIRIUM

Delirium is a common occurrence for those who have been hospitalized, have undergone surgery, or who are overmedicated. It is not common in a healthy aging population. Generally, delirium is a transient state in which the person shows extreme confusion and inability to learn new information. This state can be devastating for family members who may conclude that the person has suddenly become demented. A health care professional can ease the tense situation by explaining the temporary nature of delirium and by educating the family about the side effects of the patient's current medical procedure or medication. Various medications (especially polypharmacy or improper medication management) can cause disorientation and foggy thinking (see Chapter 6). Psychiatric illnesses, brain disorders, and lack of oxygen (for example, as a result of lung disease or emphysema) may also lead to confusion and alteration in thinking processes. Any change in mental status should to be reported to and addressed by the health care team.

---

* A&O × 1 = Alert and oriented to self only; A&O × 2 = Oriented to self and surroundings; A&O × 3 = Oriented to self, place, and time; and A&O × 4 = Oriented to self, place, time, and situation (not always used as A&O × 3 is considered "normal").

TABLE 4-1   The Cognitive Changes of Aging.

Aspect of Cognition	Changes of Aging	Helpful Hints
Orientation—knowing who one is (A&O × 1), where one is (A&O × 2), and having an adequate understanding of time (A&O × 3). A&O × 4 may include situation as well.	In the typical aging process, orientation usually remains largely intact as part of crystallized intelligence.[a] As a result of retirement lifestyle, older adults may have more difficulty remembering the exact date or day.	Use calendars and orient person as needed. If the older adult is in an institution, be sure that the orienting information available is up-to-date. Questioning people about orienting information may be intimidating.
Attention—includes being able to sustain attention or focus on one task, alternating attention between two tasks, or dividing attention between two or more tasks (simultaneously). Selective attention involves paying attention to relevant stimuli while filtering out unimportant information.	Ability to sustain attention without distractions remains intact, although older adults tend to be less able to ignore distractions during tasks. Alternating and divided attention tasks may become more difficult, for example, in the task of driving.[b]	Limit distractions, especially when older adults are completing difficult tasks (such as driving) or when they are attending to crucial information (such as health care instructions).
Memory—the different types of memory are defined in the chapter.	A decline in memory acuity at older ages has been corroborated by a number of cross-sectional studies.[c] Older people tend to have more difficulty with short-term memory and remembering more recent episodes in their lives, including the source of information or the episode (e.g., where it happened, whom they already told).[d]	Repetition is important for learning. Writing lists and other memory aids can be helpful (and may be used more spontaneously by older adults than by younger people.[e] Do not assume just by telling someone something that he or she will remember and incorporate what you said.
Crystallized intelligence—includes both basic knowledge and skills that accumulate over the course of life.	In typical aging this remains intact or may even continue to improve, especially for overlearned material and individual work-related skills. Reading comprehension, for example, is maintained well into old age, at least until age 75 or beyond.[f] Elders may see themselves as more open minded or able to see shades of gray (i.e., ambiguity), rather than black-and-white facts.[g]	This is related to the construct known as wisdom; may relate to the ninth stage of life "gerotranscendence";[h] well older adults have the potential to gain wisdom through life experience and an increased universal knowledge base.[i] Plenty of older people have wisdom to share with others, including their health care providers.

TABLE 4-1 The Cognitive Changes of Aging. *(continued)*

Aspect of Cognition	Changes of Aging	Helpful Hints
Fluid intelligence—is defined as "the ability to find meaning in confusion and solve new problems . . . [and] to draw inferences and understand the relationships of various concepts, independent of acquired knowledge."[j] Includes executive skills which involve judgment, awareness, and problem solving.	Declines with age to a degree; older adults have difficulty with more complex, multiple-step tasks.[k] Because fluid intelligence is crucial to the learning process,[l] learning may slow down but does not stop in well older adults.	Fluid intelligence may improve through practice of tasks requiring executive skills such as self-monitoring performance, completing two tasks simultaneously, and inhibiting irrelevant stimulation. However, this finding was based on respondents mostly in their 20s.[l] Challenging (not frustrating) tasks, especially novel ones, may be crucial for maintaining brain health.[m]

[a] Perlmulter, M. Cognitive potential throughout life. In JE Birren, VL Bengston (eds.), *Emergent Theories of Aging.* New York: Springer.

[b] Tun, PA, Wingfield, A. One voice too many: Adult age differences in language processing with different types of distracting sounds. *Journals of Gerontology Series B: Psychological Sciences and Social Sciences,* 1995;54B(5):P317–P327. West, R. Visual distraction, working memory, and aging. *Memory and Cognition,* 1999;27(6):1064–1072. Verhaeghen, P, Cerella, J. Aging, executive control, and attention: A review of meta-analyses. *Neuroscience and Behavioral Reviews,* 2002;26(7):849–857.

[c] Colsher, P, Wallace, R. Longitudinal application of cognitive function measures in a defined population of community-dwelling elders. *Annals of Epidemiology,* 1991;1:215–230. Hultsch, D, Hertzog, C, Small, B, McDonald-Miszcak, L, Dixon, R. Short-term longitudinal change in cognitive performance in later life. *Psychology and Aging,* 1991;7:571–584. Wheeler, MA. A comparison of forgetting rates in older and younger adults. *Aging, Neuropsychology, and Cognition,* 2000;7(3):179–193.

[d] Hoyer, WJ, Verhaeghen, P. Memory aging. In JE Birren, KW Schaie (eds.), *Handbook of the Psychology of Aging.* Burlington, MA: Elsevier, 2006, pp 209–232.

[e] Baddeley, AD. The psychology of memory. In AD Baddeley, BA Wilson, FN Watts (eds.), *The Handbook of Memory Disorders.* Chichester, UK: John Wiley and Sons, 1995.

[f] Schaie, KW. *Intellectual Development in Adulthood: The Seattle Longitudinal Study.* New York: Cambridge University Press, 1996. Salthouse, TA. Pressing issues in cognitive aging. In N Schwartz, D Park, B Knauper, S Sudman (eds.), *Cognition, Aging and Self-Reports.* Philadelphia: Psychology Press.

[g] Erikson, EH, et al. *Vital Involvement in Old Age.* New York: W. W. Norton, 1989, p 36.

[h] Erikson, EH, Erikson, JM. *The Life Cycle Completed.* New York: W. W. Norton, 1998.

[i] Ardelt, M. Intellectual versus wisdom related knowledge: The case for a different kind of learning in later years of life. *Educational Gerontology,* 2000;26:1–15.

[j] Cavanaugh, JC, Blanchard-Fields, F. *Adult Development and Aging.* 5th ed. Belmont, CA: Wadsworth Publishing/Thomson Learning, 2006.

[k] West, R. Visual distraction, working memory, and aging. *Memory and Cognition,* 1999;27(6):1064–1072.

[l] Jaeggi, SM, Buschkuehl, M, Jonides, J, Perrig, WJ. Improving fluid intelligence with training on working memory. *PNAS,* 2008;105(19). Retrieved June 24, 2008, from http://www.pnas.org/cgl/dol/10.1073/pnas.08012681056829-6833

[m] Nussbaum, PD. *Brain Health and Wellness.* Tarentum, PA: Word Association Publishers, 2003.

Source: Adapted from Robnett, RH. Client factors and their effect on occupational performance in late life. In S Coppola, SJ Elliott, PE Toto (eds.), *Strategies to Advance Gerontology Excellence.* Bethesda, MD: AOTA Press, 2008, pp 163–197.

ATTENTION

Being able to focus or concentrate does not seem to be affected by age as such.[7] Especially, simple, overlearned tasks do not become more difficult for older people. However, in a study by Tun and Wingfield,[8] older adults were questioned about their perceptions of their own abilities to complete 16 different divided-attention tasks, such as walking and talking, or driving and planning a schedule. The researchers determined that older people did not perceive routine tasks and those involving speech processing to become more challenging over time. Relative to younger adults, however, the older respondents reported increasing difficulties with simultaneous dual task performance on more demanding tasks. Therefore, it may be more difficult for older adults to divide their **attention** between two activities (e.g., driving and talking; cooking multiple courses at the same time). Objectively, older people do have more difficulty with divided-attention tasks, especially when the two or more tasks are more complex (e.g., not simple or overlearned).[9]

MEMORY

Memory is not a simple, one-dimensional construct. Although, generally speaking, memory does decline with age, it is worth taking the time to qualify exactly what the construct of memory entails and to explore the different aspects of memory in relation to the aging process. Recalling something "out of the blue" is a more complex task and is affected to a greater extent than recognition (in which one is given hints about the potential answer, for example, multiple-choice answers). Recognition, which is simpler, may be retained to a high level throughout life.[10] Other basic memory tasks, such as those requiring procedural memory (i.e., motor patterns), basic cognitive skills (mathematics or use of vocabulary), or remembering facts that have been well learned, are usually preserved throughout the typical aging process.

Several types of memory are described here, although these categories are not an exhaustive list. The description also includes how aging is associated with the type of memory in question.

The following types of memory are based on temporal aspects of remembering:

- **Primary memory**. Primary memory has limited capacity and is based on incoming information that is either used or generally forgotten in a matter of seconds. Immediate recall of seven digits (plus or minus two) has been considered normal for adults since Miller's research in the 1950s.[11] Primary memory does not seem to be affected by aging. This type of memory involves sustained attention and is of extremely short duration (unless rehearsal takes place).
- **Short-term memory**. Short-term memory involves remembering information for a short duration. An example of normal short-term memory is being able to recall a 7-digit number (for example, a telephone number) for a few minutes. Although older people do show a decline in this type of memory, the decline is more pronounced as the information increases in length or complexity.[12]

- **Working memory**. Working memory refers to being able to actively use or manipulate the information from the brain's short-term storage base. For example, it involves not only recalling the telephone number but actually dialing the number to make a call (one must retain the number while dialing). Age-related deficits, such as in reading and listening span, have been consistently significant.[12]
- **Prospective memory**. Prospective memory enables a person to remember to do something in the future (e.g., appointments, medications, meetings, chores). With regard to aging, older people may be better at spontaneously compensating for losses in prospective memory because they may learn to adjust to memory losses gradually.[13] In naturalistic or real-life settings, older people often outperform their younger counterparts.[12]
- **Long-term memory**. Long-term memory is permanent or long-term storage, for example, autobiographical information, early life experiences, or repetitive information that involves "more durable encoding and storage systems."[14(p.479)] For well-learned knowledge, this type of memory is the least affected by age, although it may be difficult to conjure up the exact facts when needed.

The following type of memory is based on information to be encoded:

- **Episodic memory**. Episodic memory is oriented toward the past and is what most people think of when they think of the global term *memory*. This type of declarative or conscious memory particularly involves remembering episodes or experiences in our lives (e.g., what we ate for lunch, our last birthday party) or as Bäckman, Small, and Wahlin state, it is the "acquisition and retrieval of information acquired in a particular place at a particular time."[15(p.354)] Episodic memory can be either short term, such as remembering that you just turned on the stove, or long term, such as remembering the very first day of school. Episodic memory is particularly vulnerable to the effects of aging.[12,16] When tested simultaneously, younger people tend to outperform older people on tests of episodic memory.[16,17]

  An analogy involving episodic memory is to imagine a bucket that holds just a certain amount (**Figure 4-1**). As time goes by, the bucket is filled by memories of life's events, and as the bucket nears capacity, more of the potential memories get sloshed out. Although this analogy has little scientific basis, it can explain the increased difficulty of retaining additional information as we grow older. (If only we could delete unimportant information to make room for additional incoming data of significance.) Another explanation for declining episodic memory skills could be disuse caused by less environmental stimulation (e.g., during retirement, especially if the older person is homebound).

- **Semantic memory**. Semantic memory involves a cumulative knowledge base about the world in general (e.g., language, including the meaning of words and the relationship of words, mathematical facts, symbols and formulas, vocational information learned during one's career, and recall of current events and worldly facts). This

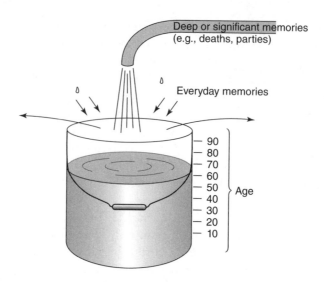

FIGURE 4-1   Episodic memory: Hypothetical bucket analogy.

"internal lexicon" is the buildup of information over the course of one's life (as part of crystallized intelligence).[15(p.352)] Semantic memory changes portray a complex picture in that elders have more word finding problems (such as the tip-of-the-tongue phenomenon) but vocabulary may even improve into old age.[12,18]

• **Procedural memory.** Procedural memory is performance based, for example, remembering how to ride a bicycle or the motoric steps to completing a recipe or self-care task. Because these tasks are often overlearned and have become automatic, this type of memory is often maintained into old age. This situation can be problematic at times, for example, when a person remembers the procedure of driving (e.g., inserting the key, turning the wheel, pushing on the gas pedal) but has forgotten how to manage the higher level aspects of driving (e.g., problem solving on the road, navigating in unfamiliar territory).

In summary, a great number of studies have been completed on memory and aging. Notable is that not all types of memory are affected equally by the typical aging process. Critical differences have been found between the various memory systems. Research in the area of episodic versus semantic memory has often demonstrated a more severe decline in memory for events (episodic memory tasks) while verbal memory such as vocabulary (semantic memory) tends to be better preserved.[19] Working memory tends to decline more sharply with age than immediate or primary memory does. Most elderly people were able to retain 7-digit telephone numbers as well as their younger counterparts (primary memory task). However, when a 10-digit number was used (e.g., a long-distance telephone number), the older participants did not perform as well.[20] Studies showing a memory decline with age have often involved more complicated tasks.[12,15] Older people also seem to have more difficulty ignoring distractions during working memory tasks, and they are less able to ignore irrelevant thoughts.[21,22]

Compensatory and adaptive techniques may be necessary to maintain quality of life if memory skills start to diminish significantly. Self-help books on this subject are readily available. For the health care professional, several tactics may be helpful when working with people who are forgetful:

- Make the material to be learned interesting (applicable to the client's life). A story, anecdote, or even a song may more easily catch and hold the client's attention.
- Use multimodal sensory input (e.g., let the person hear the information, see it, and use other senses to interact with the material as appropriate).
- Use repetition, but not to the point of boredom.
- Use cuing, but only as needed.
- Have clients work with or manipulate the information if at all possible (e.g., have them write out or input their own schedule rather than just giving them the printed schedule).
- Information perceived to be important will more likely be able to find a place in memory storage banks.
- Immediately following an instruction session, have clients paraphrase what was just conveyed or show-and-tell the information they just encountered; both can be effective techniques to enhance the learning process, applying the adage that one learns best by teaching.

Following are some tips to stimulate remembering (or compensate for decreased memory) adapted from a list by Dr. Robert Lucci of the Huffington Center on Aging at Baylor[23]:

- *Pay attention.* Information can be remembered only if it is initially acknowledged.
- *Repeat what you want to remember by rehearsing.* If you meet someone and want to remember his or her name, be sure to use the name in conversation within the next few minutes.
- *Make lists.* Write down what you want to remember (but then practice remembering without the list).
- *Establish habits.* For example, always put your keys on the hook, or always park in the same section of the parking lot at the mall.
- *Relax.* Relaxation may allow the mind to clear itself of problems, which may help to facilitate recall, whereas stress can hinder learning and memory.
- *Use self and environmental cues.* These cues can be invaluable for stimulating memory skills. Environmental cues can be as diverse as a sign on the door to remind you of what is behind the door to using a kitchen timer to remember to turn off the oven.

Problems with memory tasks, both subjective (memory complaints) and objective (actual losses), are probably the most common age-related cognitive decline.[24] Declining memory does not mean that a person has dementia. Mild forgetfulness, when it is an isolated cognitive impairment, is not a cause for alarm. Decreased memory, or **age-associated memory impairment** (AAMI), is widespread and refers to memory skills that are lower than average. AAMI is not as serious and may or may not relate to **mild cognitive impairment** (MCI). MCI refers to more serious cognitive losses that may portend the diagnosis of AD because those with MCI are at higher risk of developing AD (12% versus 1% or 2% of the general population).[24] Despite the pervasiveness of decreased memory as people get older, mild memory losses often do not interfere with day-to-day functioning.[20]

Memory remediation may be possible for those who are motivated to improve their ability to remember. An overview of websites dedicated to interventions for forgetfulness is provided by Shultz.[25] Compensating for, rather than trying to improve, decreased memory, however, seems to work best for most older people who sometimes get creative in their approaches to remind themselves. For example, putting car keys in the refrigerator to remind one to take lunch or keeping pill boxes at the dinner table to remind one to take medications can both be helpful.

One way to assess whether older people have memory impairments is simply to ask them. Yet it is worth noting that people, in general, do not have a good sense of how well they can remember. Although self-assessments are efficient and easy to use, their usefulness is questionable because the correlation between level of memory impairment per self-report and level determined through objective neuropsychological testing has typically been insignificant or low.[26-28] Keep in mind that we are asking those with less than perfect memory capabilities to make judgments about their ability to *remember*. A more objective measure is more functional, for example, noting whether the person has left the stove on, has had difficulty with medication routines, or has forgotten important appointments. Compensatory measures, including perhaps reminders from others, may be necessary.

CRYSTALLIZED AND FLUID INTELLIGENCE

Crystallized intelligence tends to remain strong in those who are aging typically and includes skills such as language comprehension, educational qualifications, and life and occupational skills. Baltes compared this type of intelligence with what we term wisdom, or "an expert knowledge system in the fundamental pragmatics of life permitting excellent judgment and advice involving important and uncertain matters of life."[29] Older adults may be more skilled at making decisions, perhaps because of their ability to take life's ambiguities into account.[30]

Despite a strong perceived link between wisdom and aging, even highly intellectual older individuals are not necessarily revered for their level of life understanding. In certain cultures, especially ancient ones, elders are expected to share historical stories, songs, rituals, and traditions with future generations. They are considered the sages of the community. On the other hand, in our modern Western society, older people rarely have such important societal roles, and therefore the wisdom of aging may often get lost in favor of individualism, materialism, and the quest for eternal youth.[31] According to do Rozario, in our developed world we may have lost "our sense of history and real wisdom."[31(p.121)] Schachter-Shalomi and Miller in their book *From Age-ing to Sage-ing: A Profound New Vision of Growing Older* (1995) put forward the idea that older people who work on expanding their consciousness and promoting their spiritual growth may demonstrate wisdom in their actions, thereby attaining "the crowning achievement of life."[32(p.17)] Rather than the "inevitable" decline and disengagement expected by many—young and old alike—older people would (again) be considered the wise stalwarts of the community. Some might say that by honoring the wise and respecting their wisdom, these elders with superior judgment would be returning to their rightful place in society. At least we could be open to the hopeful possibilities.

Fluid intelligence includes the speed and accuracy of information processing, such as discrimination, comparison, and categorization. It has been deemed to be largely evolutionarily and genetically based. Baltes researched the two types of intelligences in young and old subjects and found that only fluid intelligence, or "biologically based mechanics," showed a significant decline in older adults. He proposes that when learning potential was no longer evident (i.e., when practice or memory training no longer had an additional effect), the participant could be starting the process of pathologic rather than typical aging.[29] However, even though this study and others[18,33] have shown that the human mind has its limitations in old age, Baltes and associates[34] also point out that these limits often are not apparent because the brain is generally not used to its full potential. Baltes draws an interesting analogy of a young and an old person strolling together. Walking together works out well until the couple approaches a hill; the steeper the hill, the more difficult it may be for the older person to keep up.

Researchers in the field of gerontology have studied the cognitive changes of aging. Cross-sectional studies comparing the young to the old at one point in time tend to show definitive differences favoring the young in various aspects of thinking, with the declines more pronounced in the realm of fluid intelligence. Longitudinal studies, such as the Seattle Longitudinal Study (SLS),[18] examine individuals over time (over 50 years in the SLS). These studies generally have found less change over time within the individual than across individuals. In addition, studies have found risk factors associated with worse or better performance over time. The genetic factors (e.g., race, gender, IQ) cannot be changed, but people can influence some of the other factors related to cognitive performance. For example, physical exercise, cognitive stimulation, nutrition, smoking, and alcohol use have all been shown to correlate to cognitive functioning.[35] Making good lifestyle choices can have lasting positive effects well into old age.

LEARNING

The ability to learn new information can change as people age. Certainly, the old (and we hope outdated) adage that "an old dog can't learn new tricks" does not apply to older people who are aging well. Ongoing research, for example, at the Salk Institute, has unequivocally demonstrated that even older (middle-aged and beyond) brain cells can regenerate, an exciting finding with huge implications for stroke rehabilitation and medicine in general.[36] We have known for years that brain cells can develop new interneuronal connections and "add system capacity" to enhance learning.[37] Older individuals indeed may need more practice sessions repeated more often to master a task. They also may need to have the instructions presented in a variety of ways (e.g., verbal, written, or demonstrated) before learning can occur.

Neuropsychologist Dr. Paul Nussbaum in his book *Brain Health and Wellness* (2003) promotes the idea that learning should no longer be considered merely a means to an end, but that learning on its own ought to be seen as crucial to maintaining health, both physical and cognitive.[38] He expands on the adage "use it or lose it" by suggesting that we need not only use our brains to maintain brain health, but also we need to stimulate our brains by engaging in activities both "novel and complex" on a regular basis.[38(p.162)] By challenging our brains through new learning, we can, throughout life, enhance the process of learning. Akin to practicing a sport, we can practice new cognitive skills and improve at the learning process. Aging brains when motivated to "remain open for business" may never have to succumb to the expected ravages of aging. For example, den Dunnen and colleagues studied the brain donated to science by the oldest Dutch woman, who lived to be 115 and died in 2005.[39] Contrary to expectations, the woman's brain worked well until she died, and the autopsy revealed no significant pathology. This finding lends hope to the idea of brain preservation throughout life, even very long life.

DEMENTIA

Normal aging does include a slowing down and a gradual wearing out of bodily systems. It does not include dementia, which is considered a pathologic aging process. **Dementia** is defined as progressive cognitive impairment that eventually interferes with daily functioning. The prevalence of dementia among 60-year-olds is only 1–2%, but dementia becomes increasingly more common with advancing age.[37] Now with a much higher proportion of the population of industrialized nations living into old age, the prevalence of dementia has been increasing, with an estimated 4.9 million people in the United States with Alzheimer's disease (AD) and a new case surfacing every 72 seconds.[40] The mean age of onset is 81.[41] Although the lifetime risk of developing AD is 14–26%, those older than 85 have at least a 42% chance of getting the disease.[40] Because AD is the most common form of dementia, and therefore health care professionals are most likely to encounter people with this type, discussion here focuses on this disease specifically.

Dementia consists of persistent disturbances in cognitive functioning, including memory and intellectual ability. Certain causes of dementia may be treatable, and given the appropriate treatment, cognitive functioning may be restored. Although AD is the most common form of dementia, accounting for 50–75% of all senile dementias,[42] other causes of dementia include infections, metabolic and endocrine disturbances, alcohol and/or drug abuse, psychiatric disorders, deficiency states, trauma, Huntington's disease, Pick's disease, and Parkinson's disease.[43]

Dementia, specifically AD, encompasses multiple cognitive, psychological, and functional deficits, including memory impairment, which is always present (**Figure 4-2**). The

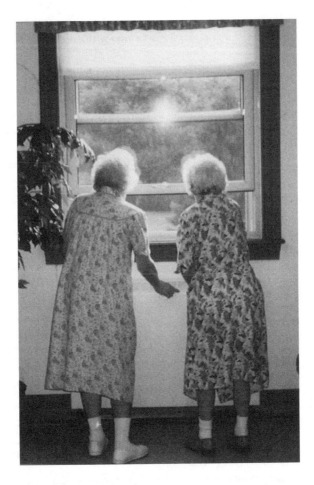

FIGURE 4-2 *(Courtesy of Darby I. Northway.)*

following signs and symptoms may be present as well:

- Difficulties with understanding or communicating through language.
- Difficulty with problem solving and other high-level cognitive tasks, such as abstract reasoning. A common cognitive test used with people who are suspected of having dementia is the Mini Mental State Examination, which is a brief and readily available cognitive screening tool.[44]
- Impaired visual spatial skills, which can impair the ability to drive safely.[45]
- Behavioral disturbances such as depression, anxiety, wandering, and neglect of personal hygiene.[41]

During the early stages of AD (usually the first few years following onset), physical symptoms are not as common. The person is able to walk and displays normal movement patterns and posture. As the disease progresses, the impairments associated with AD worsen. Those suffering from AD usually regress developmentally until, when near death, they may display some behaviors similar to a newly born infant. **Table 4-2** describes some

TABLE 4-2 Alzheimer's Disease Symptom Progression.

	Initial	End Stage
General behavior	Indifferent, may be delusional or depressed; may deny problems	Withdrawn, agitated, mood may change abruptly
Language	Normal or mild word finding difficulties	Severe impairment, words may be meaningless "word-salad"
Memory	Mild short-term deficits	Unable to test
Orientation	Fully oriented	Oriented to self only
Personal care/ADL skills[a]	Inattention to detail, but able to complete basic personal care	Dependency, may show fear of bathing
Instrumental ADLs[b]	Slight impairment, carelessness, decreased safety awareness, may need supervision	Unable to complete
Mobility	Normal	Abnormal, may not be able to walk or transfer independently
Posture	Normal	Flexed, often preferring a fetal position
Range of motion/ movement	Normal or within functional limits	Increased muscle tonus contractures[c] common

[a]ADLs include bathing, dressing, self-feeding, grooming, and so forth.
[b]IADLs include home management, money management, care of others, and so forth.
[c]A contracture is defined as a decrease of 50% or more of normal passive range of motion. It is a painful condition affecting many in long-term care settings, including more than three-quarters of patients who can no longer walk (Souren, LE, Frensses, EH, Reisberg, B. Contractures and loss of function in patients with Alzheimer's disease. *Journal of the American Geriatrics Society*, 1995;43(6):650–655).
Data from: Ham, RJ. Making the diagnosis of Alzheimer's disease. *Patient Care*, June 15, 1995, pp 104–120; Morris, JC. The Clinical Dementia Rating (CDR): Current version and scoring rules. *Neurology*, November 1993; pp 2412–2414, and Cole, SA. Behaviorial disturbances in Alzheimer's disease. *Patient Care*, June 15, 1995, pp 121–131.

of the progression of features commonly seen in AD. It needs to be pointed out that each person displays an individual course of the disease and therefore may have only a few rather than all of these traits.

AD progresses through three stages: mild, moderate, and severe. Because there is no cure, the current emphasis of medical providers is to prolong the first two stages. Medications to maintain cognitive functioning and manage agitation are constantly being tested. The Cochrane Database of Systematic Reviews provides up-to-date overviews of different medications being proposed as treatment for AD.[46,47] Scientists try to ward off the third stage because they believe that initially and into the middle stages for those with AD "most of the person is still there." Someone in the initial stages is still physically capable and can still find joy in living.[45] As health care professionals, we need to emphasize these beliefs with caregivers, who greatly need support when caring for someone with AD.

WORKING WITH THOSE WHO HAVE DEMENTIA

There are some general guidelines to follow when working with persons who have dementia. Again, remember that these are suggestions only; what works for one may have the opposite impact on another.

- Caring and respect are essential, even when the person cannot reciprocate.
- Health care professionals (or anyone) should never speak about persons with dementia in front of them as if they were not there.
- The behavior of those with AD may try your patience even as a professional, but controlling your emotions is crucial. Remember that the person is not intentionally trying to provoke you.
- Soothing music may defuse the intensity of an uncomfortable situation and foster relaxation.
- A sense of humor, so that you can laugh together, also can be extremely helpful, although it is important never to let the person think that you are laughing at him or her.
- Diversion may help to calm a stressful situation, including the following:
  - Involvement in simple (not childish) activities
  - Playing music and singing songs they have enjoyed formerly
  - Drawing, writing, or painting
  - Looking through old photograph albums; creating albums or scrapbooks for the future
  - Reminiscing
  - Involving them in tasks or parts of tasks they enjoy, for example, helping with meal preparation or taking care of a pet

Several books are available for those who want to improve their ability to work with older people who have dementia. A few examples are *A Dignified Life: The Best Friends Approach to Alzheimer's Care* by Bell and Troxel[48] and *Talking to Alzheimer's* by Strauss and Khachaturian.[49] **Table 4-3** offers some more specific, though not prescriptive, suggestions as well.

TABLE 4-3 Dementia: Problems and Potential Solutions.

Functional Problem Area	Potential Solutions
Decreased self-care skills (ADLs)	• Offer supervision • Simplify clothing/environment • Gently encourage person to do as much as possible without nagging • Remove safety hazards • Obtain an occupational therapy referral
Decreased involvement in daily activities	• Encourage involvement in what person can still do well • Praise successes and have patience • Try safe, simple repetitive chores • Offer items of interest
Wandering	• Take walks together in safe areas • Purchase identification bracelet • Alert neighbors • Remove obstacles indoors • If balance is decreased, obtain physical therapy referral
Impaired communication	• Speak slowly and calmly; do not yell • Give simple directions, one step at a time • Use repetition as needed • Obtain speech therapy referral
Sleep disturbance	• Establish a bedtime routine • Make sure person gets enough exercise during the day • Limit liquid before bedtime • Toilet immediately before bedtime • Omit obstacles in bedroom to bathroom route or purchase bedside commode • A back rub may promote restful sleep

Problem Behavior	Possible Solutions
Inappropriate behavior	• Always treat person with dignity and respect • Divert person to another activity • Watch for signs of overstimulation and try to avoid these situations • Listen and respond to the feeling behind the words being said, rather than the words themselves • Ask for help (e.g., doctors, support group, adult day care) • Use humor • Do not ignore requests for assistance

TABLE 4-3 Dementia: Problems and Potential Solutions. *(continued)*

Problem Behavior	Possible Solutions
Anxiety and/or agitation	• Structure environment
	• Establish daily routine with lots of opportunity for structured activities
	• Promote the feeling of security
Anger	• Offer a drink, a snack, or a favorite item
	• Do not confront, tease, or argue with the person
	• Listen and divert to new topic if possible
	• Limit stimulation
	• Remove from disruptive environment
	• Take care of your own safety

Data from: Cole, SA. Behavioral disturbances in Alzheimer's disease. *Patient Care,* June 15, 1995, pp 121–131; Gwyther, LP. General guidelines for caregivers and tips for communicating with your relative. *Patient Care,* June 15, 1995, pp 132–134; and Colorado State University. Guidelines for working with people with Alzheimer's disease [class handout]. Fort Collins, CO: Alzheimer's Disease and Aging Research, Department of Psychology, 1989.

RELATED DISORDERS

Sometimes what appears to be dementia is actually another medical disorder in disguise. Gaining a basic understanding of some of these common disorders may help you decide when to make referrals. Some of the more common ailments with signs and symptoms similar to dementia are briefly described here.

Malnutrition   Deficiencies of the B-complex vitamins, vitamin C, zinc, magnesium, folic acid, and protein, or **malnutrition**, can cause behavioral disturbances, including those implicated in the diagnosis of clinical depression.[50] (See also Chapter 7.)

Cerebrovascular Accident (CVA) or Stroke   **Cerebrovascular accident** (CVA) or stroke, especially small infarcts with limited accompanying functional declines, may cause behavior disturbances much like those brought about by depression or AD. In fact, a rather common type of dementia (multi-infarct dementia) is directly caused by a series of small strokes.

Hypothyroidism   Hypothyroidism slows metabolic processes, which causes the affected person to respond slowly and to be lethargic.

Failure to Thrive   A related syndrome to ones previously described is **failure to thrive** (FTT). An insidious deterioration in functioning that is not related to a specific disease, FTT can be caused by depression, dementia, chronic conditions, or drug reactions. Social isolation, low socioeconomic status, and functional dependency all are predisposing factors of FTT. Case examples are common; perhaps we all know of someone who just seemed to wither away prior to dying. Common features of FTT include weight loss resulting from lack of appetite, social withdrawal, lack of concern about appearance, memory loss, impaired ambulation, and incontinence (common in nearly half the cases described).[51] Those with this syndrome simply seem to be giving up on life.

Lack of Oxygen   Certain disorders (e.g., lung disease, pneumonia) are associated with a lowered ability of the body to complete oxygen uptake. *Hypoxemia* refers to insufficient oxygen levels in the blood. Oxygen saturation levels (O_2Sat) for most people should be 95% or higher. The saturation level is measured by a pulse oximeter that is placed on the finger. Although a physician must determine what is abnormal for any one person, in general hypoxemia can lead to tissue damage as well as mental confusion, including impaired judgment and problem-solving ability. Therefore, someone with low blood oxygen levels may appear to have dementia. Fortunately, administering oxygen, often through a nasal cannula per physician's orders, may improve mental status quickly.

Both learned helplessness and depression may exhibit symptoms similar to dementia, as well as each other, and therefore you should become familiar with them. These conditions are related and may occur together or be confused with one another.

Learned Helplessness   Another complication that has received little attention as a problem of aging is **learned helplessness**. Learned helplessness is a condition that develops when living beings "learn that their responses are independent of desired outcomes."[52] Consequently, they learn to not respond to stimulation from their environment. For example, in experiments when dogs learned that they could not control the onset of electric shocks, they eventually gave up and became helpless and apathetic. Similar results can occur in human beings, perhaps especially older people who may receive (too much) care from others.

For example, Mr. M., who came in as a patient for rehabilitation in a skilled nursing unit after rather minor surgery, was unable to complete his self-care skills, even though he had no medical or physical reason not to (other than deconditioning). It turned out that his home health aides, provided by his well-intentioned family, had taken over doing everything for him, even the most basic self-care tasks. He had learned to become compliant and helpless. Fortunately for Mr. M., he was able to unlearn learned helplessness and was actually surprised about what he could accomplish when given the chance. Caregivers, who may be overly caring, do more than necessary for their patients and therefore may inadvertently "help" them lose the ability to complete vital life tasks.

DEPRESSION IN OLDER ADULTS

At least one out of every 20 community-dwelling people older than age 65 have clinical **depression**. This number rises sharply in hospitals and long-term care facilities, where the prevalence of depression reaches at least 10% to over 30%.[53,54] Despite this high

TABLE 4-4   EBAS DEP Screening Instrument.

Question	Assessment	Rating	
1. Do you worry? In the past month?	Admits to worrying in the past month	1	0
2. Have you been sad or depressed in the past month?	Has had sad or depressed mood during past month	1	0
3. During the past month have you ever felt that life was not worth living?	Has felt that life was not worth living at some time during past month	1	0
4. How do you feel about your future? What are your hopes for the future?	Pessimistic about the future or has empty expectations (i.e., nothing to look forward to)	1	0
5. During the past month have you at any time felt you would rather be dead?	Has wished to be dead at any time during the past month	1	0
6. Do you enjoy things as much as you used to—say, like you did a year ago?	Less enjoyment in activities than a year previously *(If question 6 rated 0, then rate 0 for question 7 and skip to question 8. If question 6 rated 1, ask question 7.)*	1	0
7. Is it because you are depressed or nervous that you don't enjoy things as much?	Loss of enjoyment because of depression/nervousness	1	0
8. In general, how happy are you? Are you very happy, fairly happy, not very happy, or not happy at all?	Not very happy or not happy at all	1	0

Total Score

A score of 3 or greater indicates the probable presence of a depressive disorder that may need treatment, and the patient should be assessed in more detail or referred for psychiatric evaluation.
Source: Allen, N, Ames, D, Ashby, D, Bennetts, K, Tuckwell, V, West, C. A brief sensitive screening instrument for depression in late life. *Age and Ageing*, 1994;23:213–218. Reprinted with permission.

proportion of depression in older adults, depression often goes unnoticed and therefore undiagnosed. This is an especially heart-wrenching fact considering that depression is often amenable to treatment. The purpose of this section is to make health care professionals aware of the signs and symptoms of clinical depression and to offer guidelines for treatment and referral. The brief screening tool Briefer Assessment Scale for Depression (EBAS DEP) is shown in **Table 4-4**, because elderly persons may benefit from a quickly administered routine screening for depression.[55]

DSM-IV-TR CRITERIA FOR DEPRESSION

According to the *Diagnostic and Statistical Manual of Mental Disorders*, 4th edition (DSM-IV-TR),[56] the following are common signs and symptoms of depression:

- *Depressed mood "most of the day, nearly every day."*[56(p.356)] The person may feel sad or appear tearful. The person may complain of feeling hopeless. (This may be the easiest symptom to recognize, but because we all have "off" days it may go unnoticed.)
- ***Anhedonia***. The person has difficulty experiencing pleasure doing formerly enjoyable activities.
- *Weight gain or loss of more than 5% of body weight within 1 month.*
- *Sleep disturbances*. Either sleeping more or less than usual.
- *Psychomotor disturbances*. Either slowness in movements or agitated/hyperactive movements.
- *Feelings of worthlessness or lowered self-esteem.*
- *Decreased energy nearly every day.*
- *Cognitive changes*. These changes may include inability to concentrate or to complete cognitive tasks that were formerly successfully completed.
- *Indecisiveness nearly every day.*
- *Recurrent thoughts of death and/or suicide.*
- *Guilt*. The DSM-IV-TR also lists guilt as a symptom of depression,[56] but others claim that the expression of guilt is not a common feature of depression in older adults.[57]

In Table 4-4, the eight items of the EBAS DEP screening schedule require raters to make a judgment as to whether the proposition in the Assessment column is satisfied or not. If a proposition is satisfied, then a depressive symptom is present and raters should circle 1 in the right-hand column; otherwise 0 should be circled. Each question in the left-hand column must be asked exactly as printed, but follow-up or subsidiary questions may be used to clarify the initial answer until the rater can make a clear judgment as to whether the proposition is satisfied or not. For items that inquire about symptoms over the past month, note that the symptom need not have been present for the entire month nor at the moment of interview, but it should have been a problem for the patient or troubled him or her for some of the past month.

If several of these signs and symptoms, especially one of the first two, are present for 2 weeks or more, a referral to the older person's physician is in order because he or she may have clinical depression, a serious but generally treatable disorder.[56] As a health care professional, you may need to confer with the doctor and/or health care team to let them know of your concern, while being careful not to violate patient confidentiality. A crucial point to keep in mind is that older people do not tend to "fake" the signs and symptoms of depression.[58]

SUICIDE IN OLDER ADULTS

Despite societal beliefs to the contrary, feeling down and depressed is not a natural consequence of the aging process. Unusual mood disturbance must be taken seriously. The suicide rate in the United States is highest among those who are older than 65, with the rate increasing from 13 per 100,000 people in the 64–69 years age group, to almost 23 per 100,000 for those 80–84.[59] Men account for 85% of all suicides among older adults.[60] Fixed risk factors for **suicide** in the United States include being male (currently 4 to 1 ratio), single, older, and having a family history of suicide. Race is also a factor, with whites and Native Americans being more susceptible to suicide than blacks and Hispanic Americans.[61] Although suicide is not always a consequence of depression, death is the most definitive outcome of depression. Health care professionals need to be aware of the potential for suicide and give serious consideration to *any* indication that the person may be thinking about it. They should listen with great care to the older person's stories and make a referral if there is *any* cause to think suicide may be a possibility.

The following are common indicators of possible impending suicide:

- Past history of suicidal attempts or current/past threats of suicide, especially direct threats
- Symptoms of depression, ongoing bodily complaints, or other psychiatric disorders[61]
- Discharge from a health care facility against medical advice or recommendation
- Spontaneous recovery from a depressed mood, including sudden euphoria
- Substance abuse or dependence
- Bereavement, severe losses in life, or identifying with a person who is deceased, especially a life partner
- Giving things away or putting one's affairs in order[62]

Although it is beyond the scope of this text to discuss the ethical issues raised by suicide undertaken to escape excruciating, irreversible pain and/or terminal illness, it suffices to reiterate that depression, which often precedes a suicide attempt, is generally amenable to treatment. Through medication management, psychotherapy, and/or electroconvulsive shock treatment there is good potential for restoring the quality of life for elderly people who are depressed. Ira Katz, director of Geriatric Psychiatry at the Hospital of the University of Pennsylvania, has stated that 80% of older adults who are properly diagnosed and treated can recover and return to their usual level of functioning.[63] Depression can happen to anyone; no amount of education, money, or social status can guarantee it will stay away. According to Dr. Katz, as health care professionals our job is "to explain to patients that we think they may have an illness that is treatable, and with treatment they can feel better and function better."[63]

DEATH AND BEREAVEMENT

Dying and death are natural life events during old age. They are nonetheless events that are, at best, accepted but more often feared or dreaded for self and loved ones. Our society has done a good job of neatly tucking away the dying process into institutions, where the final event of death is sometimes forestalled for a very long time. Currently, an estimated

80% of deaths occur in institutions, whereas a century ago institutional deaths were rare.[64] Many ethical issues related to death and dying are particularly pertinent for older people. They or their loved ones are more likely to need to make a decision about the level of medical care desired for the eventual times when they would be unable to make a decision for themselves. Living wills and advance directives can outline one's wishes and everyone is encouraged to have them. They can ease the sense of uncertainty when a loved one must make those "life or death" decisions. (See Chapter 10.)

Generally people experience an increased number of losses of significant others as they age. Not only the death of spouses, but also the death of siblings and friends occur more frequently as a person reaches the end of his or her own life, especially if it is particularly long. However, just because one experiences these death events more often does not imply that **bereavement** gets any easier. The health care professional should keep in mind that grieving persons of all ages may need additional emotional support, and each grieving process is highly individualized with regard to duration and methods of coping.

Several theorists have described the stages of grief. Parkes delineates four stages: numbness, yearning/protest, disorganization, and developing a new identity.[65] Kubler-Ross, on the other hand, describes five stages: denial, anger, bargaining, depression, and finally acceptance.[66] These stages are neither set to specific timelines nor are they completely distinct from one another. However, in our society, grieving is expected to last only a short while, and then those who are grieving are encouraged to "get on with things" or "snap out of it."[67] Unfortunately, the feelings of loss, isolation, and extreme sadness may persist for years—sometimes much longer than is socially expected.[68] Health care professionals often encounter older people who are in the midst of some stage of bereavement.

Caregivers of people who are dying are enmeshed in an extremely stressful situation. Health care professionals can ease the burden of caregiving at least a little by promoting wellness practices, by setting limits, and by providing "opportunities for distraction, humor and relaxation."[64] These caregivers are already grieving the impending loss of their loved one, even if they seem to be in denial about the upcoming death event.

Several recommendations are offered for those working with bereaved individuals or families. Keep in mind that each person has his or her own way of handling grief, yet many have found the following suggestions helpful:

- As much as time allows, let the person talk about the loved one and the loss. Asking about the deceased person, even a spouse or child, is generally acceptable and may even be desired. You can assess quickly whether this is a subject the person would rather not broach. Shedding tears is a natural, healthy experience that can aid the healing process.

- Assure the bereaved person that his or her feelings are legitimate. Stating "I understand" is usually not helpful, unless you really have been in a similar situation. Euphemistic comments such as "He was quite old" or "It's all for the best" are better left unspoken. Even if the person was old, the death of a loved one is never easy.[67] Clichés and sympathizing remarks are generally regarded as not helpful.

- It is okay not to have the right words or the answers. Just being there and offering your compassion and support does help.[69]
- Allow the bereaved person to make decisions. According to Alty, well-meaning individuals often will take over decision making for grieving persons, but just because a person is grieving does not mean that he or she cannot think rationally (or that the person wants to give up decision making).[70]
- Discuss counseling or contacting their spiritual adviser for those who need additional help. Behavior that is harmful to self or others is an example of pathologic bereavement. If the person talks about suicide, tells you that his or her life is now over, or talks about or with the deceased person as if he or she were still alive, a referral is in order.[67] Social workers can be extremely helpful to the grieving individual because they can assist clients and their significant others "to cope with their feelings, . . . to recognize their choices, . . . to develop and maintain meaningful communication with one another, and to link up with people and services beyond themselves."[71] (Refer to Chapter 11 for a more complete description of the role of social workers working with older people.)

Remember, older people may have had to contend with a number of losses in a short period of time. Not only are their loved ones and friends more apt to die, but they may be dealing with other personal losses as well. For example, older people may have physical losses related to abilities in life skills, or they may need to move out of their long-term homes. In addition, the older person may be demonstrating anticipatory grief of his or her own approaching death.[70] Sensitivity and knowing one's own limits as a health care professional are necessary ingredients for working with bereaved clients effectively.

PERSONALITY DEVELOPMENT

The great thing about getting older is that you don't lose all the ages you've been.
—*Madeleine L'Engle, "Wrinkles, Wit and Wisdom"*

Personality is what makes a person a unique individual. Each one of us has a set of character traits, attitudes, habits, and emotional tendencies that distinguish us from everyone else. These dispositions can be intimated by our appearance (e.g., tattoos, clothing styles, or level of care taken in grooming) but are essentially inner characteristics causing us to behave as we do. Many studies have explored the development of personality in youth and into young adulthood, whereas fewer studies have concentrated on personality evolvement during older adulthood. The question is whether significant personality change takes place during old age (in both healthy adults and those afflicted with disease).

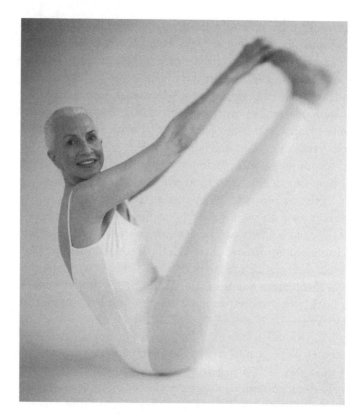

FIGURE 4-3 Both inner and outer stretching are benefical at any age. (© † *Ryan McVay/ Photodisc/Getty Images*)

There are many theories on personality, yet the well-known theorists (Maslow, Piaget, Freud) devoted little attention to the personality of older people. One theorist who may already be familiar to many readers is Erik Erikson, who initially proposed eight stages of psychosocial development.[72] Originally, the final stage was integrity versus despair. Erikson viewed those who were successful in this stage as being able to develop a sense of pride in their past accomplishments and present lives. They judge their own lives as being worthwhile. Others, who do not successfully complete this stage, experience instead a feeling of despair, not only about the course of their lives thus far, but also because they do not believe that they have enough time left to improve their life. Overall, Erikson proposed that this then-final stage of life was a time both positive and integrating for well older adults.[73] In an updated version of personality development, Erikson and Erikson include a ninth stage in their theory: **gerotranscendence**, which is associated with wisdom and a moving away from early and midlife materialism.[74] Ardelt describes this "transcendence of the self" as a move toward selflessness, compassion, and reflection, all character-istics of a truly wise person.[75]

Social scientists are beginning to show more interest in the final years of life with regard to personality development. The trait theory espoused by McCrae and Costa is perhaps the most well known.[76] Their 5-factor model of personality includes the following:

1. *Neuroticism*. Associated with hostility, depression, anxiety, and impulsiveness
2. *Extraversion*. Associated with a high level of energy and being outgoing in social situations
3. *Openness to experience*. Associated with open-mindedness, curiosity, and adjustment to change
4. *Agreeableness*. Associated with affection, compassion, and being altruistic
5. *Conscientiousness*. Associated with a strong commitment to goals and being a principled person

Each of us falls on a continuum for each of these traits. Research conducted on these traits has determined they have the greatest instability between the ages of 17 and 35 years, and then they tend to become more fixed. When these traits were studied in older people over 3- and 6-year intervals, strong stability of all five traits was found using both self and spousal reports. Even when the intervals between testing increased to as much as 50 years, stability coefficients still remained statistically significant, indicating that overall personality traits, at least in these five realms, are relatively fixed, with life events exerting little overall influence.[77] Weiss and colleagues also found few differences in the five traits based on age when looking at more than 1,000 Medicare patients from ages 65 to 100.[78] In the Weiss study, the older participants did show a higher level of agreeableness, which may be the result of a cohort effect or higher levels of mortality of those with lower levels of this trait (those with "type A" or hostile personality have proportionately more heart disease, which ultimately leads to an earlier death).

Other evidence in support of the permanence of personality traits in typically aging older adults is presented by Mitchell and Helson, who determined that people who are optimistic and manage their lives well at one stage of life tend to feel more positive about their lives at other times as well.[79] Hayflick, in citing the results of the Baltimore Longitudinal Study of Aging (BLSA), maintains that personality traits remain essentially the same throughout the life span in typically aging older adults, although most people older than age 50 do begin to prefer slower-paced activities.[80] This is a valuable piece of information for health care professionals who work with older people. Pacing health care intervention for the convenience of the client, rather than the provider, is essential for good care (and perhaps getting more difficult in these hectic times for health care).

Although overall they are stable, nonetheless personality changes can and do occur. Wood and Roberts suggest that personality traits are open systems that are plastic and can be influenced throughout life.[81] Research has shown that men, as they get older, may become more nurturing and open about their feelings, while women may become more assertive, confident, and comfortable with themselves. Social scientists believe these changes could be influenced by hormonal fluctuations perhaps causing a diminution of the character distinctions between the genders.[79] Levels of agreeableness and conscientiousness also tend to increase with age (at least until age 70) for both genders.[82]

Representations of the self such as one's goals, values, coping styles, and control beliefs are likely to change over the course of a lifetime. In a pivotal study done by Erikson and colleagues, older people described themselves as more tolerant, patient, open-minded, understanding, compassionate, and less critical than when they were younger.[72] However, many study participants viewed both themselves and the other older adults in the study as more set in their ways. This seeming contradiction was explained by the proposal that as people age they increasingly integrate their own personal style, but they also can gain a new understanding and tolerance of others' behavioral styles. Conceivably, people may be able to improve their character throughout life by simply doing what they would do if they were who they wanted to be ("acting as if"),[83] for example, if a woman wants to be an altruistic person, she simply decides to become a volunteer.

Personalities come in many flavors, and not all are compatible with one another. As health care professionals, we need to make a concerted effort to provide excellent customer service to all our clients of any age. We now have substantial evidence that old age does not equate with any specific personality traits, especially those often heard on the street (e.g., grumpy [old men], doddering [old woman], stubborn, disagreeable, closed-minded, etc.). Some people were this way their whole lives, while others may become "better all the time."[83] Others may have personality disorders associated with disease, such as AD. In these cases, it is crucial to remember the people are not necessarily still "themselves" and may be acting out the disease process rather than being self-directed. One AD sufferer even described his experience as, "Sometimes I'm me, and sometimes I don't know who I am. I don't know, it comes and it goes; I never know."[84(p.115)] Even when working with people who have challenging personality types, compassion is the path of least resistance and the most fulfillment, when all things are considered at the end of the day.

Self-efficacy is a construct that was introduced by Bandura in the 1970s.[85] It relates to the beliefs that each of us hold about the level of control we have over our future. Those who have strong self-efficacy, or internal locus of control, feel empowered to shape the future of their lives. On the other hand, those with low self-efficacy or external locus of control believe that the course of their lives is determined by the whims of the world and that they, personally, can have little influence over their own future.

The tendency has been to attribute a lower level of self-efficacy and to expect an external locus of control in older people. Because of various hardships (e.g., medical emergencies, living on fixed incomes) that usually occur more frequently as people age, it makes sense that older people would feel a diminished sense of control. Older people also may have fewer choices about their personal living arrangements and variety of physical pursuits. However, surprisingly, Rhee and Gatz drew a different conclusion.[86] Older adults in their study showed a higher level of self-perceived internal control when compared to college students. Additionally, the college students actually had even a lower level of self-perceived locus of control than attributed to them by the older adults.

The strength of one's sense of self-efficacy may be variable across time and across different domains of life.[87] For example, people may feel empowered about financial matters, yet feel that their health is beyond their personal control. Other domains besides health and finances include work or productivity, transportation, family, friends, safety, and living arrangements. McAvay and her colleagues were interested in looking at older peoples' perceptions of self-efficacy in the different domains mentioned and the potentially influencing factors of these perceptions over time.[87] They found the trait of self-efficacy in any domain was quite stable over the course of 2 months. For each domain listed, a majority of older respondents (65% to 95%) reported a high degree of self-efficacy, indicating that at least these older people believed that they have a high level of control over many aspects of their lives. The only domain in which less than half of the respondents reported a high level of self-efficacy was finances. This finding is logical; many elderly people may feel a lack of control over finances because they are on fixed incomes and no longer part of the paid workforce.

A decline in health (as evidenced by an increase in number of medical conditions) was significantly correlated to decreased self-efficacy in the domains of productivity, family, friends, and living arrangements. Perhaps somewhat expectedly, prior depression was the one factor corresponding most closely with a low level of self-efficacy across all domains. Older people who feel depressed have a tendency to feel powerless about the course of their lives, which subsequently can lead to even further social isolation. The downward spiral of depressed mood and withdrawal emphasizes the need for medical intervention for depression. In a study of perceived self-efficacy, a high level of spiritual self-efficacy was most highly predictive of lower levels of psychological distress. Low levels of self-efficacy in other domains also predicted loneliness and distress.[88] A significant correlation has been found between a high level of self-perceived self-efficacy and positive health behaviors such as healthy diet, exercise, and nonsmoking.[89,90] On the other hand, chronic illnesses may lower the level of perceived control, and this in turn may decrease one's motivation to maintain a healthy lifestyle.[89] Both McAvay and colleagues and Blazer have stressed the importance of developing and maintaining social support systems and learning coping strategies to boost self-efficacy and deal effectively with daily problems.[87,90]

Overall, in the realm of personality, there are no definitive answers with regard to aging. People who go through typical life development adhere to their personhood throughout life: they remain unique individuals with distinct features. Disease processes, especially AD, absolutely can rob people of their essential personality, leaving someone quite different in the wake. Also, extreme diversity is found even within a set cohort of people, especially as the cohort grows older. Although we can use stereotypes to explain and explore the personality of older people in general, these theories will never adequately illuminate any one person.

QUALITY OF LIFE

In spite of illness, in spite even of the archenemy sorrow, one can remain alive long past the usual date of disintegration if one is unafraid of change, insatiable in intellectual curiosity, interested in big things, and happy in small ways.

—*Edith Wharton (1862–1937)*

Quality of life is an elusive construct about which a profusion of documents have been written, but it can only truly be understood on a personal level. Each person has his or her own sense of what constitutes a high level of quality in life (**Figure 4-4**). Health care professionals must keep in mind that stereotypical information, while helpful in understanding older people as a global population, will not likely fit any one situation.

According to Schalock, quality of life is an overarching, multidimensional concept made up of several core principles[91]:

- Quality of life (QOL) is best understood from the perspective of the individual.
- QOL embodies feelings of well-being.
- A high QOL is experienced when a person's basic needs are met and he or she has opportunities to pursue and meet personal goals and challenges.

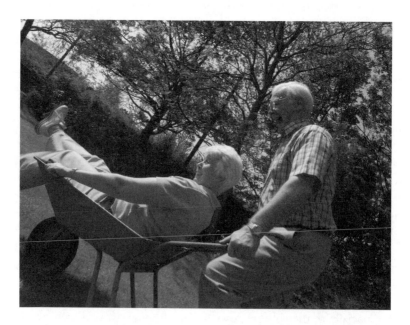

FIGURE 4-4 Enjoying time with loved ones can boost quality of life at any age. (© *abimages/ ShutterStock, Inc.*)

- QOL can be enhanced by giving people choices and encouraging them to make decisions that affect their own lives.
- A sense of community enhances QOL.
- QOL for all persons (including those with disabilities and older adults) may be composed of the same dimensions (although the level and priority of these dimensions will differ among individuals).

These dimensions are as follows:

- Basic material well-being (e.g., food and housing)
- Emotional well-being, including safety and spirituality
- Interpersonal relations
- Engagement in meaningful activities (life occupations)
- Personal development, including education, learning, and skills
- Physical well-being (health and wellness)
- Self-determination, including personal control and goals/values
- Social inclusion, including roles and supports
- Rights, such as voting and accessible housing

Among the older population, it is assumed that the degree of health or illness can have a significant impact on the level of quality of life. In a study done on life satisfaction in older adults, lack of health was listed as the biggest threat to happiness five times more frequently than any other threat, even death.[92] Kehn concluded that health status was a strong predictor of happiness.[92]

Although increasing age did have a somewhat negative correlation with robust aging, Garfein and Herzog found many members of the oldest-old group (80 years and older) fit into the "robust aging" category.[93] Therefore, older age per se should no longer be considered a "phase of waning health and declining resources," but rather we need to learn to put more emphasis on aging well. In a qualitative study of eight older people ages 85 to 100, Ward-Baker determined that ongoing engagement in productive activities such as work, resilience in the face of hardships, and a high degree of self-efficacy ("internally guided behavior") were crucial to living a satisfying life among the oldest-old.[94] Close relationships, lifelong learning, being an optimist, and accepting circumstances also came out as important contributing factors, but not for everyone. In another study on robust or successful aging (which could also be viewed as aging with a comparatively high quality of life), four factors were determined to promote well-being in these "successful agers" (and distinguish them from those who were aging less well): social contact and support, subjective satisfaction with health (note, *not* objective health status), low vulnerability scores (on the personality scale), and fewer stressful life events in the past 3 years.[93]

From a different perspective, a research effort spearheaded by Ardelt explored the impact of wisdom on life satisfaction in old age.[95] She found objective life conditions, such as health, finances, social relationships, and physical environment, could explain only a small portion of the variation of life satisfaction scores in previous studies. Her contention is that a person's level of wisdom explains much of the variability of life satisfaction in older adults. She defines wisdom as "an integration of cognitive, reflective and affective elements" including an "awareness and acceptance of human limitations" allowing us to view the human condition with humor, compassion, and detachment. This is an interesting premise because it allows those with even poor *objective* life conditions to have a great amount of *subjective* life satisfaction. One's existential sense of personal control, insight, and/or attitude may indeed affect personal quality of life more than anything else. There may even be reason to believe that the hardships of life could challenge a person in such a way as to stimulate increased wisdom and thereby improve life satisfaction. When viewed in this light, you can more easily understand why there are many older people who, despite ongoing, daily concerns and frequent losses, continue to find their lives satisfying and fulfilling. So many older people report a high level of satisfaction with life (despite ongoing losses) that this finding has been termed "the paradox of aging."[96(p.346)]

Despite ongoing research, QOL remains a nebulous construct. We need to keep in mind that each older person is unique and deserving of respect for his or her own opinions. Exploring these life meanings with clients can help promote an optimal level of life satisfaction. As health care professionals, our contributions to clients' life quality may be minimal, or through the use of keen listening skills, client-centered approaches, creative problem solving, and/or by making referrals to others who may be able to provide direct assistance, our input may be invaluable and much appreciated.

SUMMARY

Although change is inevitable throughout life, the essential core of the human being is not likely to be altered by the aging process alone. As people age, if they experience typical aging, they *tend* to exhibit the following characteristics:

- Take longer to learn new tasks
- Become more forgetful especially of short-term information
- Prefer somewhat slower paced activities
- Retain essential personhood
- Continue to perceive level of life quality as satisfactory

However, many cognitive, psychological, and personality changes can and do occur over time. These changes can be positive, such as when someone makes an effort toward self-improvement. Other times, these changes can be detrimental as wreaked by disease, misfortune, or injurious lifestyle choices. Each age cohort becomes more diverse as their ages increase. Although as a group the members tend to show the signs of aging already mentioned, within each age group there are those who continue to perform essentially as well as they ever did and those who have succumbed to the "ravages of old age."

Although no one is guaranteed a long life including a successful or happy aging process, everyone can take steps to improve their odds of living well into old age. The value of close human connections, physical and mental exercise, and ongoing involvement in occupations (in the global sense of the term) and important life roles have been written about extensively.[97–99]

By listening, being supportive and respectful, promoting a personal level of independence, and making referrals as appropriate, we can help older persons live their best potential quality of life and remain as productive or engaged as they choose to be. Our goal, as a caring, highly developed society, should be to promote meaningful involvement right up until the time of death.

Review Questions

1. The "paradox of aging" refers to
   A. A high quality of life despite the problems of aging
   B. Wisdom despite cognitive losses
   C. Lower levels of depression among older people
   D. Long life despite various medical conditions

2. Which personality trait tends to decrease in typically aging older people?
   A. Optimism
   B. Extraversion
   C. Neuroticism
   D. Agreeableness

3. Self-efficacy, or the sense that one has control over one's life
   A. Tends to remain stable over all domains over the course of adulthood
   B. Tends to be lowest in older adults for the domain of finances
   C. Increases significantly after one retires
   D. Was found to be at a lower level in older adults as compared to college students

4. Which of the following statements about attention and aging is true?
   A. Sustained attention declines significantly with age.
   B. Older people have more difficulty dividing attention between complex tasks.
   C. Attentional switching does not decline with age.
   D. Older people have difficulty paying attention for more than 5 to 10 minutes.

5. A&O × 2 means a person is alert and oriented to
   A. Self and others only
   B. Time and self only
   C. Situation and self only
   D. Self and place only

6. Compared to younger people, older people do better in real-life tasks involving which type of memory tasks?
   A. Procedural
   B. Prospective
   C. Working
   D. Short term

7. Which of the following statements about intelligence is accurate?
   A. Crystallized intelligence is less affected by aging than fluid intelligence is.
   B. Fluid intelligence is less affected by aging than crystallized intelligence is.
   C. Age-associated memory impairment is less prevalent than age-associated cognitive decline.
   D. Longitudinal studies show a decline in all cognitive test areas by age 60.

8. Which of the following tends not to be a factor in depression in older adults?
   A. Anhedonia
   B. Guilt
   C. Sleep disturbances
   D. Cognitive changes

9. Suicide among older adults
   A. Is not common
   B. Is a natural desire resulting from the aging process
   C. Is highest among older men
   D. Is highest among women

10. Alzheimer's disease
    A. Always includes memory impairment
    B. Always includes physical symptoms in the early stages
    C. Always includes language disturbances
    D. Is inevitable for those reaching 100 years old

11. Learned helplessness
    A. May develop when caregivers do more than necessary for the older person
    B. Is not a phenomenon found in older people
    C. Is caused by depression
    D. Is irreversible

12. The stages of bereavement
    A. Are indistinguishable from one another
    B. Have set timelines
    C. Last longer for older adults
    D. Are highly individualized

Learning Activities

1. Think of the role models you know who are at least 60 years old. What personality traits do you appreciate in these older people? How can you ensure that you will have some of these same traits when you are older? Do you think one can develop these traits? Why or why not?

2. It may be interesting to interview a few older people. Ask them how they think their personalities and thinking skills have changed over the course of years. How does this compare with the research data? How do you think you will change as you get older?

3. Discuss the concept of self-efficacy (having a sense of control over one's life). Do you think that for yourself your sense of self-efficacy will increase, decrease, or stay the same as you get older? In one or all domains? Explain your answer.

4. Generally the level of cognition declines as one gets older. How can you ensure that this decline will be minimal? List five things that you can do to improve your cognitive level.

5. Discuss wisdom. What is it, and what makes someone wise? Do you equate being wise with being older? Why or why not? How do we view wisdom compared to other world cultures?

6. Discuss quality of life, which means many things to different people. What aspects of your life give it a high level of quality? Share these with the group. Do you think these will change as you age? Why or why not?

7. Discuss depression in older adults. What are some of the reasons that older people become depressed? (Include life events and changes that tend to occur.)

8. Handling grief is a personal issue. Discuss with one other person what actions you think would be helpful when you are grieving for a significant other. What actions would cause you to feel worse? Discuss the themes in a larger group. Afterward discuss how this knowledge will change how you might interact with a grieving person as a friend or as a professional.

REFERENCES

1. Perlmutter, M. Cognitive potential throughout life. In JE Birren, VL Bengston (eds.). *Emergent Theories of Aging*. New York: Springer Publishing, 1988.

2. Levy, BR. Mind matters: Cognitive and physical effects of aging self-stereotypes. *Journals of Gerontology, Series B: Psychological Sciences and Social Sciences*, 2003;58B(4):P203–P211.

3. Alzheimer's Association. Alzheimer's Disease Prevalence Rates Rise to More Than Five Million in the United States. Retrieved March 15, 2008, from http://www.alz.org/news_and_events_rates_rise.asp

4. Terry, DF, Sebastiani, P, Andersen, SL, Perls, TT. Disentangling the roles of disability and morbidity in survival to exceptional old age. *Archives of Internal Medicine*, 2008;168(3):277–283.

5. Thomas, D. Do not go gentle into that good night. In D Jones (ed.). *The Poems of Dylan Thomas*. New York: A New Directions Book, 1971.

6. *Stedman's Concise Medical Dictionary for the Health Professions*. 3rd ed. Baltimore, MD: Williams & Wilkins, 1997.

7. Zec, RF. The neuropsychology of aging. *Experimental Gerontology*, 1995;30:431–442.

8. Tun, PA, Wingfield, A. Does dividing attention become harder with age? Findings for the divided attention questionnaire. *Aging and Cognition*, 1995;2(1):39–66.

9. Verhaeghen, P, Cerella, J. Aging, executive control, and attention: A review of meta-analyses. *Neuroscience and Biobehavioral Reviews*, 2002;26(7): 849–857.

10. Parkin, AJ, Java, RI. Determinants of age-related memory loss. In TJ Perfect, EA Maylor (eds.). *Models of Cognitive Aging*. Oxford, UK: Oxford University Press, 2000, pp 188–203.

11. Connor, LT. Memory in old age: Patterns of decline and preservation. *Seminars in Speech and Language*, 2001;22(2):117–125.

12. Hoyer, WJ, Verhaeghen, P. Memory aging. In JE Birren, KW Schaie (eds.). *Handbook of the Psychology of Aging*. Burlington, MA: Elsevier, 2006, pp 209–232.

13. Baddeley, AD. The psychology of memory. In AD Baddeley, BA Wilson, FN Watts (eds.). *The Handbook of Memory Disorders*. Chichester, UK: John Wiley and Sons, 1995.

14. Birren, JE, Schroots, JJF. Autobiographical memory and the narrative self over the life span. In JE Birren, KW Schaie (eds.). *Handbook of the Psychology of Aging*. Burlington, MA: Elsevier, 2006, pp 477–498.

15. Bäckman, L, Small, BJ, Wahlin, A. Aging and memory: Cognitive and biological perspectives. In JE Birren, KW Schaie (eds.). *Handbook of the Psychology of Aging*. San Diego: Academic Press, 2001.

16. Hultsch, DF, Hertzog, C, Dixon, RA, Small, BJ. *Memory Change in the Aged*. Cambridge, UK: Cambridge University Press, 1998.

17. Prull, MW, Gabrieli, JDE, Bunge, SA. Age-related changes in memory: A cognitive neuroscience perspective. In FIM Craik, TA Salthouse (eds.). *The Handbook of Aging and Cognition*. 2nd ed. Mahwah, NJ: Lawrence Erlbaum Associates, 2000.

18. Schaie, KW. *Intellectual Development in Adulthood: The Seattle Longitudinal Study*. New York: Cambridge University Press, 1996.

19. Hultsch, DF, Dixon, RA. Learning and memory in aging. In JE Birren, KW Schaie (eds.). *Handbook of the Psychology of Aging*. 3rd ed. San Diego, CA: Academic Press, 1990, pp 258–274.

20. Gorman, WF, Campbell, CD. Mental acuity of the normal elderly. *Journal of the Oklahoma State Medical Association*, March 1995;88:119–123.

21. Hasher, L, Zacks, RT. Working memory, comprehension, and aging: A review and a new view. In GH Bower (ed.). *The Psychology of Learning and Motivation*, New York: Academic Press, 1988, pp 193–225.

22. Gazzaley, A, Sheridan, MA, Cooney, JW. Age-related deficits in component processes of working memory. *Neuropsychology*, 2007;21(5):532–539.

23. Lucci, RJ. In Rosenthal, HF. Spring cleaning turns up some leftover news tidbits. *Portland Press Herald* (Portland, ME), March 26, 1997.

24. Bartrés-Faz, D, Junqué, C, López-Alomar, A, Valveny, N, Moral, P, Casamayor, R, et al. Neuropsychological and genetic differences between age-associated memory impairment and mild cognitive impairment entities. *Journal of the American Geriatrics Society*, 2001;49(7):985–990.

25. Shultz, SM. Forgetfulness. *Journal of Consumer Health on the Internet*, 2005;9(3):71–76.

26. Knight, RG, Godfrey, HPD. Behavioral and self-report methods. In AD Baddeley, BA Wilson, FN Watts (eds.). *The Handbook of Memory Disorders*. Chichester, UK: John Wiley and Sons, 1995.

27. Craik, FIM, Anderson, ND, Kerr, SA, Li, KZH. In AD Baddeley, BA Wilson, FN Watts (eds.). *Handbook of Memory Disorders*. Chichester, UK: John Wiley and Sons, 1995.

28. Ryan, EB. Beliefs about memory changes across the adult lifespan. *Journal of Gerontology: Psychological Sciences*, 1992;47:41–46.

29. Baltes, PB. The aging mind: Potential and limits. *Gerontologist*, 1993;33:580–594.

30. Kim, S, Hasher, L. The attraction effect in decision making: Superior performance by older adults. *Quarterly Journal of Experimental Psychology*, 2005;58A(1):120–133.

31. do Rozario, L. From ageing to sageing: Eldering and the art of being as occupation. *Journal of Occupational Science*, 1998;5(3):119–126.

32. Schachter-Shalomi, Z, Miller, R. *From Age-ing to Sage-ing: A Profound New Vision of Growing Older*. New York: Warner Books, 1995.

33. Schaie, KW, Hofer, SM. Longitudinal studies in aging research. In JE Birren, KW Schaie (eds.).

Handbook of the Psychology of Aging. San Diego: Academic Press, 2001.

34. Baltes, PB, et al. People nominated as wise: A comparative study of wisdom-related knowledge. *Psychology of Aging*, 1995;10:155–166.

35. Robnett, RH, Porell, FW, Turner, BF, Tun, PA. The correlates of cognitive and metacognitive stability and change in the first five waves of the Health and Retirement Study (1992–2000). Unpublished dissertation. Boston, University of Massachusetts, 2007.

36. Dana Alliance for Brain Initiatives. Stem cells and neurogenesis, progress report 2006. Retrieved July 5, 2008, from http://www.dana.org/news/publications/detail.aspx?id=4234

37. Hotz, RL. Probing the workings of hearts and minds. Research. *Los Angeles Times*, April 3, 1997.

38. Nussbaum, PD. *Brain Health and Wellness*. Tarentum, PA: Word Association Publishers, 2003.

39. den Dunnen, WFA, Brouwer, WH, Bijlard, E, Kamphuis, J, van Linschoten, K, Eggens-Meijer, E, et al. No disease in the brain of a 115-year-old woman. *Neurobiology of Aging*, 2008;29(8): 1127–1132.

40. Alzheimer's Association. *Alzheimer's Disease Facts and Figures 2007*. Chicago: Alzheimer's Association, 2007.

41. Cole, SA. Behavioral disturbances in Alzheimer's disease. *Patient Care*, June 15, 1995, pp 121–131.

42. Ebly, EM, et al. Prevalence and types of dementia in the very old: Results from the Canadian Study of Health and Aging. *Neurology*, 1994;44:1593–1600.

43. Cummings, JL, et al. Dementia. In CK Cassell et al. (eds.). *Geriatric Medicine*, 3rd ed. New York: Springer-Verlag, 1997, pp 897–913.

44. Folstein, MF, Folstein, SE, McHugh, PR. "Mini-Mental State": A practical method for grading the cognitive state of patients for the clinician. *Journal of Psychiatric Research*, 1975;12(3):189–198.

45. Ham, RJ. Making the diagnosis of Alzheimer's disease. *Patient Care*, June, 15, 1995, pp 104–120.

46. Birks, J, Grimley Evans, J, Iakovidou, V, Tsolaki, M. Rivastigmine for Alzheimer's disease. *Cochrane Database of Systematic Reviews*, 2008;2.

47. Lopez-Arrieta, JM, Schneider, L. Metrifonate for Alzheimer's disease. *Cochrane Database of Systematic Reviews*, 2008;2.

48. Bell, V, Troxel, D. *A Dignified Life: The Best Friends Approach to Alzheimer's Care*. Deerfield Beach, FL: Health Communications, 2002.

49. Strauss, CJ, Khachaturian, ZS. *Talking to Alzheimer's*. Oakland, CA: New Harbinger Publications, 2002.

50. Patenaude, J. Nutrient deficiency-related depression and mental changes in elderly persons. *Home Health Care Management and Practice*, 1996;9(1): 29–39.

51. Palmer, RM. "Failure to thrive" in the elderly: Diagnosis and management. *Geriatrics*, 1990;45(9):47–55.

52. Seligman, ME. In FD Fincham, KM Cain. Learned helplessness in humans: A developmental analysis. *Developmental Review*, 1986;6:301–333.

53. Johnson, JC. Depression and dementia in the elderly: A primary care perspective. *Comprehensive Therapy*, 1996;22:280–285.

54. National Institute of Mental Health. Older Adults: Depression and Suicide Facts. Retrieved July 7, 2008, from http://www.nimh.nih.gov/health/publications/older-adults-depression-and-suicide-facts.shtml#role

55. Callahan, CM, et al. Depression in late life: The use of clinical characteristics to focus screening efforts. *Journals of Gerontology Series A: Biological Sciences and Medical Sciences*, 1994;49:M9–M14.

56. American Psychiatric Association. *Diagnostic and Statistical Manual of Mental Disorders*. 4th ed. (Text Revision). Washington, DC: American Psychiatric Association, 2001.

57. McIntyre, LG, et al. Depression and suicide: Assessment and intervention. *Home Health Care Management and Practice*, 1996;9(1):8–17.

58. Juratovac, E. The Ohio Nurses Association presents "Anxiety and depression in older adults": An independent study. *Ohio Nurses Review*, March 1996, pp 4–13.

59. National Strategy for Suicide Prevention, Department of Health and Human Services. At a Glance—Suicide Among the Elderly. Retrieved June 24, 2008, from http://mentalhealth.samhsa.gov/suicideprevention/elderly.asp

60. Centers for Disease Control and Prevention. Web-based Injury Statistics Query and Reporting System (WISQARS). 2004. Retrieved June 25, 2008, from http://www.cdc.gov/ncipc/wisqars/

61. Welton, RS. The management of suicidality: Assessment and intervention. *Psychiatry*, May 2007, 2–12.

62. Hemphill, BJ. Depression among suicidal elderly: A life-threatening illness. *Occupational Therapy Practice*, 1992;4(1):61–66.

63. Adams, RC. Geriatric rehab treat depression to improve function. *Advance for Occupational Therapists*, December 9, 1996, p 19.

64. McCue, JD. The naturalness of dying. *Journal of the American Medical Association*, 1995;273:1039–1043.

65. Parkes, CM. *Bereavement*. London: Penguin Books, 1972.

66. Kubler-Ross, E. *On Death and Dying*. New York: Macmillan, 1970.

67. Waltman, RE. When a spouse dies. *Nursing*, 1992;92:48–52.

68. Goleman, D. Grief may not follow a predictable pattern. In W Dudley (ed.). *Death and Dying: Opposing Viewpoints*. San Diego, CA: Greenhaven Press, 1992, pp 139–144.

69. Chessler, BR. Friends can help the grieving cope with death. In W Dudley (ed.). *Death and Dying: Opposing Viewpoints*. San Diego, CA: Greenhaven Press, 1992, pp 155–160.

70. Alty, A. Adjustment to bereavement and loss in older people. *Nursing Times*, 1995;91(12):35–36.

71. Davidson, KW, Foster, Z. Social work with dying and bereaved clients: Helping the workers. *Social Work in Health Care*, 1995;21(4):3.

72. Erikson, EH, et al. *Vital Involvement in Old Age*. New York: W. W. Norton; 1989, p 36.

73. Erikson, EH. *Childhood and Society*. 2nd ed. New York: W. W. Norton; 1963.

74. Erikson, EH, Erikson, JM. *The Life Cycle Completed: Extended Version with New Chapters on the Ninth Stage of Development*. New York: W. W. Norton, 1998.

75. Ardelt, M. Self-development through selflessness: The paradoxical process of growing wiser. In HA Wayment, JJ Bauer (eds.). *Transcending Self-Interest: Psychological Explorations of the Quiet Ego*. Washington, DC: American Psychological Association, 2008, pp 221–223.

76. McCrae, RR, Costa, PT. *Personality in Adulthood*. New York: Guilford Press, 1990. Morris, JC. The

77. Clinical Dementia Rating (CDR): Current version and scoring rules. *Neurology*, November 1993, pp 2412–2414.

77. Costa, PT, Herbst, JH, McCrae, RR, Siegler, IC. Personality at midlife: Stability, intrinsic maturation, and response to life events. *Assessment*, 2000;7(4):365–378.

78. Weiss, A, Costa, PT, Karuza, J, Duberstein, PR, Friedman, B, McCrae, RR. Cross sectional age differences in personality among Medicare patients aged 65 to 100. *Psychology and Aging*, 2005;20(1):182–185.

79. Papalia, DE, Aids, SW (eds.). *Human Development*. New York: McGraw-Hill; 1995, p 505.

80. Hayflick, L. *How and Why We Age*. New York: Ballantine Books; 1994, p 145.

81. Wood, D, Roberts, BW. The effect of age and role information on expectations for big five personality traits. *Personality and Social Psychology Bulletin*, 2006;32(11):1482–1496.

82. *Harvard Mental Health Letter*. As a man (or woman) grows older. May 2006.

83. Sohn, E. Better all the time. *Health*, January 1, 2004;18(1), n.p. Retrieved June 28, 2008, from http://O-web.ebscohost.com.lilac.une.edu/ehost/detail?vid+11& hid+8&sid+063f0b6a-4740

84. Harris, PB. The sense of self in Alzheimer's disease: The person's perspective. In BM Oberg, E Nasman, E Olsson (eds.). *Changing Worlds and the Ageing Subject: Dimensions in the Study of Ageing and Later Life*. Hants, UK: Ashgate Publishing, 2004; pp 115–132.

85. Bandura, A. Self-efficacy: Toward a unifying theory of behavioral change. *Psychology Review*, 1977;84:191–215.

86. Rhee, C, Gatz, M. Cross-generational attributions concerning locus of control beliefs. *International Journal of Aging and Human Development*, 1993;37:153–161.

87. McAvay, GJ, et al. A longitudinal study of change in domain-specific self-efficacy among older adults. *Journals of Gerontology Series B: Psychological Sciences and Social Sciences*, 1996;51B:P243–P253.

88. Fry, PS, Debats, DL. Self-efficacy beliefs as predictors of loneliness and psychological distress in older adults. *International Journal of Aging and Human Development*, 2002;55(3):233–269.

89. Deeg, DJH, et al. Health behavior and aging. In JE Birren, KW Schaie (eds.). *Handbook of the Psychology of Aging*. 4th ed. San Diego, CA: Academic Press, 1996, pp 129–149.

90. Blazer, DG. Self-efficacy and depression in late life: A primary prevention proposal. *Aging and Mental Health*, 2002;6(4):315–324.

91. Schalock, RL. Reconsidering the conceptualization and measurement of quality of life. In *Quality of Life*. Washington, DC: American Association on Mental Retardation, 1995, pp 123–138.

92. Kehn, DJ. Predictors of elderly happiness. *Activities, Adaptation and Aging*, 1995;19(3):11–30.

93. Garfein, AJ, Herzog, AR. Robust aging among the young-old, old-old, and oldest-old. *Journals of Gerontology Series B: Psychological Sciences and Social Sciences*, 1995;50B:S77–S87.

94. Ward-Baker, PD. The remarkable oldest old: A new vision of aging. *Dissertation Abstracts International Section A: Humanities and Social Sciences*, 2007;67(8-A):3115.

95. Ardelt, M. Wisdom and life satisfaction in old age. *Journals of Gerontology Series B: Psychological Sciences and Social Sciences*, 1997;52B(1):P15–P27.

96. Carstensen, LL, Mikels, JA, Mather, M. Aging and the intersection of cognition, motivation, and emotion. In JE Birren, KW Schaie (eds.). *Handbook of the Psychology of Aging*. Burlington, MA: Elsevier, 2006, pp 343–362.

97. Adelmann, PK. Multiple roles and psychological well-being in a national sample of older adults. *Journals of Gerontology Series B: Psychological Sciences and Social Sciences*, 1994;49:S277–S285.

98. Ruuskanen, JM, Ruoppila, I. Physical activity and psychological well-being among people aged 65 to 84 years. *Age and Ageing*, 1995;24:292–296.

99. Netuveli, G, Wiggins, RD, Hildon, Z, Montgomery, SM, Blane, D. Quality of life at older ages. *Journal of Epidemiology and Community Health*, 2006;60(4):357–363.

FUNCTIONAL PERFORMANCE IN LATER LIFE: BASIC SENSORY, PERCEPTUAL, AND PHYSICAL CHANGES ASSOCIATED WITH AGING

REGULA H. ROBNETT, PhD, OTR/L, AND JOHN MURRAY, BS, RPSGT, RRT

Old age is not an illness—it is a stage of life.

Chapter Outline

Sensation and Perception
  Vision
  Visual Perception
  Age-Related Hearing Loss: Presbycusis
  Smell and Taste
Physical Changes and Performance
  Range of Motion
  Strength

Endurance
Praxis
Reaction Time
Work Performance
Sleep and Aging
  Normal Sleep
  The Aging Process and Its Impact on Sleep
  Sleep Disorders

Behavioral Objectives

Upon completion of this chapter, the reader will be able to:

1. List at least four recommendations for health care professionals who work with people who have diminished visual skills.
2. Define perception and describe how perceptual skills may change as one ages.
3. Describe compensatory measures related to decreased perceptual functioning.
4. Describe how sensory systems tend to change over the course of aging including the impact on life functioning.
5. List compensatory measures for each of the sensory changes related to aging.

6. List at least four recommendations for health care professionals who work with people who are hard of hearing.
7. Describe the basic physical changes of aging related to range of motion, strength, motor control, and endurance.
8. Discuss how physical changes affect performance in various life skills including self-care and work.
9. Describe how sleep patterns change with age.
10. Describe the components of cognitive behavioral therapy for sleep disorders.

Key Terms

Agnosia	Perception
Anosmia	Praxis
Apraxia	Presbycusis
Cognitive behavior therapy	Range of motion
Contracture	Reaction time
Dyspraxia	Restless leg syndrome
Endurance	Scotoma
Hyposmia	Senescence
Insomnia	Sleep hygiene
Motor coordination	Sleep restriction
Muscle strength	Stimulus control
Obstructive sleep apnea	Vision
Olfaction	

Ironically, change may be the only constant in our lives. This chapter explores the sensory, perceptual, and physical changes associated with the aging process. The intent of the chapter is to provide a brief overview of these potential changes and to provide helpful hints that may help the health care professional in assisting older people who have experienced these age-related changes. The chapter is not intended as a fully developed source book of interventions in these realms. It merely offers a springboard of ideas and information. Although there are charts and lists of potential interventions, these are suggestions only.

Health care professionals who are rehabilitation specialists, such as occupational and physical therapists and speech-language pathologists, are the experts in the realm of sensory, perceptual, and physical changes, including how to remediate these problems or compensate for the problems not amenable to restoration. They are skilled at in-depth interventions to improve functional performance based on extensive professional theories and evidence-based research and practice. This chapter, although helpful to nonrehabilitation specialists, students, and those working in the field of rehabilitation, is not a comprehensive guidebook or a cookbook for intervention. Each of the mentioned professions has textbooks (often several hundred pages long) focusing precisely on the topics in this chapter. The interested reader can view this chapter as a mere appetizer; those with the skill and motivation can go for the "full course" through additional reading and education.

In Chapter 3, the focus was on the typical physical changes taking place within the aging body. **Senescence**, or the process of physical decline, does occur, but often at a slower and, among the global older population, at a more variable rate than originally believed. This chapter discusses the concurrent sensory, perceptual, and physical changes associated with the structural changes (e.g., impairments) previously described, but from a more functional perspective. Along with the physical and sensory changes, an important aspect to consider is the associated performance. Even though the described changes related to aging are rarely outwardly encouraging, nonetheless daily functioning throughout life can remain good or even optimal given enough drive, good fortune and the right genes, and the absence of disease. The majority of older adults are likely to have one or more chronic conditions (for example, in 1999, 82% of Medicare patients reported having at least one chronic condition, with 65% reporting multiple chronic conditions),[1] and yet most of those who do have chronic conditions are still able to live well and would be able to improve their functioning with a little education or assistance.

The chapter starts with an overview of sensation including vision, perception, hearing, olfactory, taste, and touch.

SENSATION AND PERCEPTION

VISION

Sensory changes occur with aging. (See Chapter 3 for the physiologic details.) Some of these changes are quite familiar and arrive almost expectedly after a half century of life. For example, visual skills are known to decrease with age, beginning in one's 20s. The good news is that "most" older people are able to maintain an acuity level close to unimpaired (20/20) with corrective lenses at least until age 88.[2(p.138)] (see **Table 5-1**.)

Other visual skills known to show a decline with advancing age are the following:

- Visual processing speed
- Sensitivity to light
- Ability to see well in dim light
- Near vision, especially problematic for reading small print
- Upward gaze without moving head
- Contrast sensitivity, separate from visual acuity

TABLE 5-1   Common Visual Diagnoses and Functional Implications in Old Age.

Disease of the Eye	Prevalence at Age		Functional Implications
Cataracts	50–54[a] 80+[a]	5% 68%	World appears dull, as if seeing through dusty or cloudy lens; readily amenable to treatment, usually on an outpatient basis.
Age-related macular degeneration (ARMD)	50–54[a] 80+[a]	<0.05% <12%	Central field vision is impaired, affecting reading and other fine detail work.
Glaucoma	50–54[a] 80+[a]	<1% <8%	Loss of peripheral vision, usually gradually; may lead to tunnel vision or total blindness.
Diabetic retinopathy (DR)[b]	40–49 >75	7–31% 12–23%	The person with diabetes and DR has blind spots or **scotomas**; visual skills may fluctuate; may be associated with depressed mood.

[a] Schieber, F. Vision and aging. In JE Birren, KW Schaie (eds.), *Handbook of the Psychology of Aging*. Burlington, MA: Elsevier, 2006, pp 129–161.
[b] Eye Diseases Prevalence Research Group, Diabetic Retinopathy Subsection. The prevalence of diabetic retinopathy among adults in the United States. *Archives of Ophthalmology*, 2004;122:552–563.

- Color sensitivity, especially along the blue–yellow axis of color
- Dynamic vision, which includes
  - Smooth visual pursuits of a moving target (such as watching the movement of a tennis ball), especially with distractions or with increased velocity of targets
  - Visual tracking or saccades, the small ballistic eye movements needed for reading (although decline with age is less than for pursuits)[2]

Visual skills that tend to be preserved include basic color **vision** and the ability to maintain fixation on a target.[3] The health care professional working with older persons may offer several simple compensatory measures to mitigate the effects of decreased eyesight. **Table 5-2** outlines some of these measures. It is important to note that these are merely suggestions, which may be helpful, but that should not be taken as if they will work for all or as if they are the only suggestions available. If the older person is having difficulty with daily tasks because of impaired visual skills, a certified low vision therapist (CLVT; who works exclusively with blind persons and persons with visual impairment), another low vision specialist such as a behavioral optometrist, or an occupational therapist may be of assistance.

VISUAL PERCEPTION

Perception is the ability to make sense of incoming sensory information. Usually this refers to being able to interpret visual data, but it can also refer to auditory, olfactory, and

TABLE 5-2 A Few Compensations for Specific Visual Impairments.

Visual Impairment	Compensatory Measures
Decreased visual acuity	• Corrective lenses • Larger print—font size 10–12 points • Larger images/signs • Closed-circuit television (a device to magnify objects or written material)
Increased sensitivity to light	• Use nonreflective materials on walls, floors, and ceilings • Use yellow film to reduce glare • Wear protective lenses • Shield eyes from bright light bulbs • Provide overhangs on windows
Decreased ability to see in dim light	• Use task lighting directed at work area • Use nightlights • Avoid driving at night, dawn, or dusk
Decreased ability to see contrasts	• Use black with white or yellow contrasts • Highlight obstacles or changes in floor surface levels • Avoid difficult color discriminations, such as blue/green

Data from: Charness, N, Bosman, EA. Human factors design for the older adult. In JE Birren, KW Schaie, M Gatz, TA Salthouse, C Schooler (eds.), *Handbook of the Psychology of Aging*, 3rd ed. San Diego, CA: Academic Press, 1990, pp 452–453; and Zoltan, B. *Vision, Perception and Cognition.* Thorofare, NJ: Slack, 1996.

gustatory sensation as well. One must have adequate vision for visual perception to be intact. Surprisingly, visual perception skills do not show a uniform decline with aging. For example, Lindfield and colleagues researched the ability of people of varying ages to complete visual closure tasks (in which one must identify a given object when shown only fragments of the object).[4] In this study, the older adults were actually able to identify the fragmented pictures more accurately than their younger counterparts were able to, perhaps because of their experience in the world. Because of decreased sensory functioning, older people may become more proficient at inferring meanings from less sensory input.[3] However, they tend to be slower at processing the information and take in less information per unit of time.

Decreases in perceptual skills, such as not understanding what common objects are used for (**agnosia**), loss of spatial awareness (e.g., right/left, back/front), and impaired visual constructional abilities (e.g., completing puzzles, assembling common objects), are not usually associated with typical aging to any notable degree. When perception is awry, the problems are usually related to disease processes such as dementia, stroke (cerebrovascular accident), or psychiatric disorders. Because intact perceptual skills are necessary for typical or normal everyday living, deficits need to be discussed with the provider who can make referrals in this realm (for example, to an occupational therapist who can assist the person with perceptual difficulties in completing daily tasks).

AGE-RELATED HEARING LOSS: PRESBYCUSIS

As described in Chapter 3, hearing is another sensory modality with a tendency to decline with age. **Presbycusis** occurs in both genders, but men, especially, tend to lose the ability to hear higher frequencies. Consonant sounds usually become more difficult than vowel sounds to understand. Also, people in general cannot recall as much of the previous conversation if the number of words spoken per minute is increased. Both younger and older subjects were able to recall more verbal information if the words were spoken in the context of normal sentences rather than in random word strings. However, older adults' accuracy decreased more dramatically than did the younger participants' with unrelated words.[3]

Older people also tend to have more difficulty tuning out background noise. Because of the discomfort brought on by the inability to understand others at social gatherings (due to the increased noise level), a hearing impairment easily may lead to social isolation. In a large-scale population-based study, Kramer, Kapteyn, Kuik, and Deeg found that older people with hearing impairments reported feeling more symptoms of depression (including loneliness) and had lower self-efficacy scores than older people with intact hearing.[5] Not surprisingly, those with hearing loss also had fewer people in their social network.

These studies and past experiences lead to the following recommendations for working with older adults:

- Speak in a tone that can be heard. Although some older people do need you to increase your volume or decibel level, do not assume this is the case. More likely, the person who has difficulty hearing will need you to lower the pitch of your words. It is always all right to ask the person what is best for him or her.
- Make sure that your rate of speech is not too fast, but neither so slow as to sound condescending.
- Whenever possible, keep background noise to a minimum.
- Do not verbally jump from one idea to the next too quickly because older people are more likely to use the context of what is being said to understand the conversation.
- Avoid "elderspeak," which is described as baby talk for older adults (e.g., use of more diminutives, slower speech, more repetition, and simpler words with fewer syllables).[6] Even though older people may have difficulty hearing, this does not imply that they need to be talked to as if they have lost their cognitive capacity.

SMELL AND TASTE

As noted in Chapter 3, other perceptions that change with time include smell (**olfaction**) and taste. These closely related declines have psychological implications. The ability to detect smells in general and correctly identify differing odors decreases with age. The majority of people older than age 80 have impaired olfaction.[7] Studies have shown a high prevalence of **hyposmia** (decreased smell sensation) and **anosmia** (complete loss of smell) in participants age 65 and older. Additionally, in a study by Nordin, Monsch, and Murphy, 77% of the older participants with smell loss (but no other apparent disease diagnoses) reported that they had a normal sense of smell.[8] This finding corresponds with other studies. Even disregarding those who are unaware of their problem because of the onset of dementia, this sensory loss and subsequent unawareness still may constitute a serious safety issue for those wishing to remain independent in their own homes. Compensatory measures, such as natural gas/smoke detectors and having someone else with a normal sense of smell check for spoilage of food, are recommended.

Because olfaction provides a backdrop for taste sensation, decreased smell sensation can contribute to decreased pleasure in eating as well (perhaps leading to yet more social withdrawal). As people age, their ability to detect salty or bitter tastes decreases, but their capability of tasting sweet and sour foods is maintained.[9] This easily can lead to an over-reliance on sweets and an oversalting of food. Thirst sensation also declines, which increases the probability of dehydration in older persons.[10] Booth and colleagues suggest that inadequate dietary intake may actually cause a loss of taste perception, rather than the reverse being true.[11] This implication points to the extreme importance of maintaining an adequate diet, especially as we age (see Chapter 7).

PHYSICAL CHANGES AND PERFORMANCE

RANGE OF MOTION

Range of motion (ROM) refers to the ability of a joint to move through its natural pattern of movement. For example, the shoulder of a typical healthy person can flex up (toward the sky) nearly straight (or close to 180°). This amount of movement is considered normal for that joint. Every joint in the body has a typical range. Older age does relate to a decline in joint range of motion including the shoulder,[12] hip rotation, and the wrist.[13] That being said, chronological age alone may affect range of motion less than do several age-related conditions, which definitely have a negative effect on smooth movement and maximum range. For example, arthritis; muscle disuse, misuse, or overuse; injuries; stroke; Parkinson's disease; and dementia have all been associated with less than optimal movement patterns. Various forms of arthritis are the most common cause of disability in the United States, with more than 19 million people currently living with the associated functional losses.[14]

Nonresistive, repetitive range of motion exercises may be able to maintain or improve current range, or may slow down the progression of disease processes such as osteoarthritis.[15] Physicians and other professionals who are experts in movement (e.g., physical therapists) can help older persons develop optimal programs for their needs, working toward their best possible performance, staving off loss of motion secondary to disease, maintaining current range, increasing range of motion, and increasing strength. No matter what the person's life situation is, regular movement (especially by engaging in meaningful life tasks) is important if the person is at all able. Especially those who tend to be sedentary or immobile, such as those who are bedridden for a prolonged period in the hospital or in long-term care facilities, are at high risk of sustaining joint **contractures**. Contractures are generally caused by joint immobilization and result in decreased range of motion, stiffening and subsequent structural changes, and pain on movement at one or more joints. The best treatment to increase joint mobility if at all possible is a passive, active-assisted, or (best) active range of motion program established by a rehabilitation specialist. If contractures are not resolved, not only the pain but also the resulting immobility will make activities of daily living such as bathing, dressing, and grooming difficult or impossible to complete.

STRENGTH

Maximum **muscle strength** tends to occur in early adulthood, while middle age is generally a time of only slight decline. By age 65, a 20% reduction in strength is common, with losses tending to occur even more rapidly thereafter. An additional 30% reduction is common after age 70.[16] However, this potential consequence of aging is based on average losses in the population. Individuals do not necessarily get progressively weaker with age. Older people, if physically able, can still be involved in and even improve in sports requiring practice and skill such as tennis, golf, skiing, boating, and bowling (**Figure 5-1**). Also, by adding a prescribed exercise routine, people can improve their muscle strength and may even get strong enough to win competitions, like 78-year-old Marjorie Newton, who started a weight-lifting program in her 70s. After 6 years, she was leg-pressing 180 pounds and winning competitions.[17] Encouraging physical activity is almost always appropriate, although the level of exertion and duration of activity need to be determined by the person's primary health care provider.

ENDURANCE

Endurance is defined as the ability to sustain involvement in a physical activity. Although not the same as strength, the two are closely related. Several studies have noted that the decrease in muscular endurance during one's lifetime is proportionately less than the decrease in muscle strength.[18] A meta-analysis of 13 aerobic exercise training programs for older people demonstrated that long-term programs (more than 30 weeks in duration) were associated with improved endurance.[19] On a hopeful and health-related note, an active lifestyle involving stretching, aerobic activity, and strength building can improve range of motion, strength, and endurance, and in so doing may actually slow the course of physiologic aging (see Chapter 3).

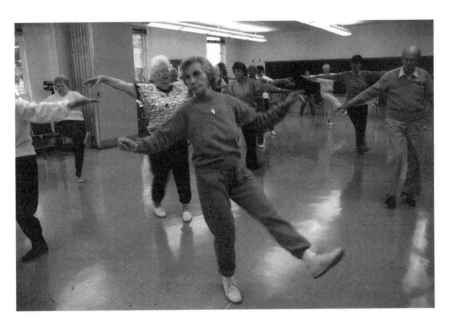

FIGURE 5-1   Physical activity can boost energy and increase brain power. (*Courtesy of Bill Branson/National Cancer Institute.*)

PRAXIS

Praxis is defined as the ability to carry out purposeful motor actions. **Dyspraxia** refers to a decreased ability to plan and/or execute purposeful movements, whereas **apraxia** refers to the total inability to carry out these motor plans. During most of our daily routines, we do not need to think consciously about our performance; we complete many tasks (such as eating or dressing) automatically. Repetition allows us to convert initially novel actions into habits over time. Goal-directed actions occur throughout the day during our self-care, work, leisure, and home management tasks. If the level of motor (or cognitive) performance significantly decreases for any reason (e.g., injury, aging, or disease), one's ability to live independently can be threatened. Also worth noting is the fact that people do not lose functional performance rapidly from one day to the next because of the aging process. However, they can have sudden physical losses caused by accidents or medical issues. Often rehabilitation, with the overall goal of regaining lost skills, is warranted.

When reviewing studies that have explored the physical performance of older people, we find cross-sectional differences between age groups, for example, when 20-year-olds are compared to 80-year-olds, as well as longitudinal changes within the same person over time (for example, from age 60 to age 80). The changes are not always in the expected direction of deterioration. Age-related performance has been measured in several domains: gross motor coordination (including balance and mobility), reaction time, strength, endurance, and work-related performance (as well as cognition and memory, discussed earlier in Chapter 4).

Reaction Time Perhaps the most straightforward trend when examining performance is the slowing of **reaction time** as people head into old age. An example of needing to take action quickly with a specific response is in driving a car: Brake lights directly ahead indicate an immediate need to step on the brake. As people age, in general, they are not able to react as quickly. In the Baltimore Longitudinal Study of Aging (BLSA), researchers determined that the slowing of behavior was a continuous process over the course of a lifetime and that increasing the complexity of task demands further increased the response time needed.[20] Stimulus–response time tends to become about 20% slower between the ages of 20 and 60, and the responses in later life are less likely to be accurate.[9] However, the BLSA study and others note that the variability within any one age group (cohort) also significantly increases with age. Therefore, at age 80, for instance, a man still can be nearly as fast in responding as he ever was and still have perfectly adequate reaction time to be successful in independent living skills such as driving. (A masculine example is used purposefully because studies have tended to show that slowed reaction time is more pronounced in older women.[20]) It is also interesting to note that when only verbal (instead of psychomotor) responses were required, the slowing has not been nearly as pronounced and may not be evident at all.[18]

Motor Coordination Gross **motor coordination** is another crucial prerequisite to complete daily tasks without assistance. Specifically, mobility, or ambulation, seems to be an extremely valued skill. Falls are more prevalent in the elderly population, with people age 65 and older having a 27% chance of falling at least once per year. Unfortunately, falling once increases the risk of the older person falling again.[21] Repeated falls generally are associated with declines in balance, coordination, and/or strength. All these areas have been studied and have generally shown age-correlated declines. Again, we must point out the increasing variability among cohorts, and the fact that the vast majority of elderly people still have adequate amounts of strength and coordination to do the tasks that they want or need to do, including walking, as part of their daily routines.

Impaired ambulation may be cause for a referral to a physical therapist, who can help remediate physical skills or possibly recommend devices for safe ambulation. Also, Area Agencies on Aging may be able to recommend local programs designed for older people who want to improve their sense of balance, for example, the Matter of Balance program started by rehabilitation specialists at Boston University.[22] There are several ways to improve postural control (for example, exercises, sports, and yoga or tai chi).[23] Also, for those with a decreased sense of balance, it is vital to make sure the home or environment is clutter-free and that obstacles (such as loose rugs, cords, and pets) are out of the way. Rehabilitation specialists such as occupational or physical therapists are good resources to contact for additional balance-related treatment strategies.

Fine motor coordination refers to hand-based skills such as writing, self-feeding, buttoning, and working with tools. Considering age alone, we see little change in a person's ability to complete fine motor tasks. Older people who are aging in a typical fashion (i.e., without disease) are just as capable as are their younger counterparts in tasks such as typing, cooking, and card playing. This maintenance of skill could be based on two potential explanations: (1) ongoing practice over the years has improved skill level over time, or (2) with ongoing repetition these tasks become more automatic and therefore require less skill for completion. Salthouse, a well-known researcher in the field of aging, has yet another explanation for the continued good performance of professionals using these types of skills (such as typing), which is explained in the following subsection. When fine motor skills are impaired, as they often are in old age, the culprit is more than likely arthritis, stroke, or another skill-robbing disease, rather than *normal* aging.

WORK PERFORMANCE

With the alleged, age-related deterioration of functional component skills, such as aspects of cognition, balance, reaction time, and muscle strength, you might surmise that the work performance of older workers would be inferior to that of their younger counterparts. However, as a group, older workers do very well (**Figure 5-2**). The following empirical evidence is offered to debunk ageist myths with regard to older workers:

- Based on actual attendance records, older workers have less absenteeism than younger workers do.[24,25]
- Age is not linked to job performance by empirical research, even on the established platform of slowed cognitive functioning in old age.[24,26]
- Older workers have proportionately fewer workplace injuries.[24,25]
- Older workers demonstrate less workplace aggression and substance abuse, and are more dependable.[24]

One employer praised older workers' stronger work ethic,[27] while others lauded the older employees' experience and sense of leadership.[28] Salthouse, who completed a series of studies on the performance of older workers, found past relevant work experience to be a more important factor than specifically tested cognitive abilities in predicting work performance.[26] After studying older architects, engineers, and secretaries, Salthouse proposed that occupation-specific experience, although it did not seem to moderate the inverse relationship between age and basic cognitive processes, did, however, contribute to successful job performance. The older secretaries, for example, had slower reaction times, but they still were able to type as proficiently as their younger counterparts through

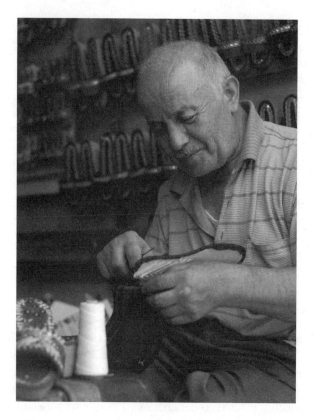

FIGURE 5-2 The diligent older worker makes a substantial contribution to society.
(page 166 © asliuzunogu/ShutterStock, Inc.; page 167 © Photodisc; page 168 © LiquidLibrary.)

the use of a phenomenon Salthouse named "anticipatory processing."[26] This developed job skill allows the older secretaries to more effectively scan ahead and maintain their speed.

Overall, although there do seem to be age-related declines in cognition, sensation, perception, and physical performance, for most typically aging older people these changes do not make a substantial impact on either their comprehensive work performance or essential daily living skills. However, any significant decreases in level of functioning, which either occurs suddenly or over the course of a few weeks or months, are not generally consistent with the typical aging process. Of course, emergency situations necessitate immediate action, but even relatively rapidly changing performance should also prompt attention. Behavioral changes should send up a warning flag to the older person, family, and friends warranting a call and probable visit to the person's physician. The physician can then make referrals for further medical care or for rehabilitation.

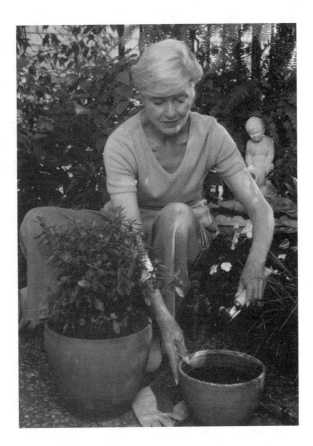

FIGURE 5-2   *continued*

SLEEP AND AGING

Sleep is considered an activity of daily living (ADL) because it is an essential part of everyday life. This daily task is completely different from other daily activities, but we cannot live without doing it regularly. Sleep has become an increasingly important and studied factor in older adults because of its central role in promoting a high quality of life. Lack of sleep can cause dramatic changes in how one feels (and acts) during the day. The National Sleep Foundation reports that 65% of people over the age of 55 have reported sleep problems at least a few times per week. Also, according to a 2003 survey by the foundation, 26% of those ages 55–64 reported that their sleep was either fair or poor, while 21% of those ages 65–84 reported fair or poor sleeping habits.[29]

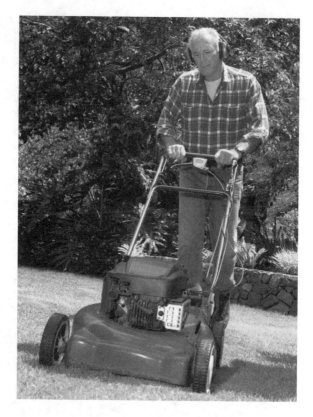

FIGURE 5-2 *continued*

NORMAL SLEEP

To discuss sleep disorders we must first have an understanding of normal sleep and the typical sleep cycle. People have a sleep–wake cycle that is known as the circadian rhythm: our 24-hour clock responsible for keeping most of us awake during the day and allowing us to feel sleepy and go to sleep at night. The stimulating effects of light through the retinohypothalmic tract control this rhythm in the hypothalamus. The light causes alerting signals to help maintain wakefulness. As the day progresses our sleep load increases and the alerting signals must get stronger for us to feel alert. When darkness falls, and we go through our evening/nighttime routines such as dinner and relaxation, the alerting signals decrease. Melatonin is released, causing further reduction in the alerting signals until the sleep load overtakes us and we fall asleep. This often happens between 9 and 11 p.m.

Once asleep, we also have a rhythm to our sleep. Sleep is broken into two states, non–rapid eye movement (NREM) and rapid eye movement (REM) sleep. Non-REM sleep consists of three stages: N1, N2, and N3. N1 is the link between consciousness and unconsciousness. In this stage of sleep we may have some awareness of surroundings and are easily aroused. We spend about 5% of our time asleep in stage N1. In stage N2, we lose consciousness, but we are still in a light stage of sleep and can be aroused easily. Approximately 50% of our sleep time is spent in stage N2. Stage N3 is considered deep sleep. When we are in deep sleep, arousal is difficult. If aroused during deep sleep, we are usually somewhat disoriented. During this stage, growth hormone is released, which continues to be needed for tissue repair as we age. The N3 stage of sleep is when we experience the most restorative sleep so essential to functional performance and feeling refreshed during the day. Unfortunately, as we age, this stage of sleep decreases and is replaced by the lighter stage N2.

Stage R, or rapid eye movement (REM), sleep is when we dream. During this stage of sleep, the brain is more active than when we are awake. REM sleep is thought to be responsible for reorganization of our thoughts similar to rebooting a computer. During stage R, we experience muscle atonia, preventing us from acting out our dreams. We also lose a degree of autonomic control, which leads to heart rate variability, irregular respiration, and fluctuations in blood pressure. Stage R comprises about 25% of our sleep.

The sleep cycle consists of four to five periods of non-REM and REM sleep, each lasting about 90 minutes. The first part of the night consists of more deep sleep and shorter REM sleep, while the latter part of the night consists of longer REM periods and shorter deep sleep (N3) periods.

THE AGING PROCESS AND ITS IMPACT ON SLEEP

Sleep requirements change over the life course; infants need approximately 16 hours per day and adults need about 8 hours per day. One longstanding misconception is that older people need less sleep. We actually need the same amount of sleep as we get older, but getting enough sleep may become more difficult to achieve. The major reasons are related to the decrease in deep sleep leading to more time spent in lighter stages of sleep. While in these lighter stages of sleep we are more able to be aroused and therefore more susceptible to sleep disruptions caused by pain or discomfort that may come with aging. Older people take more medications than any other age group, and many of these medications have a negative effect on sleep, including exhaustion,[30] hypotension, morning sedation, central nervous system overstimulation and depression, daytime drowsiness, and somnolence.[31] This leads to a more disruptive and fragmented sleep for many older people. Although their sleep requirements stay the same throughout adulthood, their sleep efficiency (time asleep to time in bed) is reduced over time, requiring older people to spend more time in bed to get the required amount of sleep.[32]

The circadian rhythm also changes as we age. The rhythm becomes phase advanced, which results in melatonin being released earlier in the evening. This leads to moving the sleep period up and very early morning awakenings. Instead of getting sleepy between 9 and 11 p.m., sleepiness may occur as early as 7 p.m. This then leads to earlier awakenings (usually between 4 and 5 a.m.). Although this is considered a normal occurrence, it can have a negative impact on one's life, for example, one's social life in the evening. The easiest way to delay the sleep period is by getting bright light (either natural sunlight or artificial light) later in the day. Artificial light of at least 2,500 lux (five times brighter than house lights) is recommended.[32]

SLEEP DISORDERS

Sleep problems/disorders include the following:

- Difficulty falling asleep (sleep-onset **insomnia**)
- Waking up often during the night (sleep maintenance insomnia)
- Waking up too early and not being able to get back to sleep (terminal insomnia)
- Waking up not feeling refreshed
- Snoring, which may be related to pauses in breathing (sleep apnea)
- Unpleasant feelings in the legs (restless leg syndrome)

Overall, about two-thirds of older adults report experiencing one or more of these symptoms at least a few nights a week, with 55- to 64-year-olds (71%) being most likely to report problems sleeping, compared to adults 65–74 years old (65%) and 75–84 years old (64%).[29]

All of these sleep disturbances lead to a decrease in sleep efficiency and an increase in symptoms of daytime sleepiness. Insomnia is the most common symptom of more than 30 different sleep disorders.[33] Acute insomnia is less than 30 days in duration whereas chronic insomnia lasts longer than a month. The onset of insomnia may begin with some type of emotional event such as the loss of a loved one or a recent stay in the hospital. During the event, the normal rhythm of sleep is disrupted and an abnormal sleep cycle ensues. The new cycle may then become the norm; many people have difficulty resuming their preevent sleep routine.

Signs and symptoms of **obstructive sleep apnea** (OSA) include snoring and witnessed apnea during sleep and/or complaints of excessive sleepiness during the day. OSA occurs because the trachea is either totally or partially obstructed, causing the body's oxygen level to drop. This in turn signals the brain to get in gear (i.e., wake up), which increases muscle tone and subsequently raises the oxygen level back to normal. This disruption of the sleep pattern can occur up to 60 times an hour, so a person may need 10–12 hours of sleep to attain just enough restorative sleep per night. Twice as many men as women, prior to menopause, are afflicted with OSA, but after people reach their 50s the gender numbers even out. Approximately 5–8% of older adults have some level of OSA. Because loss of oxygen to the brain obviously can be dangerous, this condition can have serious consequences, including heart arrhythmias. Whereas repositioning to side-lying may help (lying on one's back seems to exacerbate the problem), the use of a continuous positive airway pressure (CPAP) device is considered the leading therapy for OSA and has helped millions to overcome the negative impact of sleep apnea. The CPAP machine does not involve oxygen transmission; it simply keeps the airway path unobstructed.[34] The CPAP hoses and masks require regular maintenance and cleaning every few months. If not maintained, the buildup of bacteria can cause additional harm just by using the machine.

Restless leg syndrome (RLS) is a neurologic disorder including "creepy crawly feelings" or other unpleasant sensations in the legs usually while in bed. These symptoms lead to periodic leg movements during sleep (PLMS), which can have the serious consequence of hindering people from getting a good night's sleep. According to the National Institute of Neurological Disorders and Stroke, PLMS may occur every 10 to 60 seconds and may last the entire night.[35] This need to move almost constantly also causes the brain to wake up, disrupting the sleep cycle much like sleep apnea does. Parkinsonian-type medications have been able to afford some relief to PLMS sufferers.[35]

Treatment of Sleep Disorders There are four primary types of **cognitive behavioral therapy** (CBT) treatments for sleep disorders:

- Sleep restriction
- Stimulus control
- Sleep hygiene
- Cognitive behavioral therapy

Although the typical health care professional is not expected to help an older person in overcoming serious sleep disorders, there are nonetheless some relatively simple helpful hints that could benefit older people in their quest for regular restful sleep.

Sleep restriction does not refer to actually restricting sleep, but rather to restricting one's time in bed. The goal is to be asleep 90% of the time that one spends in bed. Often those who have insomnia will spend many hours in bed not sleeping. This leads to poor sleep habits whereby one learns (subconsciously) that a bed is not for sleeping. If people aim for the 90% rule, they can determine how long they would need to be in bed to get the desired number of hours of sleep. Whether or not they have slept enough, they get out of bed at the allotted time. The person forces himself or herself to stay awake (and out of bed) until it's time to go to sleep again. Later, time spent in bed can be gradually added back in.

Stimulus control also refers to amount of time spent in bed, in this case attempting to get to sleep or back to sleep. If someone cannot fall asleep within a half hour, it's best to get out of bed and do something relaxing. When the person is sleepy, she or he can go back to bed and try again to go to sleep. Rather than tossing and turning, consumed with worry that one will not get enough sleep, one gets out of the bedroom and does an activity. This ritual should be individualized because some find reading or puzzles relaxing, while others may have differing interests.

Sleep hygiene involves those activities and habits that are conducive to sleeping soundly. To some degree these factors are also individualized, although most find that a quiet, cool, dark room is helpful for inducing sleep, while eating, exercising, or a blaring television is more likely to keep one awake. Exercise should take place at least 2 to 3 hours before bedtime, and taking a hot bath can be helpful an hour or more before heading to bed. Some find it helpful to write down a to-do list for the next day to put the next day's demands into perspective. It can certainly be helpful for those having sleep disturbances to spend time devising their own personal sleep hygiene "dos and don'ts" list so that they can promote healthy, restful sleep patterns.

Finally, cognitive behavior therapy (CBT) has been found to be helpful for those having difficulty sleeping. A therapist who specializes in sleep disorders can teach the client about sleep and work with the person to understand that it is not necessarily catastrophic if one occasionally does not get enough sleep. Worrying about a lack of sleep only exacerbates the situation. CBT puts the daily activity of sleep into perspective, and the therapist attempts to get those with sleep disorders to relax more about their sleep patterns. This attitude adjustment along with the other techniques mentioned may be all that is needed for a person to regain sound sleeping habits. For example, Edinger, Wohlgemuth, Radke, Marsh, and Quillian completed a randomized controlled trial comparing CBT to relaxation therapy and a placebo treatment for 75 adults.[36] They determined that CBT led to better sleep outcomes not only over the 6-week study period, but also these gains were sustained over a 6-month period.

With regard to sleep, overall people need adequate amounts of varying durations, typically around 8 hours per night. As people age, various diagnoses, aches and pains, or the need to get up for toileting in the middle of the night can interfere with healthy sleep patterns. Also, medication use, which increases as one ages, affects sleep patterns in various ways. Fortunately, sleep disorders are usually treatable. The importance of normal sleep was emphasized in a large study by Ancoli-Israel (cited in *Science Daily*, June 11, 2008), who found that those with fewer sleep disturbances were more likely to be "successful agers."[37]

Although many believe the most effective treatment for insomnia is in the form of a sleeping pill, this may only rarely be true. Sleeping pills are perhaps a good short-term solution, especially for those who have had a traumatic or emotional event that is interfering with sleep (e.g., death of a spouse or a forced move). However, in the long run, the other CBT techniques such as sleep restriction, stimulus control, sleep hygiene, and therapy can offer more sustainable positive impact on the older person's overall quality of life.

SUMMARY

This chapter reviews some of the sensory and physical changes that tend to accompany the aging process, especially as these changes relate to day-to-day functioning. It also covers work performance and sleep because these are two functional areas relevant to older people. The fact is that the vast majority of older people manage their daily routines just fine. Those who are afflicted with one of the diseases associated with aging or the consequences of poor lifestyle choices may not do as well as the typically aging population, but people, even in the midst of chronic conditions or physical decline secondary to ill health, can sometimes be surprisingly resilient and outperform expectations. As health care professionals, it is at least part of our job to instill hope for the future. We can almost always make small but significant positive changes to any life situation.

Highlights of the changes addressed in this chapter are as follows:

- Common visual diagnoses include decreased acuity, cataracts, macular degeneration, glaucoma, and diabetic retinopathy, yet the majority of older people are able to maintain adequate visual skills for the completion of daily tasks.
- Visual perceptual skills, or the ability to interpret incoming visual information, is more affected by disease processes (such as stroke) than by the aging process alone.
- Physical skills such as joint range of motion, strength, endurance, reaction time, and motor coordination do change over the course of time, with older adults generally not performing as well as their younger counterparts. However, several measures can be taken to improve performance even among the oldest members of the population.
- Perhaps surprisingly, for various reasons older workers tend to perform as well as or better than their younger counterparts.
- Sleep disorders are common among older adults, and several treatment techniques for improving quality and quantity of sleep are available for those needing help in this area.

Review Questions

1. Perceptual skills in older adults
   A. Decrease dramatically with age
   B. Are more likely to be affected by disease than by the typical aging process
   C. Are more accurate and show decreased response time than for younger people
   D. Do not change with the aging process

2. Choose the *false* statement about sensation and aging:
   A. Men, more than women, lose the ability to hear high frequencies as they age.
   B. The ability to taste sweet and sour is maintained.
   C. Thirst sensation declines with age.
   D. Most older people who have hyposmia are aware of their impairment.

3. Older workers tend to
    A. Be slower and therefore less efficient
    B. Have less of a work ethic driving them
    C. Use past experience to work efficiently
    D. Withdraw from leadership roles

4. The most common visual condition (and the one most directly related to the aging process) is
    A. Cataracts
    B. Diabetic retinopathy
    C. Macular degeneration
    D. Glaucoma

5. Generally, the best way to compensate for presbycusis is by
    A. Yelling in the person's ear
    B. Speaking extra slowly and simply
    C. Decreasing background noise
    D. Raising the pitch of your voice

6. The most common causes of decreased range of motion and strength are
    A. Diabetes and dementia
    B. Old age and being female
    C. Arthritis and disuse
    D. Overuse and repetitive injuries

7. Which of the following statements about sleep and aging is *false?*
    A. Older people need about the same amount of sleep as younger adults.
    B. Restorative sleep decreases as we get older.
    C. Snoring has no significant impact on quality of sleep.
    D. Older people spend more time in lighter stages of sleep.

8. Cognitive behavioral therapy has been shown to work well for older people who are experiencing
    A. Dementia
    B. Sensory losses
    C. Loss of balance
    D. Sleep disorders

Learning Activities

1. (Do the first part of this learning activity before reading the chapter.) On the left side of a piece of paper, make a list of the following: vision, visual perception, hearing, smell, taste, range of motion, strength, endurance, work performance, and sleep. For each category, write down what you expect to happen with this factor as you get older.

Then, read the chapter and compare what you expected with what you learned in the chapter. Were you surprised about any of the results?

2. Based on what you learned in the chapter, why does driving become more difficult with advancing age? What other life tasks may be more difficult for older adults and why?

3. Two, three, or four people should choose a card game they all know how to play. One player will wear glasses smeared with petroleum jelly, another player should wear ear plugs and heavy leather gloves. The third player must keep his or her hands in a fist and wear dark sunglasses, and if there is a fourth player, he or she will cover one eye and can move her arms only by sliding them across the table (because of arm weakness, though she can move her fingers). Any time a player cheats, he or she will lose a point toward the total score. After the game, discuss how the simulated age-related changes affected your ability to play the game.

4. Review the activity in item 3. How could you make it easier for the players to enjoy their game of cards? Come up with several suggestions.

5. Make a personal list of sleep hygiene "dos and don'ts" for yourself. Discuss with the group.

REFERENCES

1. Wolff, JL, Starfield, B, Anderson, G. Prevalence, expenditures, and complications of multiple chronic conditions in the elderly. *Archives of Internal Medicine*, 2002;162(20):2269–2276.

2. Schieber, F. Vision and aging. In JE Birren, KW Schaie (eds.). *Handbook of the Psychology of Aging*. Burlington, MA: Elsevier, 2006, pp 129–161.

3. Fozard, JL. Vision and hearing in aging. In JE Birren, KW Schaie, M Gatz, TA Salthouse, C Schooler (eds.). *Handbook of the Psychology of Aging*. 3rd ed. San Diego, CA: Academic Press, 1990, pp 150–170.

4. Lindfield, KC, et al. Identification of fragmented pictures under ascending versus fixed presentation in young and elderly adults: Evidence for the inhibition-deficit hypothesis. *Aging and Cognition*, 1994;1:282–291.

5. Kramer, SE, Kapteyn, TS, Kuik, DJ, Deeg, DJH. The association of hearing impairment and chronic diseases with psychosocial health status in older age. *Journal of Aging and Health*, 2002;14(1):122–137.

6. Thornton, R, Light, LL. Language comprehension and production in normal aging. In JE Birren, KW Schaie (eds.). *Handbook of the Psychology of Aging*. Burlington, MA: Elsevier, 2006, pp 262–288.

7. Murphy, C, Schubert, CR, Cruickshanks, KJ, Klein, BEK, Klein, R, Nondahl, DM. Prevalence of olfactory impairment in older adults. *Journal of the American Medical Association*, 2002;288 (18):2307–2312.

8. Nordin, S, Monsch, AU, Murphy, C. Unawareness of smell loss in normal aging and Alzheimer's disease: Discrepancy between self-reported and diagnosed smell sensitivity. *Journals of Gerontology Series B: Psychological Sciences and Social Sciences*, 1995;50B:P187–P192.

9. Hayflick, L. *How and Why We Age*. New York: Ballantine Books, 1994, p 145.

10. Smolowe, J. Older, longer. *Time*, Fall 1996; 148(14):76–80.

11. Booth, DA, et al. Measurement of food perception, food preference and nutrient selection.

Annals of the New York Academy of Sciences, 1989;561:226–242.

12. McIntosh, L, McKenna, K, Gustafsson, L. Active and passive range of motion in healthy older people. *British Journal of Occupational Therapy,* 2003;66(7):318–324.

13. Beal, MF, Lang, AE, Ludolph, Clinical aspects of normal aging. In *Neurodegenerative Diseases.* Cambridge, UK: Cambridge University Press, 2005.

14. Arthritis Foundation. Arthritis Prevalance, Activity Limitations to Skyrocket, Act Now to Reduce Future Disability, Arthritis Foundation Warns, USA. Retrieved September 18, 2008, from http://www.medicalnewstoday.com/articles/71007.php

15. King, OS, Halpern, BC. An exercise plan for older patients with arthritis: Keeping joints moving can stabilize or slow the degenerative process. *Journal of Musculoskeletal Medicine,* 2002;19(4):147–149.

16. American College of Sports Medicine. Position stand of exercise and physical activity for older adults. *Medicine and Science in Sports and Exercise,* 1998;30:992–1008.

17. Noel-Bassior, J. Sure, you'll get older, so what? *Parade Magazine,* November 22, 1998, pp 20–22.

18. Spirduso, WW, MacRae, PG. Motor performance and aging. In JE Birren, KW Schaie (eds.). *Handbook of the Psychology of Aging.* 3rd ed. San Diego, CA: Academic Press 1990, pp 183–200.

19. Huang, G, Shi, X, Davis-Brezette, JA, Osness, WH. Resting heart rate changes after endurance training in older adults: A meta-analysis. *Medicine and Science in Sports and Medicine,* 2005; 37:1381–1386.

20. Fozard, JL, et al. Age differences and changes in reaction time: The Baltimore Longitudinal Study of Aging. *Journals of Gerontology Series B: Psychological Sciences and Social Sciences,* 1994; 49:P179–P189.

21. Ganz, DA, Bao, Y, Shekelle, PG, Rubenstein, LZ. Will my patient fall? *Journal of the American Medical Association,* 2007;297(1):77–86.

22. Maine Health. A Matter of Balance: Managing Concerns About Falls. Retrieved January 20, 2009, from http://www.mmc.org/mh_body.cfm?id=432

23. Gillespie, LD, Gillespie, WJ, Robertson, MC, Lamb, SE, Cumming, RG, Rowe, BH. Interventions for preventing falls in elderly people. *The Cochrane Library,* 2006;(1):CD000340.

24. Prenda, KM, Stahl, SM. The truth about older workers. *Business and Health,* May 2001, pp 30–38.

25. Ng, TWH, Feldman, DC. The relationship of age to ten dimensions of job performance. *Journal of Applied Psychology,* 2008;93(2):392–423.

26. Salthouse, TA. Age-related differences in basic cognitive processes: Implications for work. *Experimental Aging Research,* 1994;20:249–255.

27. Gunn, EP. Retire today, find a new job tomorrow. *Fortune,* July 24, 1995;132(2):102–106.

28. Lieberman, S, McCray, J. The coming of age(ism): Newsrooms should be wary of the generation gap. *The Quill,* April 1994;82(3):33–34.

29. National Sleep Foundation. *Sleep in America Poll.* Retrieved August 3, 2008, from http://www.kintera.org/atf/cf/%7BF6BF2668-A1B4-4FE8-8D1A-A5D39340D9CB%7D/2003SleepPollExecSumm.pdf

30. National Institute of Health. Conference, Workshops, and Meetings: Unexplained Fatigue in the Elderly [workshop]. June 25–26, 2007. Retrieved September 22, 2008, from http://www.nia.nih.gov/ResearchInformation/ConferencesAndMeetings/UnexplainedFatigue.htm#summary

31. Ringdahl, DM, Snively, CG, Carney, PR. Pharmacological treatments. In PR Carney, RB Berry, JD Geyer (eds.). *Clinical Sleep Disorders.* Philadelphia: Lippincott Williams & Wilkins, 2005, pp 485–486.

32. Phillips, B. Sleepiness. In PR Carney, RB Berry, JD Geyer (eds.). *Clinical Sleep Disorders.* Philadelphia: Lippincott Williams & Wilkins, 2005, pp 101–112.

33. Nau, SD, Lichstein, KL. Insomnia: Causes and treatment. In PR Carney, RB Berry, JD Geyer (eds.). *Clinical Sleep Disorders.* Philadelphia: Lippincott Williams & Wilkins, 2005, pp 157–190.

34. Berry, RB, Sanders, MH. Positive airway pressure treatment for sleep apnea. In PR Carney, RB Berry, JD Geyer (eds.). *Clinical Sleep Disorders.*

Philadelphia: Lippincott Williams & Wilkins, 2005, pp 290–310.

35. National Institute of Neurological Disorders and Stroke. Restless Legs Syndrome Fact Sheet. Retrieved September 22, 2008, from http://www.ninds.nih.gov/disorders/restless_legs/detail_restless_legs.htm#106073237

36. Edinger, JD, Wohlgemuth, WK, Radke, RA, Marsh, GR, Quillian, RE. Cognitive behavioral therapy for treatment of primary chronic insomnia. *Journal of the American Medical Association*, 2001;285(14):1856–1864.

37. Ancoli-Israel, S. Normal sleep linked to successful aging. *Science Daily*. June 11, 2008. Retrieved September 29, 2008, from http://www.sciencedaily.com/releases/2008/06/080611071051.htm

GERIATRIC PHARMACOTHERAPY

THOMAS D. NOLIN, PharmD, PhD, AND
LISA A. WENDLER, PharmD

Medicine sometimes snatches away health, sometimes gives it.

—*Ovid, Roman poet*

Chapter Outline

Behavioral Objectives

Upon completion of this chapter, the reader will be able to:

1. List the four pharmacokinetic parameters, all of which change in older persons.
2. Describe the primary alterations occurring with each of the parameters listed in objective 1.
3. List five drugs/drug classes that require dosage adjustment in older persons.
4. Contrast pharmacokinetic and pharmacodynamic changes.
5. Describe factors contributing to polypharmacy and explain why polypharmacy is not desirable.

6. Define the term *medication-related problem*, and describe three common types.
7. Define the term *adverse drug reaction*, and differentiate it from side effect.
8. Identify the drug most likely to be abused by older persons.
9. Define the term *medication adherence*, describe barriers to it, and suggest possible strategies for maintenance of adherence.
10. Discuss an effective means of medication management in older persons.

Key Terms

Adverse drug reaction	Medication-related problems
Adherence	Pharmacodynamics
Health literacy	Pharmacokinetics
Hydrophilicity	Polypharmacy
Lipophilicity	

The continued increase in life expectancy has translated to a growing number of older people worldwide. The percentage of the world's population over the age of 60 years doubled during the last century and is projected to double or triple during the next century.[1] Moreover, older adults have become the fastest growing segment of the U.S. population. Individuals over age 65 currently represent 13% of the U.S. population and are expected to double in number to 70 million by 2030.[2,3] The majority of older people have at least one chronic disease and consequently use more medications than younger people do, taking on average two to five medications concurrently.[1] As such, seniors consume approximately 25% of prescribed medications and spend nearly $3 billion per year in the United States alone.[3,4]

Older persons undergo well-documented age-related physiologic changes that directly influence drug disposition and response, a phenomenon that makes them susceptible to often preventable drug-related problems, particularly adverse drug reactions (ADRs).[5] An increased number of chronic illnesses contributes to polypharmacy, which may in turn lead to the development of ADRs and poor **adherence** to prescribed medication regimens.[1,4] An understanding of each of these issues is important in ensuring safe and effective pharmacotherapy. Clinicians familiar with them are better prepared to evaluate and individualize drug therapy in older adults.

PHARMACOKINETIC CHANGES

Pharmacokinetics is the study of how drugs travel through the body over time. It deals with all aspects of drug disposition in the body, including *absorption* from the administration site, *distribution* into various body compartments, and *clearance* from the body. Drug clearance is composed primarily of *metabolism* to active and inactive metabolites (by-products of drug metabolism) and renal *excretion* of parent drug and metabolites.

TABLE 6-1   Physiologic Changes Affecting Drug Disposition in Older Adults.

Physiologic Change	Pharmacokinetic Parameter Affected
↑ Gastric pH	Absorption
↓ Gastric emptying time	
↓ GI motility	
↓ GI blood flow	
↓ Lean muscle mass	Distribution
↑ Total body fat	
↓ Total body water	
↓ Serum albumin	
↓ Cardiac output	
↓ Liver mass	Clearance (metabolism)
↓ Hepatic blood flow	
↓ Enzyme activity	
↓ Renal blood flow	Clearance (excretion)
↓ Glomerular filtration rate	
↓ Renal tubular function	

In short, clinical pharmacokinetics strives to reduce drug toxicity without compromising efficacy and/or to increase efficacy while avoiding toxicity. This is accomplished by maintaining blood concentrations of drugs within a proven therapeutic range. Age-related physiologic, and hence pharmacokinetic, changes affect the manner in which the body responds to medications (**Table 6-1**).[6,7] Careful consideration of these changes, combined with knowledge of which drugs are affected and how those drugs are influenced, allows estimation of the most appropriate dosing regimen.

ABSORPTION

Drugs are administered most frequently via the oral route, so changes in the gastrointestinal tract may translate into altered drug absorption and response. Age-related changes in the gastrointestinal tract include increased gastric pH, delayed gastric emptying time, and decreases in both intestinal motility and blood flow.[6] An increase in gastric pH can interfere with the dissolution or breakdown and subsequent pharmacologic response of some drugs. For example, the antifungal agent ketoconazole requires a low gastric pH to be broken down and subsequently available for systemic absorption.[1] When used in the setting of an increased gastric pH, the drug exhibits lowered therapeutic responses because of incomplete dissolution.

The delay in gastric emptying allows more contact time between drugs and the stomach. This can be problematic with potentially ulcer-causing drugs such as the non-steroidal anti-inflammatory agents (e.g., ibuprofen, naproxen). Increased drug–drug inter-actions are also possible, as is the case with antacids and other compounds containing a cation or positively charged element (e.g., calcium carbonate, magnesium hydroxide, aluminum hydroxide, iron, ferrous sulfate), as a result of increased binding (chelation) of the cation to other medications, such as tetracycline and quinolone antibiotics. Generally, this can be avoided by administering them at least 2 hours apart from one another.

Decreased cardiac output and blood flow may slightly affect the rate of absorption of drugs administered orally, as well as those administered topically, intramuscularly, and subcutaneously, as a result of reduced regional blood perfusion.[8] In general, however, despite the preceding changes, the *extent* of absorption and resulting bioavailability of most drugs are not significantly affected in older adults.[4,8] Because of the delay in gastric emptying and decreased motility, the *rate* of absorption may potentially be reduced, but any reduction is usually minor.

DISTRIBUTION

Various changes in the composition of the aging body influence the distribution of drugs. The *volume of distribution* is a term that refers to the extent to which a drug distributes throughout bodily tissues. It does not represent a specific body fluid or volume per se, but a virtual volume in which a given amount of drug would have to distribute to gener-ate the measured concentration.[5] It is dependent on several factors, including the extent of water solubility (**hydrophilicity**), fat solubility (**lipophilicity**), and plasma protein binding. Body composition changes with age, affecting each of these factors, so the volume of distribution of many drugs also changes.

The ratio of lean body mass to total body fat changes with age. Total body fat increases up to 45% as we grow older.[1,8] As a result, lipophilic drugs, which distribute extensively into fat tissue, may exhibit increased volumes of distribution. This is the case with the tranquilizing agent diazepam and the cardiovascular drugs amiodarone and verapamil. Consequently, lipophilic drugs often accumulate over time, resulting in a prolonged dura-tion of action and longer elimination half-lives as a result of delayed release from fat tissues.

Other drugs are hydrophilic (i.e., distribute primarily into water), and their volumes of distribution are proportional to lean body weight. Lean body weight reflects primarily skeletal muscle mass and total body water, which falls up to 15% by the age of 80 years compared to young healthy adults.[1,8] The decrease in both of these as we age reduces the volume of distribution of water-soluble compounds, resulting in higher plasma concentra-tions and more frequent toxicity than in younger people given the same dose.[8] Examples of hydrophilic drugs include ethanol, the antibiotics gentamicin and tobramycin, the antiulcer drug cimetidine, and lithium, a common antipsychotic medication.

As one ages, decreases in serum albumin concentrations may occur secondary to chronic disease states, malnutrition, and severe debilitation.[9] Because only the free, non-protein–bound fraction of a drug is active, a reduction in serum albumin concentrations may result in higher free drug concentrations and intensified pharmacologic effects. Acidic compounds, including oral antidiabetic agents, the antiepileptic agents phenytoin and phenobarbital, and the anticoagulant warfarin, bind primarily to albumin and should be used cautiously in patients with hypoalbuminemia.[9] Generally speaking, however, age-related changes in protein binding do not affect many drugs and are not clinically relevant.[8,9]

METABOLISM

Enzymatic metabolism or biotransformation by organs such as the liver and intestine is a crucial step in the elimination of drugs from the body. It serves to convert drugs through various metabolic pathways to more hydrophilic metabolites, which can then be excreted by the kidneys.[5] Hepatic metabolism of drugs is dependent on the organ's mass, microsomal enzyme activity, and blood flow. Hepatic mass decreases by approximately 1% per year after the age of 40, and blood flow to the liver may be reduced by up to 40% in older individuals.[1] This reduction in blood flow results in less of the drug being presented to the liver and decreased drug metabolism.

In addition to changes in blood flow, age influences the hepatic clearance of drugs by causing alterations in the intrinsic activity of selected microsomal enzymes. Drug metabolism occurs primarily via two enzyme pathways: phase I functional reactions (e.g., oxidation, reduction, hydrolysis) and phase II conjugation reactions (e.g., glucuronidation, acetylation, sulfation).[5] The cytochrome P450 superfamily of enzymes is responsible for the overwhelming majority of phase I metabolism. Phase I reactions are typically reduced in older adults, whereas phase II pathways generally remain unaffected.[4] As depicted in **Table 6-2**, the clearance of numerous drugs substrates of phase I and II metabolic enzymes is affected by age. For example, the benzodiazepine anxiolytic and hypnotic agents chlordiazepoxide, diazepam, and alprazolam all undergo phase I metabolism and have prolonged elimination half-lives in older adults.[5] Conversely, oxazepam, lorazepam, and temazepam undergo phase II conjugation, are not affected by age, and are preferred for use in older adults.[5]

EXCRETION

Kidney function is the most predictable and quantifiable determinant of drug clearance from the body. Reduction in kidney mass, the number of functioning nephrons, renal blood flow, glomerular filtration rate (GFR), and the rate of tubular secretion account for the decreased renal excretory capacity observed with aging.[1] Between the ages of 30 and 80 years, kidney mass decreases by about 25% and renal blood flow and GFR decline approximately 1% per year after the age of 40 years.[1,8] An otherwise healthy 70-year-old

TABLE 6-2 Representative Drugs with Reduced Clearance in Older Adults.

Clearance Pathway	Drugs	
Phase I metabolism	Chlordiazepoxide	Diazepam
	Alprazolam	Midazolam
	Diltiazem	Verapamil
	Propranolol	Theophylline
	Amiodarone	Cyclosporine
	Imipramine	Amitriptyline
Phase II metabolism	Morphine	
Renal excretion	Gentamicin	Vancomycin
	Nitrofurantoin	Ciprofloxacin
	Imipenem	Penicillins
	Fluconazole	Acyclovir
	Digoxin	Atenolol
	Lithium	Sotalol
	Glyburide	Ranitidine

person may have a 50% decrease in renal function, even in the absence of kidney disease.

Many drugs are renally excreted and require dosage adjustments in older adults to avoid toxicity (Table 6-2). Drug dosage adjustments are typically based on an individual's kidney GFR. GFR is easily estimated based on age, sex, race, and serum creatinine concentration.[10] This must be done with caution in older adults, however. Serum creatinine is a by-product of muscle that is almost completely excreted by the kidneys, so it is an excellent endogenous marker of kidney function. In normal young individuals, a decline in kidney function results in a predictable rise in serum creatinine concentration. However, because muscle mass decreases with aging, creatinine production and presence in the serum also decrease so that the serum creatinine value may not accurately reflect the true level of renal function in older adults. It is not uncommon for older adult patients with markedly reduced kidney function to have apparently normal serum creatinine concentrations.

Renally excreted drugs requiring dosage adjustments in older adults include numerous antimicrobials, the cardiovascular drug digoxin, lithium, and several antiulcer medications such as cimetidine, famotidine, and ranitidine (Table 6-2). Many drugs also require dose adjustment because of the production of active metabolites that are renally eliminated. These include the narcotic agents morphine, meperidine, and propoxyphene, the antiarrhythmics procainamide and disopyramide, and allopurinol, a drug used to prevent gout.

PHARMACODYNAMIC CHANGES

Pharmacodynamics refers to the biological effects resulting from the interaction between a drug and its receptor site, and generally describes the relationship between plasma drug concentrations and an observed effect or response.[11] Most age-related changes in drug response are a result of pharmacokinetic changes that alter the concentration of drug reaching the site of action or receptor site rather than changes at the site of action itself. In the setting of altered pharmacokinetics, target drug concentrations remain the same, and the dose or dosing interval is adjusted to compensate for the alteration to achieve the desired plasma concentration. However, despite these dosage adjustments and attainment of the desired drug concentrations, altered drug responses may still occur because of age-related pharmacodynamic changes.[11] The interrelationship between pharmacokinetics and pharmacodynamics is depicted in **Figure 6-1**.

Equal concentrations of drug at the site of action produce different effects in the young and the old. Although poorly studied, age-related pharmacodynamic changes in older adults can greatly influence drug response, usually leading to increased sensitivity or an exaggerated pharmacologic response to a given drug.[11] This is seen with benzodiazepines (e.g., alprazolam, lorazepam, midazolam), narcotic analgesics (e.g., morphine), anticoagulants (e.g., warfarin), and many antihypertensive agents.[8,11] Diminished pharmacologic responses may also be seen with certain cardiovascular drugs including beta-blocking (e.g., propranolol), beta-adrenergic (e.g., isoproterenol), and calcium channel blocking agents (e.g., verapamil).[1,8,11] Altered responses may be the result of depletion of neurotransmitters and changes at the receptor site, including a decreased number of receptors and a decreased affinity or sensitivity of receptors overall. Changes in the sensitivity of older adults to drug therapy often require new target drug concentrations and more aggressive or alternative means of monitoring drug response to achieve the desired effects. In an effort to minimize adverse outcomes, it is always best to "start low and go slow" when initiating treatment with new drugs—that is, start new drug therapy with low doses and slowly titrate doses upward until the desired effects are achieved.

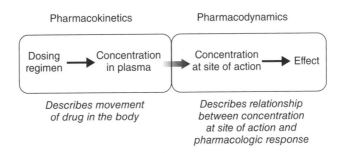

FIGURE 6-1 **The interrelationship between pharmacokinetics and pharmacodynamics.**

POLYPHARMACY

Polypharmacy, in simple terms, refers to the use of multiple medications in one individual.[12,13] In older adults, polypharmacy is often the rule rather than the exception.[14] Although the use of multiple medications may often be perfectly appropriate, the term *polypharmacy* usually connotes the use of more drugs than are clinically indicated or the excessive and unnecessary use of drugs, which in turn may lead to increased patient morbidity.[15] Indeed, as the number of medications taken increases, the likelihood of adverse drug reactions and drug–drug interactions also increases.[14,16] Furthermore, as the complexity of the drug regimen increases, the ability of older adults to adhere to the prescribed regimen diminishes.[17] As mentioned previously, age-related pharmacokinetic and pharmacodynamic changes in older persons make them uniquely susceptible to medication-related problems. For these reasons, the added element of polypharmacy is often detrimental to geriatric patients.

There are many possible reasons for polypharmacy. These include an increased number of chronic illnesses or physical ailments, a lack of one primary health care provider to coordinate medical care and drug use, subsequent use of multiple physicians (i.e., specialists), use of multiple pharmacies, and self-treatment, primarily with over-the-counter drugs, herbal remedies, or supplements.[13,18,19] More than 40% of ambulatory adults older than 65 years of age use at least 5 medications per week, and 12% use at least 10 medications per week.[19] It is not surprising that polypharmacy increases with advancing age.[20] In any age category, 50% of patients expect their physician to prescribe a drug at each office visit, and simultaneously, physicians often think that patients desire a prescription because it is seen as acknowledging the patient's ailment.[21] Ultimately, the final prescribing decision may result from the interaction of the patient, prescriber, and in some cases the family or caregiver.[22]

Studies have focused on establishing and quantifying the use of inappropriate medications in older persons and on discouraging their use.[12,15,23,24] One strategy to minimize polypharmacy requires shifting attention from specific inappropriate medications and refocusing on the appropriate use of medications.[16,22,25] It is important to distinguish between excessive and unnecessary drug use and a well-controlled drug regimen that appropriately and justifiably contains several agents. There is no magic number of drugs that equates to polypharmacy. We must resist the temptation simply to count the number of drugs a patient is receiving, determine it to be polypharmacy, and pass judgment on providers or the patient.

Strategies for reducing polypharmacy have been suggested.[14–16,21,26,27] A pharmacotherapeutic plan should be devised for every patient for whom drugs are prescribed.[16,22] Initially, nondrug therapies should be considered. Medications should only be prescribed with clear therapeutic goals in mind. Those with minimal side effects, the simplest dosing schedules, and the lowest cost should be selected whenever possible. Patients need to be educated regarding their drug regimens, and these should be routinely reevaluated every health care visit. Polypharmacy can be managed if the prescriber assesses each patient's drug regimen every time a patient is seen.[16,28] It is entirely possible for a drug that was appropriately prescribed initially to subsequently become inappropriate for various reasons, including the development of adverse effects or therapeutic failure.[16] If these situations are identified, older patients will receive maximal benefits from the fewest number of medications.

MEDICATION-RELATED PROBLEMS

Drugs, if used inappropriately, may cause more harm than good.[29] It has been estimated that up to 200,000 people may die in the United States each year from **medication-related problems** (MRPs), which are defined as "events or circumstances involving a patient's drug treatment that actually, or potentially, interfere with the achievement of an optimal outcome."[30] If adverse drug reactions, one type of MRP, were classified as a distinct disease, it would rank as the fifth leading cause of death in the United States.[31] Moreover, MRPs also have a significant financial impact in this country, costing us at least $200 billion annually.[29] Half of the morbidity and mortality caused by MRPs may be preventable.[32] By identifying, resolving, and preventing medication-related problems, a patient's medications are more likely to be appropriate, the most effective available, and correctly used. Common types of MRPs include untreated indications, drug use without indications, improper drug selection, incorrect dose, adverse drug reactions, drug interactions, and nonadherence. Each of these is described in the following subsections.

UNTREATED INDICATIONS

Untreated indications occur when the patient does not receive the therapy indicated for some medical condition or prophylactic need, such as immunizations.[33] Underuse of potentially beneficial medications is an increasingly recognized problem in older patients,[15,25,33] with some concluding that undertreatment of older persons is a problem equivalent to or of greater magnitude than that of medication overuse.[25,33,34] One example is the undertreatment of osteoporosis, a common condition resulting in significant adverse outcomes and an enormous economic burden.[27]

DRUG USE WITHOUT INDICATION

One of the primary goals of medication management in older adults is to eliminate medications being used without appropriate indications.[16] These include prescription and over-the-counter products for which there is currently no valid medical indication, the use of multiple drugs for a condition for which single-drug therapy is indicated, and drug therapy to treat an avoidable adverse effect caused by another medication. Use of unnecessary antihypertensive agents is a frequent example of this problem.[27] Frequent medication reassessment and cautious withdrawal of agents that do not have clearly defined indications improve the quality of pharmacotherapy in older adults.[35,36]

IMPROPER DRUG SELECTION

Improper drug selection occurs when the patient has a medical indication for which the prescribed drug is ineffective or less effective than alternatives, or if the patient has risk factors for which the medication is contraindicated, that is, prescribing a medication to which a patient is allergic.[27]

INCORRECT DOSE

The interindividual variability of drug response increases with age, so finding the optimal dose is not always straightforward in older individuals.[6] Adjusting doses to match appropriate physical attributes and organ function is essential; however, it is often overlooked. The start low and go slow drug dosing strategy is typically recommended. That said, whereas clinicians are usually concerned about excessive medication dosing, occasionally an inadequate dosage of medication may be prescribed.[16] For instance, antidepressant therapy is typically initiated at a low dose and titrated upward to response. Failure to titrate upward in the event that a favorable response is not achieved (i.e., an inadequate dosage) may lead to therapeutic failure.[27] Documenting response to therapy provides a rational basis for the modification, continuation, or discontinuation of a drug.

ADVERSE DRUG REACTIONS

An **adverse drug reaction** (ADR) is defined as an "undesirable response associated with use of a drug that either compromises therapeutic efficacy, enhances toxicity, or both."[37] The U.S. Food and Drug Administration approves drugs on the basis that their benefits outweigh their risks. All drugs have the ability to cause problems, from minor side effects to permanent disability and even death.[38-40] It is important to differentiate ADRs from normal side effects of drugs, which are extensions of the known pharmacologic activity of the drug in question and are therefore expected and predictable. The clinical picture can often be so complex that this differentiation may be extremely difficult to determine. ADRs typically have the following characteristics[39]:

- Require a modification in drug therapy (e.g., drug discontinuation or dosage change)
- Cause or prolong admission to the hospital
- Require supportive treatment
- Negatively affect prognosis
- May result in disability or death

ADRs may go undetected because the presenting symptoms may mimic problems commonly associated with older age, such as forgetfulness, weakness, or tremor.[2] ADRs also can be misinterpreted as a new medical condition and lead to drug use without indication.[2] A 2-year study of nursing home residents found that 74% had an ADR during their stay and at least 61% of the ADRs were preventable.[41] Common drug categories implicated in ADRs in older patients include cardiovascular drugs, antibiotics, diuretics, anticoagulants, hypoglycemic drugs, steroids, opioids, anticholinergics, benzodiazepines, and nonsteroidal anti-inflammatory drugs.[32,42,43] In fact, adverse events stemming from use of only three drugs—warfarin, insulin, and digoxin—have been shown to be responsible for up to one-third of emergency department and outpatient care visits in people at least 65 years of age.[44]

DRUG INTERACTIONS

Older patients are at high risk of drug interactions. This risk may be because of patient factors (e.g., concurrent use of many drugs, numerous comorbidities), prescriber factors, or difficulties within the health care system such as inefficient communication between health care professionals and patients.[45] Several types of interactions exist, including drug–drug interactions, drug–disease interactions, drug–food interactions, and drug–alcohol interactions.[45–51] Drug–drug interactions can be pharmacokinetic or pharmacodynamic in nature. The understanding and management of these varied types of interactions can be challenging. Common drug interactions are often detected by commercial drug interaction software systems; however, the detection of complex interactions is often difficult. The individual choice of drugs for each disorder is usually appropriate, but when combined with several other agents in the same patient, this can yield unwanted results.[45] Older patients have been shown to benefit by having their care managed by interdisciplinary teams that practice the principles of geriatric care focused on individualized pharmacotherapy.

NONADHERENCE

Nonadherence with prescribed drug regimens is a prevalent medication-related problem. In people age 60 years or older, rates of adherence to medication regimens range from 41% to 74%.[52] The term *adherence* more accurately reflects a therapeutic alliance or agreement between the patient and prescriber and is currently preferred over the now outdated term *compliance*, which suggests the passive following of the prescriber's orders.[53] Adherence also reflects the persistence, or length of time, with which regimen compliance has occurred.[54] Numerous potential barriers to adherence, depicted in **Figure 6-2**, need to be considered when devising strategies for improvement.[55] These take into account factors under the patient's control, as well as interactions between the patient and the health care provider and between the patient and the health care system.[55]

Medication adherence and health outcomes are affected by **health literacy**, defined as "the degree to which people have the capacity to obtain, process, and understand basic health information and services needed to make appropriate health decisions."[56] Health literacy has been found to be significantly lower among older persons, even after adjusting for various types of cognitive impairments.[57] Knowledge of the patients' health literacy and efforts to enhance it may improve adherence rates and subsequent health outcomes. Methods to improve health literacy, and thus adherence, have been grouped into four general categories[55]:

- Patient education
- Improved dosing schedules
- Increased access to clinic or office visits, such as longer open hours
- Improved communication between patients and health care providers

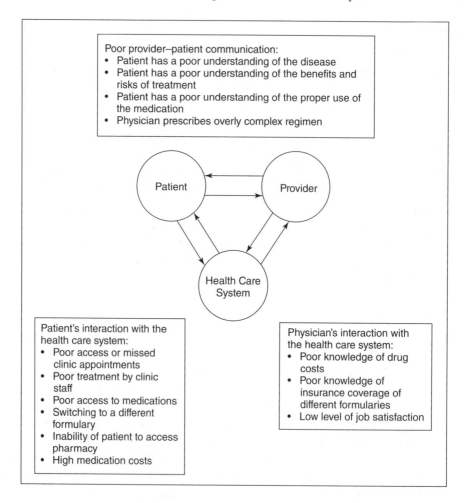

FIGURE 6-2   Barriers to adherence.

The interactions among the patient, health care provider, and health care system depicted are those that can have a negative effect on the patient's ability to follow a medication regimen.

Source: Osterberg, L, Blaschke, T. Adherence to medication. *New England Journal of Medicine,* 2005;353(5):492. Reprinted with permission. © 2000 Massachusetts Medical Society. All rights reserved.

Despite use of these methods, low adherence is generally not "cured." So, efforts to improve adherence must be maintained for as long as the treatment is needed.[58]

DRUG ABUSE

Drug abuse among older adults may not be as prevalent as in younger age groups, but it does exist. Of the drugs abused by older adults, alcohol is the most common.[59] With age-related physiologic changes, older adults may experience unfavorable health effects even from relatively low levels of alcohol consumption.[60] Older patients are more likely to use multiple alcohol-interactive medications, as well as have interactive medical conditions and diminishing functional status.[50] Screening for alcohol use is essential, as well as the provision of warnings to patients regarding potential detrimental effects, to minimize adverse reactions.[50,51,60]

MEDICATION MANAGEMENT

Medication management generally involves periodic review of a patient's medications (prescription, nonprescription, vitamin supplements, herbal remedies, and nutritional products) to assess whether they are medically necessary, tailor prescriptions accordingly, and consult with patients to ensure that they understand the purpose and use of their medications.[61] Before initiating new drug therapy, nondrug treatments such as lifestyle modifications (e.g., diet and exercise programs), occupational and/or physical therapy, and psychotherapy should be employed first if possible. When medically justified, drugs should be prescribed with clear therapeutic goals in mind for each agent, including dosing schedule, monitoring parameters, duration of therapy, and desired outcome or endpoint. Medications should be stopped when desired goals or outcomes are not met. Individual patients should be evaluated for issues that may contribute to poor adherence. Factors to consider when initiating new drug treatment include the drug's efficacy and side effect profile, cost, perceived and actual affordability, dosing schedule, and ease of administration. The effect of pharmacokinetic and pharmacodynamic changes and the likelihood of developing medication-related problems should be considered. The lowest possible effective dose should be the starting point. Patients should be well informed regarding their new medications and provided with opportunities to express concerns or questions. The indications, benefits, potential adverse effects, and directions for use should be clearly explained. Well-written instructions should also be provided (see Chapter 13). During subsequent visits, monitoring parameters should be reviewed and endpoints or outcomes desired initially should be assessed to determine whether they have been met.

Communicating the pharmaceutical care plan across all settings is essential to prevent medication-related problems as old prescriptions are discontinued and new drugs are initiated. Effective communication with family members and caregivers is especially important to prevent hospitalizations because of side effects from unintended drug combinations.

PORTABLE PERSONAL MEDICATION RECORDS

An up-to-date medication list that is readily accessible to the patient and all caregivers is a critical component of medication management. This list should include all prescription medications, over-the-counter medication, herbals, and dietary supplements. This comprehensive medication list allows efficient and ongoing drug regimen review and evaluation. A majority of patients do self-medicate with nonprescription alternatives, making it essential for these to be included in any medication list. For example, one-third of over-the-counter drugs sold in the United States are used by patients older than 65 years,[62] and more than half of all older adults have reported using dietary supplements within the past 6 months.[63]

MEDICATION THERAPY MANAGEMENT SERVICES

The prevention and resolution of medication-related problems can be addressed through medication therapy management (MTM) services. This is a recognized covered service in the Medicare Part D drug benefit, some state Medicaid programs, and other private pay plans. MTM services are usually provided directly to the patient by licensed pharmacists, but may also be performed by other qualified health care providers. Taking into account the individual needs of the patient, MTM services include but are not limited to the following[64]:

- Performing or obtaining necessary assessments of the patient's health status
- Formulating a medication treatment plan
- Selecting, initiating, modifying, or administering medication therapy
- Monitoring and evaluating the patient's response to therapy, including safety and effectiveness
- Performing a comprehensive medication review to identify, resolve, and prevent medication-related problems, including adverse drug events
- Documenting the care delivered and communicating essential information to the patient's other primary care providers
- Providing verbal education and training designed to enhance patient understanding and appropriate use of his or her medications
- Providing information, support services, and resources designed to enhance patient adherence with his or her therapeutic regimens
- Coordinating and integrating medication therapy management services within the broader health care management services being provided to the patient

Further information regarding MTM services may be viewed at the website of the American Pharmacists Association.

SUMMARY

Drug therapy offers tremendous benefits to older people when used appropriately. However, inherent risks associated with suboptimal drug use in this tenuous population create challenges for professionals working with them. The effective management of medication regimens in older adults requires knowledge of the relevant issues. Pharmacokinetic and pharmacodynamic changes necessitate unique dosing and the careful selection of medications to minimize polypharmacy, minimize adverse effects, and improve adherence. We must become attuned to reviewing medication regimens with these issues in mind and develop a high index of suspicion for medication-related problems. In doing so, we will ensure that older patients receive maximal benefits from drug therapy while minimizing potential adverse outcomes.

Review Questions

1. Despite numerous pharmacokinetic changes in older adults, the extent of drug _____ is not significantly affected in older adults.
   A. Absorption
   B. Distribution
   C. Hepatic metabolism
   D. Renal excretion

2. Which of the following is the most predictable pharmacokinetic change in older adults?
   A. Absorption
   B. Distribution
   C. Hepatic metabolism
   D. Renal excretion

3. *Pharmacodynamics* refers to
   A. Movement of drugs through the body
   B. The inability of drugs to move through the body
   C. The biological effects of drugs on the body
   D. Constantly changing pharmacokinetic parameters

4. Pharmacodynamic changes in older adults usually result in _____ pharmacologic responses.
   A. Diminished
   B. Unchanged
   C. Exaggerated
   D. Absent

5. Possible reasons for polypharmacy include which of the following?
   A. Lack of chronic illnesses
   B. Self-medication
   C. Use of a primary care physician
   D. Financial wealth

6. Medication-related problems often include
   A. Adherence to medications
   B. Accurate medication doses
   C. Adverse drug reactions
   D. Appropriate medication indications

7. Which of the following answers includes only potential barriers to adherence?
   A. Poor provider knowledge of drug costs, use of simple drug regimens, poor provider–patient communication
   B. Poor provider knowledge of drug costs, use of complex drug regimens, improved provider–patient communication
   C. Overly complex drug regimens, poor understanding of the proper use of the medication, low medication costs
   D. Poor provider–patient communication, poor access to medications, poor provider knowledge of drug costs

8. Commonly observed ADRs that often mimic common complaints or symptoms in the older patient include
   A. Confusion, irritability
   B. Forgetfulness, weakness, tremor
   C. Diarrhea, constipation, bladder obstruction
   D. Leukopenia, thrombocytopenia

9. An essential component of medication management includes
   A. Reviewing the patient's drug regimen every other visit
   B. Continuing medications that are no longer medically indicated
   C. Educating patients regarding their medications
   D. Taking no notice of patient's complaints

10. The prevention of medication-related problems can be addressed through MTM services. Which of the following statements is *false*?
    A. These services are usually provided by licensed pharmacists.
    B. Evaluating the patient's response to therapy is a component of this service.
    C. MTM services are not recognized by the Medicare Part D drug benefit.
    D. Integration of MTM services within patients' broader health care management services is important.

Learning Activities

1. Role-playing; two individuals required. One person plays an older adult patient with several chronic diseases, including arthritis and visual impairment, and limited income. Another plays a health care provider counseling the patient on how to take the medications. Generally speaking, what are the problems encountered by each individual and how can they be minimized?
2. Design a pharmacotherapeutic plan for the patient in activity 1. What strategies can be used by the health care provider to improve adherence?
3. Assume each of the following scenarios occurs in an older adult patient. Describe what the primary problem is and how it may be avoided or corrected.
   A. A patient taking an expensive medication every other day versus daily as prescribed so that it will "last longer."
   B. A patient started on a new H_2 antagonist for a peptic ulcer at normal dosing a few days later develops confusion.
   C. A patient receiving multiple medications, all of which are taken at different times of the day. When asked, he or she has no idea what each medication is, what it is used for, or when to take it.

REFERENCES

1. McLean, AJ, Le Couteur, DG. Aging biology and geriatric clinical pharmacology. *Pharmacological Reviews*, 2004;56(2):163–184.
2. Linnebur, SA, O'Connell, MB, Wessell, AM, et al. Pharmacy practice, research, education, and advocacy for older adults. *Pharmacotherapy*, 2005;25(10):1396–1430.
3. Williams, CM. Using medications appropriately in older adults. *American Family Physician*, 2002; 66(10):1917–1924.
4. Schwartz, JB. The current state of knowledge on age, sex, and their interactions on clinical pharmacology. *Clinical Pharmacology and Therapeutics*, 2007;82(1):87–96.
5. Bressler R, Bahl, JJ. Principles of drug therapy for the elderly patient. *Mayo Clinic Proceedings*, 2003;78(12):1564–1577.
6. Mangoni, AA, Jackson, SH. Age-related changes in pharmacokinetics and pharmacodynamics: Basic principles and practical applications. *British Journal of Clinical Pharmacology*, 2004;57(1): 6–14.
7. Cusack, BJ. Pharmacokinetics in older persons. *American Journal of Geriatric Pharmacotherapy*, 2004;2(4):274–302.
8. Turnheim, K. When drug therapy gets old: Pharmacokinetics and pharmacodynamics in the elderly. *Experimental Gerontology*, 2003;38(8): 843–853.
9. Grandison, MK, Boudinot, FD. Age-related changes in protein binding of drugs: Implications for therapy. *Clinical Pharmacokinetics*, 2000;38(3):271–290.
10. Levey, AS, Bosch, JP, Lewis, JB, Greene, T, Rogers, N, Roth, D. A more accurate method to estimate glomerular filtration rate from serum creatinine: A new prediction equation. Modification of Diet in Renal Disease Study Group. *Annals of Internal Medicine*, 1999;130(6):461–470.
11. Bowie, MW, Slattum, PW. Pharmacodynamics in older adults: A review. *American Journal of Geriatric Pharmacotherapy*, 2007;5(3):263–303.

12. Chutka, DS, Takahashi, PY, Hoel, RW. Inappropriate medications for elderly patients. *Mayo Clinic Proceedings*, 2004;79(1):122–139.

13. Stewart, RB. Polypharmacy in the elderly: A fait accompli? *Drug Intelligence and Clinical Pharmacy*, 1990;24(3):321–323.

14. Hayes, BD, Klein-Schwartz, W, Barrueto, F Jr. Polypharmacy and the geriatric patient. *Clinics in Geriatric Medicine*, 2007;23(2):371–390.

15. Hanlon, JT, Schmader, KE, Ruby, CM, Weinberger, M. Suboptimal prescribing in older inpatients and outpatients. *Journal of the American Geriatrics Society*, 2001;49(2):200–209.

16. Shrank, WH, Polinski, JM, Avorn J. Quality indicators for medication use in vulnerable elders. *Journal of the American Geriatrics Society*, 2007;55(Suppl 2):S373–S382.

17. Eisen, SA, Miller, DK, Woodward, RS, Spitznagel, E, Przybeck, TR. The effect of prescribed daily dose frequency on patient medication compliance. *Archives of Internal Medicine*, 1990;150(9):1881–1884.

18. Anderson, GF. Medicare and chronic conditions. *New England Journal of Medicine*, 2005;353(3):305–309.

19. Kaufman, DW, Kelly, JP, Rosenberg, L, Anderson, TE, Mitchell, AA. Recent patterns of medication use in the ambulatory adult population of the United States: The Slone survey. *Journal of the American Medical Association*, 2002;287(3):337–344.

20. Jyrkka, J, Vartiainen, L, Hartikainen, S, Sulkava, R, Enlund, H. Increasing use of medicines in elderly persons: A five-year follow-up of the Kuopio 75+Study. *European Journal of Clinical Pharmacology*, 2006;62(2):151–158.

21. Rollason, V, Vogt, N. Reduction of polypharmacy in the elderly: A systematic review of the role of the pharmacist. *Drugs and Aging*, 2003; 20(11):817–832.

22. Spinewine, A, Schmader, KE, Barber, N, et al. Appropriate prescribing in elderly people: How well can it be measured and optimised? *Lancet*, 2007;370(9582):173–184.

23. Buetow, SA, Sibbald, B, Cantrill, JA, Halliwell, S. Appropriateness in health care: Application to prescribing. *Social Science and Medicine*, 1997;45(2):261–271.

24. Fick, DM, Cooper, JW, Wade, WE, Waller, JL, Maclean, JR, Beers, MH. Updating the Beers criteria for potentially inappropriate medication use in older adults: Results of a U.S. consensus panel of experts. *Archives of Internal Medicine*, 2003;163(22):2716–2724.

25. Higashi, T, Shekelle, PG, Solomon, DH, et al. The quality of pharmacologic care for vulnerable older patients. *Annals of Internal Medicine*, 2004;140(9):714–720.

26. Montamat, SC, Cusack, B. Overcoming problems with polypharmacy and drug misuse in the elderly. *Clinics in Geriatric Medicine*, 1992;8(1): 143–158.

27. Simonson, W, Feinberg, JL. Medication-related problems in the elderly: Defining the issues and identifying solutions. *Drugs and Aging*, 2005;22(7):559–569.

28. Sherman, FT. Medication nonadherence: A national epidemic among America's seniors. *Geriatrics*, 2007;62(4):5–6.

29. Cameron, KA. Preventing medication-related problems among older Americans. *Managed Care Interface*, 1998;11(10):74–76, 78, 83–85.

30. Hepler, CD, Strand, LM. Opportunities and responsibilities in pharmaceutical care. *American Journal of Health-System Pharmacy*, 1990;47(3):533–543.

31. Lazarou, J, Pomeranz, BH, Corey, PN. Incidence of adverse drug reactions in hospitalized patients: A meta-analysis of prospective studies. *Journal of the American Medical Association*, 1998; 279(15):1200–1205.

32. Gurwitz, JH, Field, TS, Harrold, LR, et al. Incidence and preventability of adverse drug events among older persons in the ambulatory setting. *Journal of the American Medical Association*, 2003;289(9):1107–1116.

33. Sloane, PD, Gruber-Baldini, AL, Zimmerman, S, et al. Medication undertreatment in assisted living settings. *Archives of Internal Medicine*, 2004;164(18):2031–2037.

34. Bain, K. Prevalence and predictors of medication-related problems. *Medicare Patient Management*, 2006:14–27.

35. Monane, M, Matthias, DM, Nagle, BA, Kelly, MA. Improving prescribing patterns for the elderly through an online drug utilization review

intervention: A system linking the physician, pharmacist, and computer. *Journal of the American Medical Association*, 1998;280(14): 1249–1252.

36. Tamblyn, R, Huang, A, Perreault, R, et al. The medical office of the 21st century (MOXXI): Effectiveness of computerized decision-making support in reducing inappropriate prescribing in primary care. *Canadian Medical Association Journal*, 2003;169(6):549–556.

37. Joint Commission. Sentinel Event Glossary of Terms. 2007. Retrieved February 5, 2008, from http://www.jointcommission.org/Sentinel Events/se_glossary.htm

38. Kelly, WN. Potential risks and prevention, Part 2: Drug-induced permanent disabilities. *American Journal of Health-System Pharmacy*, 2001;58(14):1325–1329.

39. Kelly, WN. Potential risks and prevention, Part 1: Fatal adverse drug events. *American Journal of Health-System Pharmacy*, 2001;58(14):1317–1324.

40. Marcellino K, Kelly, WN. Potential risks and prevention, Part 3: Drug-induced threats to life. *American Journal of Health-System Pharmacy*, 2001;58(15):1399–1405.

41. Cooper, JW. Adverse drug reaction-related hospitalizations of nursing facility patients: A 4-year study. *Southern Medical Journal*, 1999;92(5):485–490.

42. Hajjar, ER, Hanlon, JT, Artz, MB, et al. Adverse drug reaction risk factors in older outpatients. *American Journal of Geriatric Pharmacotherapy*, 2003;1(2):82–89.

43. Routledge, PA, O'Mahony, MS, Woodhouse, KW. Adverse drug reactions in elderly patients. *British Journal of Clinical Pharmacology*, 2004; 57(2):121–126.

44. Budnitz, DS, Shehab, N, Kegler, SR, Richards, CL. Medication use leading to emergency department visits for adverse drug events in older adults. *Annals of Internal Medicine*, 2007;147(11): 755–765.

45. Mallet, L, Spinewine, A, Huang, A. The challenge of managing drug interactions in elderly people. *Lancet*, 2007;370(9582):185–191.

46. Charrois, TL, Hill, RL, Vu, D, et al. Community identification of natural health product-drug interactions. *Annals of Pharmacotherapy*, 2007; 41(7):1124–1129.

47. Elmer, GW, Lafferty, WE, Tyree, PT, Lind, BK. Potential interactions between complementary/ alternative products and conventional medicines in a Medicare population. *Annals of Pharmaco- therapy*, 2007;41(10):1617–1624.

48. Fugh-Berman, A. Herb–drug interactions. *Lancet*, 2000;355(9198):134–138.

49. Juurlink, DN, Mamdani, M, Kopp, A, Laupacis, A, Redelmeier, DA. Drug–drug interactions among elderly patients hospitalized for drug toxi- city. *Journal of the American Medical Association*, 2003;289(13):1652–1658.

50. Pringle, KE, Ahern, FM, Heller, DA, Gold, CH, Brown, TV. Potential for alcohol and prescrip- tion drug interactions in older people. *Journal of the American Geriatrics Society*, 2005;53(11): 1930–1936.

51. Tanaka, E. Toxicological interactions involving psychiatric drugs and alcohol: An update. *Journal of Clinical Pharmacy and Therapeutics*, 2003;28(2):81–95.

52. van Eijken, M, Tsang, S, Wensing, M, de Smet, PA, Grol, RP. Interventions to improve medica- tion compliance in older patients living in the community: A systematic review of the literature. *Drugs and Aging*, 2003;20(3):229–240.

53. Steiner, JF, Earnest, MA. The language of medication-taking. *Annals of Internal Medicine*, 2000;132(11):926–930.

54. Gold, DT. Medication adherence: A challenge for patients with postmenopausal osteoporosis and other chronic illnesses. *Journal of Managed Care Pharmacy*, 2006;12(6 Suppl A):S20– S25.

55. Osterberg, L, Blaschke, T. Adherence to medica- tion. *New England Journal of Medicine*, 2005; 353(5):487–497.

56. Parker, RM, Ratzan, SC, Lurie, N. Health liter- acy: A policy challenge for advancing high- quality health care. *Health Affairs* (*Millwood*), 2003;22(4):147–153.

57. Baker, DW, Gazmararian, JA, Sudano, J, Pat- terson, M. The association between age and health literacy among elderly persons. *Journal of Gerontology Series B: Psychological Sciences and Social Sciences*, 2000;55(6):S368–S374.

58. Haynes, RB, Yao, X, Degani, A, Kripalani, S, Garg, A, McDonald, HP. Interventions to enhance medication adherence. *Cochrane Database of Systematic Reviews*, 2005(4):CD000011.

59. Office of Applied Studies, Substance Abuse and Mental Health Services Administration. Substance use among older adults: 2002 and 2003 update. 2005. Retrieved March 10, 2008, from http://www.oas.samhsa.gov/2k5/olderadults/olderadults.cfm

60. Fink, A, Elliott, MN, Tsai, M, Beck, JC. An evaluation of an intervention to assist primary care physicians in screening and educating older patients who use alcohol. *Journal of the American Geriatrics Society*, 2005;53(11):1937–1943.

61. Alkema, GE, Frey, D. Implications of translating research into practice: A medication management intervention. *Home Health Care Services Quarterly*, 2006;25(1–2):33–54.

62. Consumer Healthcare Products Association. OTC Facts and Figures. 2000. Retrieved January 22, 2009, from http://www.chpa-info.org/pressroom/OTC_FactsandFigures.aspx

63. Consumer Healthcare Products Association. Dietary Supplement Facts and Figures. 2006. Retrieved January 22, 2009, from http://www.chpa-info.org/pressroom/DS_FactsandFigures.aspx

64. Academy of Managed Care Pharmacy. Appendix A. In *Sound Medication Therapy Management Programs: 2006 Consensus Document*. Retrieved January 22, 2009, from http://www.amcp.org/data/nav_content/websiteMTMdocument.pdf

NUTRITION AND AGING

LOUISE D. WHITNEY, MS, RD, AND
SHEFALI AJMERA, MS, RD, LD

Thanks in old age—thanks ere I go,
For health, the mid-day sun, the
Impalpable air for life, mere life.

—*Walt Whitman,* Leaves of Grass, *1892*

Chapter Outline

Behavioral Objectives

Upon completion of this chapter, the reader will be able to:

1. Demonstrate knowledge of current research on the impact of aging on nutrition status for healthy individuals and individuals with chronic diseases.

2. Describe the importance of early screening and intervention for nutrition risk in older adults.
3. Describe knowledge of available screening tools.
4. Understand the multiple factors that affect nutrition status in older adults (physiologic, social, psychological, economic, and environmental).
5. Describe the physiologic impact of aging on nutrition.
6. Understand the essential nutrients, the Modified MyPyramid for older adults, and special considerations regarding nutrition for older adults.
7. Understand the impact of polypharmacy on nutritional status and drug and nutrient interactions in older adults.
8. List the indications for supplemental nutrition in older adults.

Key Terms

Antacids

Antidepressants

Anti-inflammatory

Carbohydrates

Cholesterol

Diabetes

Dietary fiber

Diuretics

Essential nutrients

Exchanges for meal planning

Gastrointestinal

Glucose tolerance

Lactose intolerance

Lipid

Monounsaturated fat

Polyunsaturated fat

Saturated fat

Supplemental nutrition

The importance of good nutrition throughout the life span and its contribution to health and quality of life cannot be overestimated. Optimum nutrition is equally important during the elderly years, when the myriad changes caused by aging can compromise health. Good nutrition optimizes health and promotes wellness. A prudent diet strengthens the immune system and helps prevent the onset of many chronic diseases, such as cardiovascular disease, diabetes, renal disease, osteoporosis, and cancer. Not surprisingly, 9 out of 10 people with chronic diseases have health problems that could be managed successfully through nutrition intervention to prevent future complications. To improve the health of older people, the Older Americans Act of 2006 places special emphasis on integrated health promotion and disease prevention through delivering nutrition education to older adults.[1,2]

Poor diet is among the major root causes for almost 35% of older adults' deaths in the United States. Malnutrition is a serious health problem, and many times it is underdiagnosed in elderly individuals.[3] The prevalence of malnutrition is 5–44% in those who are homebound, 20–66% among hospitalized older adults, and even higher, 23–85%, among nursing home residents.[4]

Despite these dietary concerns, the average life span of individuals has increased drastically over the past few decades. In 1940, only 7% of Americans age 65 years were expected to live to age 90. Now, more than 27% are expected to become nonagenarians, and by 2050, given life circumstances similar to today, nearly 50% of 65-year-olds will reach this milestone.[5] In the next 20 years, the older population is predicted to reach 71 million, which will account for nearly 20% of the total U.S. population. The cost of providing health care to the older American population is three to five times greater than providing health care to those younger than 65 years of age.[3]

Proper nutrition is important to ensure good health, not only to prevent chronic diseases but also to manage these chronic conditions and help prevent future complications.[2] This chapter discusses the nutritional needs of older people, the importance of early nutrition screening and intervention, the physiologic effects of aging on nutritional status, and special dietary considerations related to aging. This chapter also briefly discusses the needs for supplemental nutrition and the impact of drugs on the nutritional status of older adults.

SCREENING AND INTERVENTION

THE NUTRITION SCREENING INITIATIVE

One of the best ways to achieve high-quality nutrition care for older adults is to promote early screening and intervention. Since 1989, the American Dietetic Association, the National Council on Aging, and the American Academy of Family Physicians have collaborated in an effort called the Nutrition Screening Initiative (NSI) to encourage early and routine screening and intervention for nutrition risk in older adults.[6] The premise of the initiative is that nutrition status is a "vital sign" just as important in evaluating a person's health and well-being as the traditional vital signs of blood pressure and pulse.

The result of the Nutrition Screening Initiative is a self-assessment checklist that can be used in a variety of settings to help identify whether an individual is at risk for compromised nutritional well-being. In addition to the self-assessment checklist, the acronym DETERMINE is an educational device that can be used along with the checklist to help identify the warning signs of poor nutritional status in older adults. The self-assessment checklist and meaning of DETERMINE are presented in **Boxes 7-1** and **7-2**.

The Subjective Global Assessment (SGA; available at http://www.hospitalmedicine. org/geriresource/toolbox/pdfs/subjective_global_assessmen.pdf) and Mini Nutrition Assessment (MNA; available at http://www.mna-elderly.com/mna_forms.html) are similar to the NSI and are reliable tools to determine nutrition risk and presence of malnutrition.

MULTIPLE FACTORS AFFECTING NUTRITION STATUS

For many, the late-life years are a time of great change socially, economically, psychologically, and physically. With the death of a spouse and/or friends, many older adults find

BOX 7-1 NUTRITION SCREENING INITIATIVE SELF-ASSESSMENT CHECKLIST.

Answer the following questions as carefully as you can. If you answer yes, add up the points and compare with the point evaluation scale. This checklist will help you determine if you are nutritionally at risk.

Question	Yes
I have an illness or condition that has recently made me change the kind and/or amount of food I eat.	2 pts
I eat fewer than two meals per day.	3
I rarely eat fruits, vegetables, and milk products.	2
I have three or more glasses of beer, liquor, or wine almost every day.	2
I have tooth or mouth problems that make it hard for me to eat.	2
I don't always have enough money to buy the food I need.	4
I eat alone most of the time.	1
I take three or more different prescription or over-the-counter drugs a day.	1
Without wanting to, I have lost or gained 10 pounds in the past 6 months.	2
I am not always physically able to shop, cook, and/or feed myself.	2
Total Score	

Point Evaluation Scale

0–2	Good! Recheck your score in 6 months.
3–5	You are at a moderate nutritional risk. See what can be done to improve your eating habits and lifestyle. The Area Agency on Aging, senior nutrition programs, senior citizen centers, or health departments may be able to help. Recheck your score in 3 months.
6+	You are at nutritional risk. Bring this checklist the next time you see your doctor, dietitian, or other qualified health care giver. Ask for nutrition counseling.

Adapted from: The Nutrition Screening Initiative, a project of the American Academy of Family Physicians, the American Dietetic Association, and the National Council on Aging; 1989.

themselves living alone and eating meals alone. Changes in income as a result of retirement can mean fewer resources are available for food purchases. Older adults may also experience more limited mobility related to various joint, muscular, and other health problems. Individually or in combination, these factors interact and influence nutritional

BOX 7-2   DETERMINE.

Use this to help you remember the warning signs of nutrition risk.

D   **Disease**—The presence of any disease causing a change in eating habits may make it harder to eat right and will increase risk. Four of five adults have chronic diseases affected by diet. Confusion and memory loss may make it harder to plan healthy diets and even to remember what and when you last ate. Depression and loneliness can cause changes in appetite, digestion, energy level, weight, and well-being.

E   **Eating poorly**—Both eating too little or eating too much can cause a decline in health status. Lack of variety, poor quality foods, and poor balance of food types all lead to poor nutritional health. Many older adults skip meals and eat fewer than the recommended five servings daily of fruits and vegetables. Alcohol consumption is a concern, with one in four adults drinking too much.

T   **Tooth loss or mouth pain**—Healthy mouth, gums, and teeth are essential to good nutrition. When dental health is compromised, so is nutritional well-being.

E   **Economic hardship**—Although Social Security and Medicare have made great progress in combating poverty among older adults (approximately 35% were below the poverty level in 1959, whereas in 2003 only 10.2% fell below the poverty level; U.S. Department of Commerce, Bureau of the Census, 2003), financial struggles may make it harder to eat right and stay healthy.

R   **Reduced social contact**—Approximately one-third of all older people live alone. For a variety of reasons, aging brings with it fewer meaningful social contacts. This too can affect nutritional well-being.

M   **Multiple medicines**—Polypharmacy, the use of multiple drugs, can also compromise nutritional well-being. Almost half of older Americans take multiple medicines daily. Some of the side effects include changes in appetite and taste, constipation, weakness, and nausea.

I   **Involuntary weight gain or loss**—Changes in weight (more than just a few pounds) should always be seen as a warning sign that a person's nutrition status may be compromised.

N   **Needs assistance in self-care**—Older people who need help with walking, shopping, cooking, and feeding are at risk for decreased nutritional status.

E   **Elder years past age 80**—Increasing age brings increased risk of health problems. Be sure to see your physician regularly, at least on an annual basis.

Adapted from: The Nutrition Screening Initiative, a project of the American Academy of Family Physicians, the American Dietetic Association, and the National Council on Aging; 1989.

status in older adults. Health care professionals should show great sensitivity to the wide variation of physiologic, socioeconomic, environmental, and psychological changes that accompany aging. Various factors and their interactions are summarized in **Box 7-3**.

PHYSIOLOGIC IMPACT OF AGING ON NUTRITION

DECREASED APPETITE, DECREASED FOOD INTAKE, AND WEIGHT LOSS

One of the critical physiologic changes accompanying aging can be declining appetite, resulting in decreased food intake and subsequent loss of body weight. Decreases in body weight are common in adults ages 65 to 90, and this should always be seen as a warning sign that the individual may be at nutritional risk. There are several explanations for a decrease in appetite and food intake that may lead to weight loss.

First, aging brings about changes in the endocrine system, which regulates hunger, appetite, and satiety. In addition, loss of lean tissue because of decreased physical activity and the normal aging process reduces metabolic rate, and this too may result in decreased appetite. Changes in taste and smell, which begin around age 60 and become more pronounced after age 70, may also account for reduced appetite. Reduced taste and smell acuity can also be caused by certain drugs and medications. Additionally, zinc deficiencies can also lead to loss of taste. **Table 7-1** presents a summary of the effects of certain categories of drugs.

When an older adult loses 5% or more of his or her weight in 1 month or 10% or more in 6 months, health care providers need to pursue ways to aggressively stimulate appetite and increase food intake. Sensitivity to the possible causes of the weight loss aids in finding ways to make foods appealing and attractive. New food combinations and new and stronger seasonings may make old favorites more palatable. Modifying food preparation techniques may also help stimulate interest in eating. Great care should be taken to ensure that nutrient-dense foods are eaten. To encourage weight gain, healthy snacking and a high-calorie nutritional supplement might be in order. (For additional information, see the section titled "Liquid Nutrition Supplements" later in this chapter.)

Following are suggestions to increase appetite:

- Suggest regular moderate exercise, which will stimulate appetite and hunger.
- Encourage testing of new recipes, the use of fresh herbs, and communal food preparation gatherings.
- Encourage eating with friends and neighbors.
- Locate assistance if financial needs are limiting intake of food (a referral to a social worker may be in order).

Refer the person to a physician to determine whether drugs or zinc deficiency is the cause and suggest increased intake of zinc-rich foods. (**Table 7-2** lists food sources of zinc.)

BOX 7-3 SUMMARY OF FACTORS THAT CAN INFLUENCE NUTRITION STATUS IN OLDER ADULTS.

Physiologic
  Health status
  Presence of chronic diseases
  Changes in appetite
  Physical disability
  Sensory functioning
  Physical activity
  Alcohol use
  Medication or drug use
  Lifelong dietary habits

Socioeconomic
  Culture/ethnicity
  Income
  Education
  Lifestyle
  Nutrition knowledge and practice
  Cooking skills
  Susceptibility to food fads
  Institutionalization

Psychological
  Belief systems
  Motivation
  Self-image
  Mental status
  Degree of independence
  Feeling of usefulness
  Presence or absence of spouse
  Social contacts
  Loneliness

Environmental
  Type and location of housing
  Adequacy of cooking facilities
  Proximity of family and friends
  Availability of transportation
  Availability, accessibility, and adequacy of food supply
  Availability of health services

Adapted from: Boyle, M, Zyla, G. *Personal Nutrition.* Minneapolis, MN: West Publishing; 1996:400.

TABLE 7-1   Drugs That Affect Appetite.

Examples of Drugs That Increase Appetite	Examples of Drugs That Decrease Appetite
Alcohol	Antibiotics
Antihistamines	Bulk agents
Corticosteroids	Indomethacin
Insulin	Digoxin
Thyroid hormone	Glucagon
Psychoactive drugs	Morphine
	Fluoxetine

Source: Beers, MH, Porter, RS, Jones, TV, Kaplan, JL, Berkwits, M. Nutrition: general considerations. *The Merck Manual* (18th ed.). Whitehouse Station, NJ: Merck & Co., Inc.; 2006.

TABLE 7-2   Dietary Requirements and Examples of Food Sources of Zinc.

Recommended Dietary Allowances:
Females 51+: 12 mg (7.9 mg/1,000 kcal)
Males 51+: 15 mg (8.2 mg/1,000 kcal)

Source	Portion	Amount of Zinc
Oysters	6 medium	77 mg
Beef shank steak	3 ounces	8.9 mg
Alaska crab	3 ounces	6.5 mg
Chicken	1 leg	2.7 mg
Yogurt	1 cup	1.6 mg
Cashews	1 ounce	1.6 mg
Chickpeas	½ cup	1.3 mg
Swiss cheese	1 ounce	1.1 mg

Sources: Fosmire, GJ. Trace Metal Requirements. In R Chernoff (ed.), *Geriatric Nutrition.* 2nd ed. Sudbury, MA: Jones and Bartlett; 2003. National Institute of Health. *Dietary Supplement Fact Sheet: Zinc.* Retrieved November 21, 2008, from http://ods.od.nih.gov/FactSheet/Zinc.asp#h3

DENTAL HEALTH

Although over the past few decades more people have been able to retain their natural teeth, a significant portion of older people are still edentate (having total loss of teeth). The percentage varies among states in the United States, from 13% having lost all their teeth in California and Hawaii to 42% in Kentucky.[7] Changes in dentition can be a real challenge for many older adults. Mouth pain, loss of teeth, ill-fitting dentures, and difficulty in chewing and swallowing all can make eating less enjoyable. Obviously, this too can lead to decreased food intake.

When modifications can be made to improve dental health by early intervention, many of the problems listed here can be avoided. Otherwise, health care professionals need creativity to assist older adults in finding foods that can be eaten with little difficulty and that also meet their nutritional needs. Modifications in consistency can help, as can choosing nutrient-dense foods such a yogurt and custards, bananas, and peanut butter. Often, just being patient and encouraging more time for chewing and swallowing are helpful.

THIRST

With aging comes a change in sense of thirst and diminished activity in the hormonal regulation of fluid balance. Together these changes may make dehydration more likely, and this can lead to confusion and hospitalization.[8]

Older adults may need assistance remembering to drink enough fluids, especially during illnesses and hot weather. The recommended amount of fluid per day is the same as for younger adults—at least 8 cups a day (2,000 ml). Water, juices, milk, decaffeinated coffee, and teas all contribute to fluid needs, but it is also good to encourage drinking water frequently to ensure adequate intake of fluids.

Dehydration   Dehydration causes several specific signs and symptoms:

- Dry lips
- Sunken eyes
- Swollen tongue
- Increased body temperature
- Decreased blood pressure
- Constipation
- Decreased urine output
- Nausea

GASTROINTESTINAL TRACT

The primary change in the **gastrointestinal** tract for older adults is constipation. Many complain of decreased frequency of bowel movements, painful defecation, stools that are hard and difficult to pass, or a feeling of incomplete evacuation. The causes include reduced motility in the gut, reduced intake of fiber-rich foods, insufficient fluid intake, physical inactivity, and medications.

The best way to remedy this is to encourage more **dietary fiber** intake with the goal being 25–30 grams daily. Most American gets only 15–20 grams daily. Fiber, although not an essential nutrient, aids in moving waste material through the large intestine. It acts to soften the stools and make them much easier to pass.[9,10] Ensuring adequate fiber intake also reduces the incidence of diverticulosis and may also lessen the risk of certain types of colon cancer.[6] Foods rich in fiber include whole grains, nuts, seeds, legumes, fruits, and vegetables. Some of the foods that are high in fiber are listed in **Table 7-3**. (See the section titled "Fiber" later in this chapter for additional information.)

In addition to adequate fiber, regular physical activity stimulates regularity, as does heeding the call of nature when the urge is felt. Adequate hydration also is important, as discussed earlier.[11] Mineral oil as a laxative should be taken with care because it binds the fat-soluble vitamins A, D, E, and K and can limit their absorption. Other types of over-the-counter laxatives should be used with caution, too, because they can foster dependence and may do little to resolve the problem.

Other changes in the gastrointestinal tract include **lactose intolerance** resulting from decreased lactase production. Lactase enzymes can be added to milk products, or specially treated milk can be used to alleviate the problem. These products are available at most grocers and pharmacies. (See also the section titled "Carbohydrates" later in this chapter.)

Acid production in the stomach decreases with age, and this can contribute to reduced absorption of vitamin B_{12}. It is important to note that vitamin B_{12} deficiencies can take some time to develop, but early diagnosis can prevent the anemia that may result. Less acid in the stomach also impairs the absorption of iron. In addition, chronic aspirin use may cause blood loss in the stomach, and chronic **antacid** use possibly binds iron. Ulcer, hemorrhoids, and colon cancer can also increase blood loss and the risk of anemia. If iron-deficiency anemia is diagnosed, supplements can be taken with vitamin C–rich foods, which will increase absorption.

TABLE 7-3   High-Fiber Foods.

½ cup cooked navy beans—9.5 g

½ cup baked beans, canned—10 g

½ cup dates—7.1 g

1 cup Raisin Bran™ cereal—7 g

½ cup tomato paste—5.9 g

½ cup frozen raspberries—5.5 g

½ cup cooked artichoke—4.5 g

½ cup peas—4.4 g

½ cup canned pumpkin—3.5 g

1 apple with skin—3.3 g

1 cup broccoli—2.5 g

1 slice whole grain bread—2 g

Source: USDA National Nutrient Database. Standard Reference Release 18. Retrieved March 1, 2009, from http://www.nal.usda.gov/fnic/foodcomp/Data/SR18/nutrlist/sr18a291.pdf.

LIVER, GALLBLADDER, AND PANCREAS

As with other systems, there are age-associated changes in the liver, gallbladder, and pancreas.

The liver functions less efficiently with age. This is further complicated if there is a history of alcohol abuse. There may be fatty buildup or outright cirrhosis of the liver that greatly diminishes function and makes it harder for the liver to metabolize alcohol. Continued use and abuse of alcohol in later life may be brought on by the many social changes that older adults experience, such as death of a spouse, loss of friendship, and feelings of loneliness and isolation.

Health care professionals need to be sensitive to these problems and be ready to make referrals to other appropriate health care professionals and community support groups. Nutritionally speaking, alcohol abuse compromises health and leads to malnutrition for several reasons. First, alcohol replaces food in the diet. Alcohol is a source of empty calories, and when older people spend their limited resources on alcohol instead of healthy foods, they definitely compromise their health. Second, alcohol interferes with the normal absorption of vitamin B_{12}, folic acid, and vitamin C. Alcohol also interferes with the metabolism of vitamins D and B_6 and increases the need for B vitamins and magnesium. All of these may result in multiple deficiencies that require a multivitamin and mineral supplement.

In contrast, diminished liver function may also result in vitamin A toxicity. Elderly people with liver disease should be warned not to take excessive amounts of vitamin A because their livers are less able to manage large doses.

Changes in the function of the gallbladder may lead to the formation of gallstones, which may result in fat malabsorption. A low-fat diet or surgery may be required to correct the situation.

One of the first signs of diminished function of the pancreas is a high blood glucose level. The pancreas secretes insulin, which controls the amount of glucose in the blood. With diminished pancreatic function, people may require oral hypoglycemic agents, exogenous insulin, and dietary modification to control blood glucose.

CARDIOVASCULAR HEALTH

Cardiovascular health can decline in older adults as a result of long-standing atherosclerosis, hypertension, and physical inactivity. The best way to maintain heart health is a lifelong commitment to a heart-healthy diet and regular exercise. Even in later years, encouraging clients to follow a diet low in fat, saturated fat, and cholesterol, to control salt intake, and to eat adequate amounts of fruits, vegetables, and fiber helps them keep cholesterol levels down and high-density lipoprotein (HDL) levels within a desirable range. In addition, make sure older people eat foods containing sufficient vitamin B_6, vitamin B_{12}, and folate to help avoid elevated homocysteine levels, which are a known risk factor for heart disease.[12]

Care needs to be taken, however, whenever extremely low-fat diets are used by older people as a means of controlling hyperlipidemia (high levels of fats in the blood that can lead to atherosclerosis). A diet too low in fat could cause weight loss and a lack of variety in the types of food eaten. This could easily compromise nutritional status. Careful evaluation of the individual's current diet usually reveals opportunities for moderate changes to help correct concerns with hyperlipidemia.

Hypertension in older adults is usually treated with medication, sodium restriction, weight loss (if overweight), and moderate exercise (if possible). Encourage older people to avoid high-sodium foods such as fast foods, snack foods (chips, salted popcorn, and nuts), salty meats (cured pork products, salted fish), pickles, and cheese, and to not add salt at the table.

NUTRITION NEEDS AND GUIDELINES

This section reviews the essential nutrients and nutrition guidelines that are helpful to maintain nutrition status and prevent chronic health problems over time.

ESSENTIAL NUTRIENTS

There are six classes of nutrients humans need for optimum health: **carbohydrates**, proteins, fats, vitamins, minerals, and water. Although water and fiber do not provide any nutrients necessarily, because of their multitude of health benefits, they are considered as important as other **essential nutrients**. They are discussed along with essential nutrients in the text. We must have them all because they are crucial for our growth, development, and for our bodies to function normally. No matter what age, these nutrients are essential for promoting growth, maintenance, and repair of our bodies.

Carbohydrates, protein, and fat are the macronutrients that provide us energy. Vitamins and minerals are the micronutrients that do not yield energy, but they play an important role in various chemical reactions, immunity, and healthy aging. Carbohydrates are the preferred source of energy and are the ideal fuel for the body. Proteins, too, can be used as energy, but they are expensive and offer no physiologic advantage over carbohydrates when used for energy. Fats are a dense source of calories but are not used efficiently by the brain and central nervous system. In addition, diets high in fat are associated with increased risk of several chronic diseases. Measured in calories, 1 gram of carbohydrate yields 4 calories, 1 gram of protein yields 4 calories, and 1 gram of fat yields 9 calories.

Carbohydrates Carbohydrates are found in bread, rice, grains, popcorn, starchy vegetables, fruits, milk, sugar, cakes, pastries, and other food products made of any of these items. Carbohydrates are made up of one or more sugar molecules. Carbohydrates are classified as simple, which means made of fewer than three sugar molecules, and complex, which means made up of three or more sugar molecules. Simple carbohydrates are usually sweet in taste. Examples of simple carbohydrates are glucose (corn or grape sugar), fructose (fruits), and sucrose (table sugar). Complex carbohydrates contain fiber. Examples are whole grains, whole-grain cereals, oatmeal, whole wheat or brown bread, brown rice, and whole-grain pasta. At least one-half of the grains eaten should be from whole grains because they are nutrient rich and have fiber in them.[13]

Foods high in added sugars such as cakes, candies, cookies, and regular sodas are called empty-calorie foods because they are high in calories and low in nutrient value. The aim while consuming carbohydrates is to get most carbohydrates in their complex forms because of the health benefits of fiber.

Individuals should consume 6 ounces of carbohydrates based on a 2,000-calorie diet. Requirements can vary depending on caloric needs. One ounce is equal to one slice of bread or one-half cup of cooked cereal, rice, or pasta.

Protein   Proteins are found in meat, beans, dairy products, and nuts. Proteins are the primary substances that the body uses to build and repair tissues such as muscle, blood, internal organs, hair, nails, and bones. Proteins are part of hormones, antibodies, and enzymes. Enzymes are proteins that catalyze the biochemical reactions that take place in the metabolism of the body.

The building blocks of proteins are amino acids. There are 20 amino acids used by the body, but only 9 of them are essential because the body cannot make them. The other 11 can be formed in the body. The presence or absence of the essential amino acids determines the quality of the protein. All animal protein is of high quality, containing all the essential amino acids. Vegetable proteins are all incomplete, meaning that they are missing one or more of the essential amino acids. Therefore, vegetable proteins should be eaten in combination with one another to ensure that the body receives all the essential amino acids.

How much protein do we need each day? Protein should comprise anywhere from 15–20% of total calorie intake. But certain physiologic situations may dictate that protein intake be higher or lower.

Whereas intake of protein at 0.8 g/kg of body weight is sufficient for younger adults, older people are encouraged to increase their protein intake slightly to 1 g/kg of body weight. This increased need is a result in part of reduced protein digestion and absorption with aging. In addition, stressful situations for the body, such as infection, wounds, or chronic disease, reduce the efficiency of protein use. Increased protein intake may also help stave off the lean tissue loss accompanying aging. Protein deficiency can result in chronic eczema, fatigue, muscle weakness, reduced resistance to disease, slower wound healing, and tissue wasting. It is easy to get protein from low-fat dairy (milk, yogurt, and cheese), beans, tofu, and nuts. However, it may become difficult to meet protein needs in the case of reduced appetite and food intake. Along with reduced protein intake, several vitamins and minerals may be lacking as well.

Fats The primary function of fats, or **lipids**, in the body is as a rich source of energy. Fat helps insulate and regulate body temperature, it surrounds internal organs and protects them from external injury, and it is the carrier of the fat-soluble vitamins A, D, E, and K. The two essential fatty acids, linoleic and linolenic acid, are widely distributed in plant foods, oil, and fish.

In recent years, there has been a heightened interest and awareness of the amount and type of fat in our diets. In our zeal to reduce the amount of fat we eat, we sometimes forget that fat is a nutrient and that we do need it—the right type and in the right quantity. Currently, trans fats have been in the news as the type of fat we should avoid. Trans fats are made by manufacturers to add shelf life and flavor stability to food products; the process of hydrogenation, or adding hydrogen to vegetable oils, changes the liquid to a solid. Although recommendations may vary slightly, most health promotion organizations urge a reduction in fat intake, especially intake of trans fat and saturated fat, both of which increase the risk of heart disease.[14] Fat calories should account for no more than 30% of total calories.

About 95% of the fat in the foods we eat and the fat in the human body is known as triglycerides. A triglyceride is made up of three units of fatty acids and one unit of glycerol. Other types of fats are phospholipids (e.g., lecithin) and sterols (e.g., cholesterol).

Fatty acids can be further divided into three categories: saturated, polyunsaturated, and monounsaturated. **Saturated fats** are solid at room temperature and are primarily found in animal foods. Beef fat, lard, and butter are all examples of saturated fats. **Polyunsaturated fats** are liquid at room temperature and are found in plant products; examples are corn, safflower, and sunflower oils. **Monounsaturated fats**, such as olive, peanut, and canola oils, also tend to be more liquid at room temperature. There are a couple of exceptions: Palm and coconut oils are from plants, but they are highly saturated fats.

These distinctions regarding types of fat are important because of the effects these fats have on cholesterol. **Cholesterol** is a waxy substance that is found in animal products and not in plant products. It is made by the human body and is necessary in making cell membranes, is a building block of some hormones, and is involved in the digestion of fats via bile. Polyunsaturated and monounsaturated fats tend to lower blood cholesterol, and saturated fats tend to elevate blood cholesterol, thereby elevating the risk for cardiovascular disease.

Another type of lipid important in determining risk for cardiovascular disease is lipoproteins. Lipoproteins are compounds involved in carrying fats around the body. Research has shown that total cholesterol, though important, is not the only predictive risk factor for heart disease. Knowing the amounts of the two types of lipoproteins is also essential. High-density lipoproteins (HDLs) are associated with reduced risk for heart disease, and low-density lipoproteins (LDLs) are associated with increased risk.[15]

When cholesterol levels are high, the health of the arteries and veins is in jeopardy because elevated cholesterol levels cause plaque to build up in the inner lining of the vessel wall. This plaque can harden and restrict the flow of blood. When blood supply is cut off to the heart, part of the heart tissue dies, resulting in a heart attack. When blood supply is cut off to the brain, a stroke occurs.

The general guidelines recommended by the National Cholesterol Education Program (2008) are to keep total blood cholesterol levels below 200 mg/dL. LDL cholesterol should be less than 100 mg/dL, and HDL cholesterol should be at or above 40 mg/dL for men and at or above 50 mg/dL for women.

A Summary of Fats

Monounsaturated Fats
- Are more liquid at room temperature
- Help lower cholesterol levels
- Examples include olive, peanut, and canola oils

Polyunsaturated Fats
- Are liquid at room temperature
- Are from plants
- Help lower cholesterol levels
- Examples include corn and safflower oils

Saturated Fats
- Are solid at room temperature
- Are of animal origin
- Elevate cholesterol levels
- Examples include lard, tallow, butter, and animal fats

The following are some suggestions for a heart-healthy diet:

- Cut back on fat in general and in particular try to substitute more monounsaturated and polyunsaturated fat.
- Get the required 30 g of fiber daily.
- Choose lean cuts of meat; trim all the fat you can see, and throw away the fat that cooks out of the meat during cooking.
- Use no more than a total of 5 teaspoons of fats and oils per day for cooking, baking, and salads.
- Use low-fat or nonfat dairy products.
- Try main dishes featuring pasta, rice, beans, and/or vegetables, or create new dishes by mixing small amounts of meats with legumes and/or grains.
- Use egg substitutes or egg whites instead of egg yolks in cooking.
- Limit your intake of high-fat meats and organ meats.
- Control the amount of butter, margarine, and cream cheese you add to bread, pasta, and rice.

- Use cooking oil spray when possible.
- Use small amounts of olive oil in cooking, and use oil and vinegar dressings for salads. Also try reduced-fat or fat-free salad dressings.

Vitamins   Vitamins are substances needed by the body to maintain metabolism, growth, and development. There are 13 vitamins, which are divided into two categories. The *water-soluble* vitamins include vitamins C and B complex. *Fat-soluble* vitamins include A, D, E, and K. The best way to ensure adequate vitamin intake is through a well-balanced and varied diet. Fruits and vegetables are loaded with vitamins, but vitamins are found in the other food groups, too. See **Table 7-4** for a summary of the vitamins, their functions, and food sources.

TABLE 7-4   Guide to Vitamins.

Vitamin (Chemical Name)	Best Sources	Chief Roles	Deficiency Symptoms	Toxicity Symptoms
		Water-Soluble Vitamins		
Thiamin	Meat, pork, liver, fish, poultry, whole-grain and enriched breads, cereals, pasta, nuts, legumes, wheat germ, oats.	Helps enzymes release energy from carbohydrate; supports normal appetite and nervous system function.	Beriberi: edema, heart irregularity, mental confusion, muscle weakness, impaired growth.	Rapid pulse, weakness, headaches, insomnia, irritability.
Riboflavin (vitamin B_2)	Organ meats, milk, dark green vegetables, yogurt, cottage cheese, liver, meat, whole-grain or enriched breads and cereals.	Helps enzymes release energy from carbohydrate, fat, and protein; promotes healthy skin and normal vision.	Eye problems, skin disorders around nose and mouth.	None reported, but an excess of any of the B vitamins could cause a deficiency of the others.
Niacin	Meat, eggs, poultry, fish, milk, whole-grain and enriched breads and cereals, nuts, legumes, peanuts, nutritional yeast, all protein foods.	Helps enzymes release energy from energy nutrients; promotes health of skin, nerves, and digestive system.	Pellagra: skin rash on parts exposed to sun, loss of appetite, dizziness, weakness, fatigue, mental confusion, indigestion.	Flushing, nausea, headaches, cramps, ulcer, irritation, heartburn, abnormal liver function, low blood pressure.

TABLE 7-4   Guide to Vitamins. (continued)

Vitamin (Chemical Name)	Best Sources	Chief Roles	Deficiency Symptoms	Toxicity Symptoms
Vitamin B$_6$	Meat, poulty, fortified cereal/soy products, organ meats.	Protein and fat metabolism; formation of antibodies and red blood cells; helps convert tryptophan to niacin.	Nervous disorders, skin rash, muscle weakness, anemia, convulsions, kidney stones.	Depression, fatigue, irritability, headaches, numbness, damage to nerves, difficulty walking.
Folate	Green leafy vegetables, liver, legumes, seeds.	Red blood cell formation; protein metabolism; new cell division.	Anemia, heartburn, diarrhea, smooth tongue, depression, poor growth.	Diarrhea, insomnia, irritability, may mask a vitamin B$_{12}$ deficiency.
Vitamin B$_{12}$ (cobalamin)	Animal products: meat, fish, poultry, shellfish, milk, cheese, eggs.	Helps maintain nerve cells; red blood cell formation; synthesis of genetic material.	Anemia, smooth tongue, fatigue, nerve degeneration progressing to paralysis.	None reported.
Pantothenic acid	Widespread in foods.	Coenzyme in energy metabolism.	Rare: sleep disturbances, nausea, fatigue.	Occasional diarrhea.
Biotin	Liver, fruits, meats.	Coenzyme in energy metabolism; fat synthesis, glycogen formation.	Loss of appetite, nausea, depression, muscle pain, weakness, fatigue, rash.	None reported.
Vitamin C (ascorbic acid)	Citrus fruits, cabbage-type vegetables, tomatoes, potatoes, dark green vegetables, peppers, lettuce, cantaloupe, strawberries, mangoes, papayas.	Synthesis of collagen (helps heal wounds, maintains bone and teeth, strengthens blood vessels); antioxidant; strengthens resistance to infection; helps body absorb iron.	Scurvy: anemia, atherosclerotic plaques, depression, frequent infections, bleeding gums, loosened teeth, pinpoint hemorrhages, muscle degeneration, rough skin, bone fragility, poor wound healing, hysteria.	Nausea, abdominal cramps, diarrhea, nosebleeds, deficiency symptoms may appear at first upon withdrawal of high doses.

TABLE 7-4   Guide to Vitamins. (continued)

Vitamin (Chemical Name)	Best Sources	Chief Roles	Deficiency Symptoms	Toxicity Symptoms
		Fat-Soluble Vitamins		
Vitamin A	*Retinol*: Liver, dairy products, dark fruits and vegetables. *Beta-carotene:* Spinach and other dark leafy greens, broccoli, deep orange fruits (apricots, peaches, cantaloupe), and vegetables (squash, carrots, sweet potatoes, pumpkin).	Vision; growth and repair of body tissues; reproduction; bone and tooth formation; immunity; hormone synthesis; antioxidant (in the form of beta-carotene only).	Night blindness, rough skin, susceptibility to infection, impaired bone growth, abnormal tooth and jaw alignmnent, eye problems leading to blindness, impaired growth.	Red blood cell breakage, nosebleeds, abdominal cramps, nausea, diarrhea, weight loss, blurred vision, irritability, loss of appetite, bone pain, dry skin, rashes, hair loss, cessation of menstruation, growth retardation, liver disease.
Vitamin D (calciferol)	Self-synthesis with sunlight; fortified milk, fortified margarine, eggs, liver, fish.	Calcium and phosphorus metabolism (bone and tooth formation); aids body's absorption of calcium.	Rickets in children; osteomalacia in adults; abnormal growth, joint pain, soft bones.	Raised blood calcium, constipation, weight loss, irritability, weakness, nausea, kidney stones, mental and physical retardation.
Vitamin E	Vegetable oils, green leafy vegetables, wheat germ, whole-grain products, butter, liver, egg yolk, milk fat, nuts, seeds.	Protects red blood cells; antioxidant.	Muscle wasting, weakness, red blood cell breakage, anemia, hemorrhaging.	General discomfort, no evidence of adverse effects in natural food sources.
Vitamin K	Bacterial synthesis in digestive tract, liver, green leafy and cabbage-type vegetables, milk.	Synthesis of blood-clotting proteins and a blood protein that regulates calcium.	Hemorrhaging.	May cause jaundice.

Sources: National Research Council, Subcommittee on the Tenth Edition of the RDAS. *Recommended Dietary Allowances*, 10th *Edition.* Washington, DC: National Academy Press; 1989; Boyle, M, Zyla, G. *Personal Nutrition.* Minneapolis, MN: West Publishing; 1996; Institute of Medicine of the National Academies updated 5/13/2008, retrieved 11/22/2008, from http://www.iom.edu/CMS/54133/54377/5411.aspx

Minerals   There are 23 minerals essential for human nutrition. They perform numerous functions in the body, including metabolism, maintenance of fluid balance, bone and teeth formation, blood clotting, muscle and nerve function, and formation of red blood cells.

The three most commonly discussed minerals are sodium, because of its association with hypertension; calcium, because of its association with bone health; and iron, because of its association with anemia. See **Table 7-5** for a summary of minerals, their functions, and food sources.

TABLE 7-5   Guide to Minerals.

Mineral	Best Sources	Chief Roles	Deficiency Symptoms	Toxicity Symptoms
		Major Minerals		
Calcium	Milk and milk products, small fish (with bones), tofu, certain green vegetables, almonds, legumes, pinenuts, herbs, fortified orange juice.	Principal mineral of bones and teeth; involved in muscle contraction and relaxation, nerve function, blood clotting, blood pressure.	Bone loss (osteoporosis) in adults; stunted growth in children.	Intestinal gas, kidney stones, constipation; hypercal-cemia; renal insufficiency.
Phosphorus	All animal products.	Part of every cell; involved in acid–base balance.	Weakness.	Can create relative deficiency of calcium, tetany, and convulsions.
Magnesium	Nuts, legumes, whole grains, dark green vegetables, seafoods, chocolate, cocoa.	Involved in bone mineralization, protein synthesis, enzyme action, normal muscular contraction, nerve transmission, lung function.	Weakness, confusion, depressed pancreatic hormone secretion, growth failure, behavioral disturbances, muscle spasms.	Occurs only from nonfood sources.
Sodium	Salt, soy sauce; processed foods: cured, canned, pickled, and many boxed foods.	Helps maintain normal fluid and acid–base balance.	Muscle cramps, mental apathy, loss of appetite (rare).	High blood pressure (in salt-sensitive persons).

TABLE 7-5 Guide to Minerals. (continued)

Mineral	Best Sources	Chief Roles	Deficiency Symptoms	Toxicity Symptoms
Chloride	Salt, soy sauce; processed foods.	Part of stomach acid, necessary for proper digestion, fluid balance.	Growth failure in children, muscle cramps, mental apathy, loss of appetite.	Normally harmless (the gas chlorine is a poison but evaporates from water); disturbed acid–base balance; vomiting.
Potassium	All whole foods: vegetables, milk, fruits (bananas), grains, legumes.	Facilitates many reactions, including protein synthesis, fluid balance, nerve transmission, and contraction of muscles.	Muscle weakness, paralysis, confusion; can cause death; accompanies dehydration.	Causes muscular weakness; triggers vomiting; if given into a vein, can stop the heart.
Sulfur	All foods containing protein.	Component of certain amino acids; part of biotin, thiamin, and insulin; acid–base balance, drug detoxyifying pathways.	Rare: protein deficiency would occur first; impaired mental function.	May depress growth. May cause pseudoallergic reaction (1–5% of asthmatics).

Trace Minerals

Mineral	Best Sources	Chief Roles	Deficiency Symptoms	Toxicity Symptoms
Iodine	Iodized salt, seafood, bread.	Role in thyroid hormone regulation; part of thyroxine, which regulates metabolism.	Goiter, cretinism, retarded growth.	Very high intakes depress thyroid activity.
Iron	Beef, fish, poultry, shellfish, eggs, legumes, dried fruits, fortified cereals.	Oxygen transport and storage; electron transport; hemoglobin formation; part of myoglobin; energy utilization.	Fatigue, dizziness, anemia, weakness, pallor, headaches, reduced immunity, inability to concentrate, cold intolerance.	Iron overload: infection, liver injury, possible increased risk of heart attack.

TABLE 7-5   Guide to Minerals. *(continued)*

Mineral	Best Sources	Chief Roles	Deficiency Symptoms	Toxicity Symptoms
Zinc	Oysters, nuts, protein-containing foods, meats, fish, poultry, grains, vegetables.	Part of many enzymes; present in insulin; involved in making genetic material and proteins, immune system function, vitamin A transport, taste, wound healing, making sperm, normal fetal development.	Growth failure in children, delayed development of sexual organs, loss of taste and smell in adults; poor wound healing; hair loss; skin lesions; susceptibility to infections.	Associated with low toxicity; fever, nausea, vomiting, diarrhea.
Copper	Organ crustaceans, meats, drinking water, widespread in food.	Antioxidant system and electron transport; absorption of iron; part of several enzymes.	Anemia, bone changes (rare in human beings).	Low toxicity; except as part of a rare hereditary disease (Wilson's disease).
Fluoride/fluorine	Drinking water (if naturally fluoride containing or fluoridated), tea, seafood.	Formation of bones and teeth; helps make teeth resistant to decay and bones resistant to mineral loss.	Susceptibility to tooth decay and bone loss.	Fluorosis (discoloration of teeth).
Selenium	Seafood, meats, grains.	Helps protect body compounds from oxidation.	Anemia (rare). (Keshan disease in China.)	Rarely observed, digestive system disorders, hair loss.
Chromium	Liver and kidney; meats, unrefined foods, vegetables, whole grains.	Associated with insulin and required for the release of energy from glucose.	Diabetes-like condition marked by inability to use glucose normally (postulated).	Unknown as a nutrition disorder. Occupational exposures damage skin and kidneys.
Manganese	Widely distributed in foods, especially plants.	Facilitates with enzymes, many cell processes.	Rare in humans, skeletal/CNS abnormalities.	Rarely observed; CNS damage.

TABLE 7-5 **Guide to Minerals.** *(continued)*

Mineral	Best Sources	Chief Roles	Deficiency Symptoms	Toxicity Symptoms
Molybdenum	Legumes, cereals, organ meats.	Facilitates with enzymes, many cell processes.	Unknown (rare).	Enzyme inhibition.
Cobalt	Meats, milk, and milk products.	As part of vitamin B_{12}, involved in nerve function and blood formation.	Unknown except in vitamin B_{12} deficiency.	Unknown as a nutrition disorder.

Sources: National Research Council, Subcommittee on the 10th Edition of the RDAs. *Recommended Dietary Allowances, 10th Edition.* Washington, DC: National Academy Press; 1989; Boyle, M, Zyla, G. *Personal Nutrition.* Minneapolis, MN: West Publishing; 1996; Biesalksi, HK, Grimm, P. *Pocket Atlas of Nutrition.* Stuttgart: Tieme Electronic Book Library; 2006.

Recommended Dietary Allowances (RDA) for Vitamins and Minerals   Research has led some to suggest that the RDA for several vitamins and minerals may need to be modified to meet the changing needs of older adults. The following is a summary of the recommended changes in vitamin and mineral needs with aging:[10]

- *Vitamin A:*   Use caution with vitamin A supplements because with older age there is increased absorption and toxic levels may occur.
- *Vitamin D:*   Increase intake to 400–800 IU. Current RDA is 200 IU. Older people may have less exposure to sunlight, resulting in reduced dermal synthesis of vitamin D and reduced metabolism of vitamin D in the kidney.
- *Vitamin B_6:*   Current RDA for vitamin B_6 (for those older than 50) is 2 mg per day for older men and 1.6 mg per day for older women. There is a reduction in blood levels of vitamin B_6 that accompanies aging.
- *Vitamin B_{12}:*   Increase to 3 μg. Current RDA is 2 μg. There is debate in this area. Some researchers think that increasing intake will not change serum levels because there is decreased absorption resulting from changes in gastric acidity in older age. Therefore, researchers recommend aggressive screening for low serum levels of vitamin B_{12} followed by intramuscular injections to correct the problem.
- *Calcium:*   Increase to 1,500 mg. Current RDA is 800 mg. There is decreased absorption of calcium in women especially after menopause. Additional calcium intake will help prevent bone loss in nonvertebral bones such as the hip.
- *Sodium:*   As per MyPyramid 2005 guidelines, the maximum sodium recommendation for everyone is 2,300 mg/day, which is approximately 1 teaspoon of salt. Most Americans consume 4,000 mg of salt per day, nearly double the recommended level. Sodium intake in older adults may need to be monitored related to the presence of chronic diseases such as hypertension, renal disease, or heart problems. With elevated

blood pressure, physicians will recommend specific guidelines for sodium restriction. Consulting with a registered dietitian can help people establish the DASH (Dietary Approaches to Prevent Hypertension) diet.[10]

The RDA guidelines are set by the National Academy of Sciences/National Research Council and are based on the latest scientific evidence regarding health and diet. They are recommendations, not requirements, and are not intended to be used by individuals in planning meals to meet nutrient needs.

Water   Water is the most important nutrient and is involved in almost every vital body process. As discussed, older adults are at high risk of developing dehydration. The row of glasses near the base of the Modified MyPyramid for older people reminds us of the importance of consuming adequate fluids throughout the day. Everyone is encouraged to drink at least eight 8-ounce glasses of fluid a day.[10] Emphasis should be placed on getting enough fluids from variable sources such as 100% fruit or vegetable juices, fruits, tea, and decaffeinated coffee to prevent dehydration.

Water intake needs or recommendations may change related to presence of other health problems (e.g., reduced kidney function). The older person's physician may suggest specific guidelines for water intake depending on the individual's health status.

Fiber   Dietary fibers are not nutrients; however, they are considered important as part of a healthy balanced diet because of their crucial role in health maintenance, disease management, and as a component of medical nutrition therapy. According to the American Dietetic Association, the RDA for fiber is 25–30 g for healthy adults. Average dietary fiber intake in a typical American diet (14–15 g per day) has been consistently less than what has been recommended.[9]

Following are sources of the dietary fibers:

- Fruits
- Vegetables
- Whole grains
- Legumes
- Nuts

Following are the benefits of fibers:

- Regulating digestion and preventing constipation
- Lowering cholesterol levels
- Controlling blood sugar levels in type 2 diabetes
- Preventing or reducing various stomach and colon-rectal cancers
- Providing the feeling of early satiety
- Potential weight management

Health professionals should encourage older adults to consume fruits, vegetables, and whole grains to prevent and manage common health problems such as constipation, diabetes, high cholesterol levels, various other cardiovascular and digestive diseases, and cancer.[13] A valuable source of fiber can be obtained from eating nuts such as almonds and peanuts; however, these are also high in fat, and therefore should be eaten in moderation, especially by overweight and obese older people.

MODIFIED MYPYRAMID FOR OLDER ADULTS

In 2005, the USDA released the new MyPyramid food guidance system. MyPyramid is an interactive, multifaceted Web-based tool that provides individual dietary guidelines. The multicolored MyPyramid emphasizes that one nutritional style does not fit all, and therefore, personalized meal planning is necessary. When the MyPyramid 2005 was unveiled, it was difficult for older adults to use because of issues related to Web access, computer availability, and computer and Internet efficiency. There are special dietary needs associated with older age (older than age 70). Various reasons prompted researchers to develop a graphic version of the Modified MyPyramid for older adults. (See **Figure 7-1**.)

The Modified MyPyramid for older adults does not intend to be a substitute for the original USDA pyramid. The Modified MyPyramid was developed by a Tufts University research team and was published in January 2008 in the *Journal of Nutrition*. It highlights the importance of regular physical activity and adequate fluid intake, along with an updated graphic version of each food group. The importance of regular physical activity, moderation, proportionality, and variety are all approaches suggested to promote a healthy lifestyle. There are five major food groups.[11]

Physical Activity The base of the Modified MyPyramid is made up of graphics showing physical activity. There tends to be a reduction in activity level as we age; hence, emphasis should be placed on encouraging older adults to participate in regular light to moderate physical activity. Engagement in physical activity reduces the risk of various chronic diseases, helps with weight management, and may reduce symptoms of depression.

Water Near the base of the Modified MyPyramid, there is a row of glasses. As discussed, older adults are at high risk of developing dehydration because of the various physiologic changes of aging. The row of glasses reminds viewers of the importance of consuming adequate fluids throughout the day.[11]

On the solid foundation of good hydration and physical activity, various graphic forms of food groups are displayed to help the viewer understand the importance of eating a healthy variety of foods.

Grains The first (orange) food group is the grain group. Grains include bread, cereal, rice, and pasta. These are the foods that should form the basis of our diets. Consumers are asked to choose 6 to 11 servings a day, based on caloric needs, and to choose at least

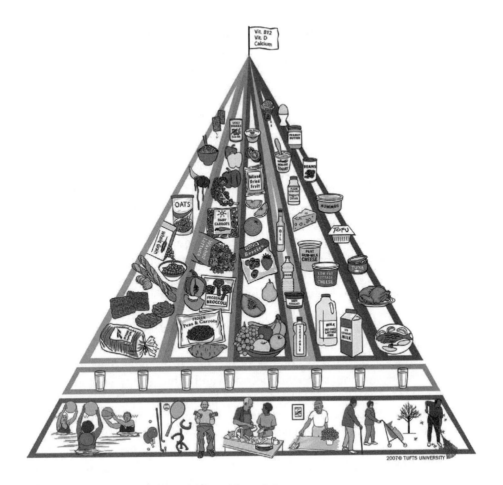

FIGURE 7-1 Modified MyPyramid for older adults.
Source: Copyright 2007 Tufts University. Reprinted with permission from Lichtenstein, AH, Rasmussen, H, Yu, WW, Epstein, SR, Russel, RM. Modified MyPyramid for Older Adults. *J Nutr.* 2008;138:78–82.

half of their grains as "whole" grains. Most grains are milled and refined; therefore, checking the ingredients list to find the words *whole grain* or *whole wheat* is important. Whole grains are good source of complex carbohydrates, fibers, vitamins, and minerals.

Vegetables and Fruits   The next groups are the vegetables and the fruits. Everyone should eat at least 5 servings of fruits and vegetables every day. The aim is to get different colors and varieties of seasonal fruits and vegetables as part of a balanced diet. Fruits and vegetables provide fibers, vitamins, minerals, and antioxidants. Consuming the recommended level of fruits and vegetables may reduce the risk of various cancers, heart problems, and hypertension. Older adults with diabetes should consider fruits as a source of carbohydrates. The assistance of a registered dietitian can be helpful for those needing to learn carbohydrate counting and in planning healthy meals.

Milk   The next group is dairy (in blue) including milk, yogurt, and cheese. The recommended number of servings is 2 or 3, and the best choices are low in fat or fat free. Food in the dairy group provides calcium, potassium, vitamin D, and protein.

Meat and Beans   The last group (in purple) is the meat, poultry, fish, dry beans, eggs, and nuts group. To reduce fat intake, choose low-fat or lean meats and try legumes. Healthy individuals not on a protein restriction diet should have 2 to 3 servings daily from the meat and beans group.

Oils   The very little area of yellow suggests limiting fats, oils, and sweets in the diet. These should be used sparingly. Most of the fat consumed should be in the form of monounsaturated (MUFA) or polyunsaturated (PUFA) form. MUFA and PUFA supply essential fatty acids and vitamin E to the body and do not raise LDL cholesterol, while solid-form saturated and trans fats raise the level of LDL cholesterol; therefore, one should avoid the use of these "bad" fats. Oils are also calorie dense. One tablespoon of oil has 120 calories; hence, fat intake should be limited to only a small portion of total caloric intake.

Flag of Vitamin D, B₁₂, and Calcium at the Top of the Modified MyPyramid   After 50 years of age, older adults need more calcium, vitamin D, and vitamin B_{12} to maintain bone mineral density and to reduce the risk of fracture. It becomes challenging to meet this need especially when one's appetite decreases and subsequently food and caloric intake goes down. Consuming fortified food products, such as juice and cereals, and using dietary supplements may be encouraged to meet these special nutrient requirements. This age group may not be able to depend on exposure to sunlight for vitamin D because of potentially decreased sun exposure and the reduced ability of the kidney to synthesize this vitamin. Sometimes deficiency of vitamin B_{12} may be caused by malabsorption. Therefore, the flag at the top of MyPyramid serves as a reminder of these specific vitamin and mineral needs.

PLANNING MEALS WITH GOOD NUTRITION IN MIND

One of the challenges of nutrition is applying the knowledge of what is necessary to eat on a day-by-day and meal-by-meal basis. There are some essential nutrition concepts to apply when planning meals. Keeping these meal-planning principles in mind helps ensure that good nutrition is achieved:

- *Adequacy*: A diet that provides enough of the essential nutrients, fiber, and energy
- *Balance*: A diet that does not overemphasize one food at the expense of another
- *Calorie control*: A diet that has just enough calories to maintain a healthy weight
- *Moderation*: A diet that does not contain excess amounts of unwanted items such as sugar, salt, and fat
- *Variety*: A diet that has many different nutrient-rich foods

BOX 7-4   SUGGESTED SERVINGS BASED ON A 2,000-CALORIE DIET FOR HEALTHY ADULTS.

Grain group	6
Vegetable group	3
Fruit group	2
Milk group	2–3
Meat group	2 (total of 5–6 ounces)

Note: 2,000 is the calorie requirement for typical healthy adults. Specific caloric requirements can be calculated depending on height, weight, age, and activity levels. Go to the MyPyramid website to get a personalized meal plan using the interactive tool (for example, one website for MyPyramid can be found at http://www.oznet.ksu.edu/dp_fnut/dietaryguide.htm).
Source: Based on USDA MyPyramid 2005.

Box 7-4 lists the number of servings of the major food groups based on a 2,000-calorie diet.

FOOD PREPARATION TIPS FOR OLDER ADULTS

Following are several suggestions for food preparation specifically for older people:

- Eat regular meals. Small, frequent meals may be best. Use nutrient-dense foods as the basis for each meal.
- Put the focus on foods that are low in fat, sugar, cholesterol, and salt. Read labels so that you know what you are buying.
- Do not hesitate to check out convenience foods as long as they are healthy and tasty. Many grocers now carry already prepared fruits and vegetables in single portions. Look for meats that have already been trimmed and cut up and are ready for cooking. However many processed foods are high in salt.
- Keep some quick and easy snacks on hand for times when you do not feel like cooking. There is nothing wrong with making a meal of snacks, as long as they are healthy.
- Keep food preparation simple. This will make cleanup easier, too.
- Keep moving. Engage in regular exercise because it will help stimulate your appetite.
- Consider shopping, preparing, and eating cooperatively with neighbors and friends. It can put some excitement back into your mealtimes.
- Steam vegetables or fruits (rather than boiling). This will make them easier to chew.
- When you do cook, prepare a larger portion and freeze some for later use.

SPECIAL CONSIDERATIONS

ENERGY NEEDS

When considering energy needs for the older adult, changes in metabolic rate resulting from decreasing physical activity and loss of lean tissue translate into decreased calorie needs. Therefore, the RDA for energy is lower for adults beginning at age 51. The estimated average energy allowance for men 51 years and older is 2,300 kcal, and for women, 1,900 kcal. These figures are only estimated averages and cannot be applied to every individual in every situation. Coming to specific conclusions regarding daily calorie needs requires knowledge of an individual's recent weight history, current goals, activity levels, lifestyle, eating habits, and the presence or absence of conditions that might affect energy needs. In general, older adults need to be mindful that it is important to choose nutrient-dense foods and limit their intake of high-calorie, low-nutrient foods.

If, however, the older adult chooses to participate in regular physical activity, calorie needs may be adjusted upward, allowing for more flexibility in meal planning. Increased calorie intake also provides more opportunities to ensure adequate nutrient intake.

When weight loss is indicated, under no circumstances should caloric intake fall below 1,200 kcal/day unless the individual is under the direct supervision of a physician. Intakes of less than 1,200 kcal/day make it very difficult to meet basic nutrient needs. Weight loss should always be undertaken under the guidance of a dietitian and/or a physician and should include regular moderate activity as well as a balanced diet. Weight loss should not exceed 1–2 pounds per week.

If weight is below healthy weight range, then calories need to be increased to reestablish a healthy body weight. This could mean increasing daily calorie intake. A dietitian can help to plan out meals with healthy high-calorie options to promote weight gain. It is often more difficult to gain weight than it is to lose it, so creativity is called for in helping an individual to increase calorie intake.

LIQUID NUTRITIONAL SUPPLEMENTS

As has been discussed, there is a myriad of changes that occur with aging that affect nutritional well-being. When weight loss occurs or food intake is compromised, or if multiple vitamin or mineral deficiencies are suspected because of poor appetite, liquid nutrition supplements are often an ideal way to correct the situation.

Supplemental nutrition products such as Ensure, Boost, and Glucerna are available in the market as liquid nutrition supplements that can help correct inadequacies in several areas. They are flavored and are easy to use. Various snacks, juices, and powders are available that may also help with meeting nutritional needs.

These companies all have consumer hotline numbers with staff available to answer questions about composition. A physician or dietitian should be consulted for getting advice and recommendations on these products.

DIABETES

Aging may also bring reduced **glucose tolerance**. Older adults may be more susceptible to temporary hyperglycemic and hypoglycemic episodes. With a high sugar load, glucose levels return to normal much more slowly in older people. High-sugar treats and sweets should be limited so as to avoid these sugar highs and lows. The older person who has **diabetes** needs regular help in adhering to a diet to manage blood glucose levels, whether or not she or he is insulin dependent. The individual needs to work with his or her physician and dietitian to formulate a diet plan and to learn carbohydrate counting. The dietitian and older person need to collaborate to develop workable menus that provide good control and take into consideration the person's food preferences and lifestyle habits.

Exchange List   One of the best ways to plan a healthy diet for those with diabetes is to use **exchanges for meal planning**. This allows some freedom of choice for the person while at the same time controlling calories and carbohydrate intake. The exchange method was developed in 1950 by the American Diabetic Association, the American Dietetic Association, and the U.S. Public Health Service. The method sorts foods into groups according to their carbohydrate, protein, fat, and calorie content.

The exchange groups include the following:

- *Milk*: Milk products and yogurt
- *Vegetables*: Fresh, frozen, and canned vegetables
- *Fruit*: Fresh, frozen, canned, and dried fruits, and fruit juices
- *Breads*: Breads, cereals, grains, legumes, and crackers
- *Meat*: Lean, medium-fat, and high-fat meat
- *Fats*: Butter, margarine, bacon, cream cheese, olives, oils, and dressings
- *Beverages, seasoning, condiments, and foods allowed as desired*

Within each group, specific foods and their portions are specified. So, for example, if an individual is allowed 2 bread exchanges, 1 fruit exchange, and 1 milk exchange for breakfast, she could have a serving of cereal, bread, or muffins; a serving of a fruit or juice; and a serving of milk or yogurt. An exchange list can be purchased from the American Diabetes Association (1-800-DIABETES or https://www.diabetes.org/nutrition-and-recipes/nutrition/overview.jsp).

Nutrition education is required to assist the person in learning how to use the exchanges to plan meals. Dietitians can work with the person to develop flexible meal planning depending on food preferences and lifestyle. The American Dietetic Association can provide physicians and patients with the names and telephone numbers of registered dietitians in their area.

LACTOSE INTOLERANCE

Another common concern for many older individuals (especially black people) is lactose intolerance, an inability to break down milk sugar, lactose, which is the carbohydrate found in many dairy products. Lactose intolerance can cause intestinal disturbances such as gas, bloating, diarrhea, and cramping. Alternative sources of calcium are available including yogurt with active cultures, soy milk (fortified with calcium), Lactaid (lactose-free milk), and acidophilus milk (which promotes the conversion of lactose to lactic acid). All are advancements in food technology easily tolerated by most individuals.

VEGETARIAN DIET

People who are vegetarians must plan their meals carefully to include enough protein of adequate quality and quantity. The primary sources of protein for vegetarians are legumes, grains, nuts, and seeds. But because each of these protein foods lacks one or more of the essential amino acids, they must be combined so that all essential amino acids are eaten. The basic rule is to combine grains with legumes, legumes with nuts or seeds, or grains with nuts or seeds. In addition, any animal protein complements any plant protein. For example, cereal (a grain) is complemented with milk (an animal protein). A good example of a high-quality nonanimal protein source is red beans and rice. Other examples include pasta and low-fat cheese sauce, tofu and sesame seeds, or tortillas and black beans.

MULTIVITAMIN SUPPLEMENTS

Do older people need a multivitamin supplement? In certain circumstances, a multivitamin supplement might be used to ensure adequate intake of nutrients. This is particularly true if the health care practitioner suspects poor or inadequate food intake, if laboratory results reveal a deficiency, or if there is some other reason why an individual may not be getting enough nutrients through diet. Vitamin supplements are not intended to be used in place of eating healthy foods, and neither should they be taken carelessly. Older patients should always inform their physician or dietitian if they use a multivitamin (and/or mineral supplement). Regardless of age, it is always best to eat a balanced and varied diet that is planned with an eye to ensuring adequate intake of essential nutrients instead of relying on supplements.

ANTIOXIDANTS

Of interest in the issue of aging are vitamins that act as antioxidants: betacarotene (a water-soluble precursor of vitamin A), and vitamins C and E. Antioxidants are thought to help diminish the effects of aging by preventing damage to cells and tissues by free radicals (by-products of metabolism). They may also be involved as a protective factor in reducing risk for heart disease and cancer.[8] Antioxidants also recently have been linked to positive changes in visual capacity and improvements in macular degeneration.[16,17] Good food sources of antioxidants include citrus fruits, green peppers, cantaloupe, apricots, carrots, sweet potatoes, and vegetable oils.

DRUG AND NUTRIENT INTERACTIONS

Older people regularly take prescription medications, and many take six or more at one time. The most widely used drugs by older adults are cardiac medications, followed by arthritis, psychiatric, respiratory, and gastrointestinal drugs.[18] Long-term use of medications can interfere with nutritional well-being. **Diuretics** (for example, furosemide [Lasix]) used to promote fluid excretion may increase need for potassium. Antacids reduce stomach acidity, which decreases absorption of calcium, vitamin B_{12}, and iron. **Antidepressants** such as monoamine oxidase (MAO) inhibitors (such as tranylcypromine [Parnate]) can lead to hypertension as a result of changes in lysine metabolism. **Anti-inflammatory** analgesics such as aspirin may induce anemia because of blood loss. These are only a few examples. See **Table 7-6** for more drug–nutrient interactions. Older adults should consult

TABLE 7-6   Examples of Drug–Nutrient Interactions in Older People.

Precipitating Factor	Affected Object	Finding	Recommendation
Foods containing vitamin K (e.g., green leafy vegetables, broccoli, spinach, cauliflower)	Warfarin (Coumadin)	Altered anticoagulant effect	Consistent intake of foods containing vitamin K
Antacids, multi-vitamins, iron, dairy products	Tetracyclines, quinolones (e.g., ciprofloxacin, moxifloxacin, levofloxacin)	Poor absorption. Potential treatment failure	Space ingestion 2 hours apart
Proton pump inhibitors (e.g., Prilosec, Protonix, Nexium)	Vitamin B_{12}	Poor absorption from dietary sources, due to lowered gastric acidity	With chronic acid suppressive therapy, evaluate need for vitamin B_{12} supplementation
Food	Levothyroxine (Synthroid)	Poor absorption	Consistent intake on an empty stomach
Atypical anti-psychotics (e.g., Zyprexa, Clozaril)	Nutritional status	Unintentional weight gain	Monitor effect of weight gain on disease states (e.g., diabetes, cardiovascular disease)
Food	Bisphosphonates (Fosamax, Boniva)	Significant reduction in absorption. Potential treatment failure	Adhere to administration in fasting state, 30 minutes before intake of any food or fluid, other than plain water. Remain upright for 30 minutes after swallowing

Source: Boullata, JI, Knight-Klimas, TC. Drug-nutrient interactions in the elderly. In: Boullata JI, Armenti VA (eds). *Handbook of Drug–Nutrient Interactions.* Totowa, NJ: Humana Press, 2004:363–410.

a physician, dietitian, and/or pharmacist to avoid complications related to drug and nutrient interactions.

SUMMARY

The value of appropriate nutrition screening and intervention cannot be underestimated in providing quality care for older adults. Good nutrition not only optimizes health and well-being, it helps prevent the onset of many chronic diseases.

It is imperative that health care providers be sensitive to the many changes that occur with aging and to the ways in which nutrition can affect the quality of life of older people. The first step is to understand the basic principles of nutrition and how these can be applied in encouraging healthy eating. Second, health care professionals need to be aware of how the aging process can alter nutrition status. With careful screening, counseling, and referral, if necessary, health care professionals can be certain that older persons' nutritional well-being is optimal. Ensuring quality nutrition is a crucial component of providing the best health care possible for the older population.

Review Questions

1. What are the essential nutrients?
   A. Protein, carbohydrates, vitamins, fiber, water
   B. Protein, carbohydrates, fat, water
   C. Protein, carbohydrates, fat, vitamins, minerals, water
   D. Protein, carbohydrates, fat, vitamins, minerals, water, fiber

2. What type of fat is associated with increasing blood cholesterol?
   A. Polyunsaturated
   B. Monounsaturated
   C. Saturated
   D. Glycerol

3. What is the current amount of protein that is recommended for older adults?
   A. As much as a person can consume.
   B. 0.8 g per kilogram of body weight.
   C. 1 g per kilogram of body weight.
   D. There is no current recommendation regarding protein intake.

4. How many servings each day from the fruit and vegetable group are recommended for older adults?
   A. 5
   B. 10
   C. 3
   D. 2

5. If a person is lactose intolerant, it means that
    A. He or she cannot digest the carbohydrate in milk.
    B. He or she can digest the protein in milk in limited quantities.
    C. He or she cannot digest the fiber in plant materials.
    D. He or she cannot eat any animal protein.

6. Some of the warning signs of nutrition risk in older adults include which of the following?
    A. Obesity, loss of weight, chronic disease
    B. Mental confusion, recent surgery, loss of appetite
    C. High intake of alcohol, limited nutrition knowledge
    D. All of the above

7. Which foods are good sources of fiber?
    A. Meat, fish, and poultry
    B. Fruits, vegetables, and whole grains
    C. Whole-fat dairy products
    D. Cakes and cookies

8. If you are older and want to diet to lose weight, which of the following recommendations should you follow?
    A. Eat as little as possible and keep calories down to about 800–1,000 kcal/day.
    B. Eat a balanced diet, get regular moderate exercise, and limit fats and sweets.
    C. Use appetite suppressants and liquid diet formulas to ensure rapid weight loss.
    D. Cut back on carbohydrates because they are fattening.

9. A diabetic is an individual who has
    A. Abnormal heartbeat
    B. Inadequate intake of protein
    C. Insufficient lean body mass
    D. Abnormal glucose levels

10. The water-soluble vitamins include
    A. Vitamin B_{12}, folic acid, and vitamin E
    B. B-complex vitamins and vitamin C
    C. Vitamins K, A, and C
    D. Vitamins A, D, E, and K

Learning Activities

1. You have just met with an older patient who will be included in your caseload. The patient is an 82-year-old man whose wife died last year. He has no family members who live in the community. He was referred to you by his physician, who is concerned because the patient has lost 20 pounds in the past year. The patient is

5'10" and his current weight is 158 lb. What additional information do you need to assist this patient? What do you believe is the cause of his weight loss? What are your recommendations?

2. You have just met with a new patient at the practice where you work as a medical assistant. Your new patient is a 75-year-old woman who is 5'4" and weighs 105 lb. She has a medical history of chronic pain caused by arthritis. She reports that she has recently lost interest in cooking for herself and her husband. She adds that she has a poor appetite and often forgets to eat. What would you suggest?

3. You have just interviewed an 80-year-old man who has high cholesterol. His total cholesterol is 255 mg/dL, his HDL is 40 mg/dL, and the LDL component is 155 mg/dL. Does this indicate risk for heart disease? If so, what would your recommendations be?

4. You are asked by your employer to give a presentation to a senior citizen women's group that regularly meets at their local church for evening meals financed by the church and prepared by volunteers. You agree to join them and note that the meal consists of roast beef, mashed potatoes and gravy, biscuits with butter, coffee, and apple pie. During dinner you ask and find that most of their meals are similar to this one. You present your talk on osteoporosis and agree to come back in a month for another talk. What would you want to focus on next time? Why?

REFERENCES

1. U.S. Department of Health Human Services, Administration on Aging. Older Americans Act. 2006.

2. Institute of Medicine. *The Role of Nutrition in Maintaining Health in the Nation's Elderly: Evaluating Coverage of Nutrition Services for the Medicare Population.* Washington, DC: National Academy Press; 2000.

3. Centers for Disease Control and Prevention, Merck Company Foundation. *The State of Aging and Health in America 2007.* Whitehouse Station, NJ: Merck Company Foundation; 2007.

4. Hajjar, RR, Kamel, HK, Denson, K. Malnutrition in Aging. *Internet Journal of Geriatrics and Gerontology,* 2004;1(1).

5. Allen, JE. *Assisted Living Administration: The Knowledge Base.* 2nd ed. New York: Springer; 2004:300.

6. Dwyer, JT. *Screening Older Americans' Nutritional Health: Current Practices and Future Pos-*
sibilities. Washington, DC: Nutrition Screening Initiative; 1991.

7. Centers for Disease Control and Prevention. Public Health and Aging: Retention of Natural Teeth Among Older Adults—United States, 2002. *JAMA,* 2004;291(3):292–293.

8. Glore, SL, et al. Soluble Fiber and Serum Lipids: A Literature Review. *Journal of the American Dietetic Association,* 1994;94:425–436.

9. Position of American Dietetic Association: Health Implications of Dietary Fiber. American Dietetic Association, June 2002;102(7):993–1000.

10. U.S. Department of Health and Human Services, U.S. Department of Agriculture. *Dietary Guidelines for Americans,* 2005. Washington, DC: USDHHS & USDA.

11. Lichtenstein, AH, Rasmussen, H, Yu, WW. Modified MyPyramid for Older Adults. *Journal of Nutrition,* 2008;138:78–82.

12. West, S, et al. Are Antioxidants or Supplements Protective for Age-Related Macular Degeneration? *Archives of Ophthalmology*, 1994;112:222–227.

13. United States Department of Agriculture. MyPyramid. 2005. Retrieved February 16, 2009, from http://mypyramid.gov.

14. Shannon, JB. Saturated Fat, Trans Fat, and Cholesterol. In *Diet and Nutrition Sourcebook*. 3rd ed. Detroit: Omnigraphics; 2005.

15. Giovannucci, E, et al. Relationship of Diet to Risk of Colorectal Cancer Adenoma in Men. *Journal of the National Cancer Institute*, 1992; 84:91–98.

16. Eastwood, MA. The Physiological Effects of Dietary Fiber: An Update. *Annual Review of Nutrition*, 1992;12:19–35.

17. Wardlaw, G, Insel, P. *Perspectives in Nutrition*. St. Louis: Mosby; 1996:410–411, 673.

18. Weisburger, JH, Williams, GM. *Causes of Cancer. American Cancer Society Textbook of Clinical Oncology*. Atlanta, GA: American Cancer Society; 1995.

Chapter 8

SEXUALITY AND AGING

NANCY MACRAE, MS, OTR/L, FAOTA

The two great needs for vital aging are control over one's own life and those bonds of intimacy.
—*Betty Friedan,* The Fountain of Age

Chapter Outline

Behavioral Objectives

Upon completion of this chapter, the reader will be able to:

1. Recognize the importance of intimacy in feelings of sexuality.
2. Define sexuality.
3. Describe gender differences in sexual functioning caused by aging.
4. Recognize complications from common diseases that can interfere with expression of sexuality.
5. List techniques to ameliorate complications in the expression of sexuality.
6. Understand the causes of inappropriate client/patient sexual behavior and be able to choose appropriate responses.
7. Recognize the role prescription drugs can play in sexual expression.
8. Identify two approaches to deal with sexuality issues.

Key Terms

Estrogen replacement therapy	Menopause
Gay	PLISSIT model
Intimacy	Sexuality
Lesbian	

The demographics of the United States underscore the graying of the American population with 70 million older adults (those 65 years or older) predicted in 2030; this is projected to be 20% of the population.[1] Issues of aging must be faced. Providing accurate information about the effects of time and development on the body, mind, and spirit is crucial to keep people informed about what to expect and perhaps, more important, what can be done to prolong health and to become a successful ager. Health care practitioners need to be vigilant about remembering the fact that only a small portion of older adults are institutionalized. The vast majority of older adults are leading active lives. Each succeeding cohort has benefited from more education and better health care practices. It will be fascinating to see what more knowledgeable and demanding older adults will require of themselves and their health care practitioners in terms of health in the future decades.

With a high quality of life potentially continuing longer, we can expect older adults to remain active in each significant area of their life. One wellness perspective[2] artificially divides life into occupational, intellectual, spiritual, social, physical, and emotional (includes sexuality and relationships) dimensions. The individually determined balance among these areas dynamically changes as people mature. Physical activities may decrease in importance as spiritual and social ones increase, for example. Changes likely will occur in the sexual area, if only because of decreased opportunities.

However, an awareness of each of these areas and how one can participate in each throughout life can enrich life. This chapter provides information about sexuality and aging, knowledge about specific acute and chronic conditions older adults experience, and information on inappropriate client/patient sexual behavior, and how these topics can be combined using two recommended approaches to help health care practitioners deal with the sexuality issues of their older clients. Addressing these issues may well help such clients regain intimacy and a sense of autonomy or control in their lives, both crucial for a meaningful existence.

SEXUALITY

Sexual innuendo pervades our society. We see sexual images and stereotypes portrayed in our daily lives in advertisements, in print, in song, in movies, and on television. Jokes with sexual connotations are also a frequent occurrence in our day-to-day activities. Yet as prevalent as sex is within our society, little time or attention is devoted to sexuality.

Sexuality is much more than an eight-letter word. It is a core characteristic of who we are; it is a state of mind; it is a holistic concept. We can be sexual without engaging in sex. Learning about sexuality is a lifelong process, a lifelong adventure. What we learn about sexuality, whether explicit or not, frames how we perceive ourselves and can greatly influence how we act. Taking stock of what constitutes sexuality can help us realize how very basic it is to our sense of self.

Sexuality includes the ability to be intimate with another person in a mutually satisfying manner. Obvious components of sexuality are our feelings and beliefs about what it is to be male or female, how we relate to people of our own or the opposite gender, how we establish relationships, especially close and intimate ones, and how we express our feelings. The familial, cultural, and religious environments in which we develop influence the growth of sexuality. If we were loved and nurtured and our sense of competence was fostered and strengthened by those we love, it is likely we have healthy self-images and a fair amount of success in both initiating and sustaining personal relationships. If abuse of any sort was present in our background, conversely, it is likely that we will not develop a positive sense of self-worth and may have difficulty with trusting relationships.

How our first exposure to overtly sexual feelings was handled by others also colors our perception of ourselves as sexual beings. Embarrassment, ridicule, or censure as reactions to sexual expressions can leave lasting scars. Acceptance, encouragement, and enjoyment of such feelings obviously lead to a different conclusion. Fostering the ability to say "no" and accept the responsibility that accompanies the expression of sexuality can only strengthen one's feeling of self-efficacy.

AGING AND SEXUALITY

Deeply embedded in our youth-oriented society is the assumption that sex and sexuality are provinces of only the young. Aging men are depicted as "dirty old men" if they show any interest in sex, while aging women are characterized as sexless old hags. Yet the feelings of sexuality do not disappear as the years pass. Hopefully, these feelings change and grow as we change and grow.

Betty Friedan, in her book *The Fountain of Age*,[3] challenges us to look at how social values victimize both sexes: women by the feminine mystique; men by a lifetime of machismo. Images of youthful erection always leading to intercourse and an excessive emphasis on performance are a heavy burden for both men *and* women to bear, as these youthful sexual measures impose barriers to intimacy for those who are aging. Pleasuring, cuddling, and touching have been found to be more important among older adults,[4] who tend to view the total sexual experience through a qualitative rather than a quantitive lens.

A 2007 study of sexuality by Lindau et al.[5p. 762] in the *New England Journal of Medicine* defines sexual activity as "any mutually voluntary activity with another person that involves sexual contact, whether or not intercourse or orgasm occurs." Successful sexuality experiences are more than meeting or exceeding a standard of performance. First, the two people involved in a sexual relationship define the parameters. Second, there is an infinite variety of possibilities that may prove satisfying to one or both partners.

Lindau's[5] groundbreaking national representative probability study of sexuality and health among older American community-dwelling adults found a strong association between physical health and sexual activity. This association is stronger than age alone with sexual activity. The majority of surveyed older adults reported sexuality to be an important component of their lives and engaged regularly in spousal or other intimate sexual relationships. Despite sexual problems, sexual activity only began to substantially decrease after the age of 74. The difficulty of women having a partner/spouse with whom to be intimate was substantiated. Older adults involved in this study welcomed the opportunity to discuss sexuality, something rarely brought up by their physicians. Fifty percent of the sexually active older adults indicated at least one "bothersome" problem, often erectile dysfunction for males and low desire and vaginal lubrication and climax difficulties for females.

A British study by Gott and Hinchliff[6] on the views of older adults about the importance of sex in their lives relied on a combination of quantitative and qualitative data. Again, these adults welcomed the chance to discuss sex. Findings underscore sex as an important part of a close relationship. Health problems and widowhood can lead to a reprioritization of the role of sex in their lives, and maintaining physical intimacy, even when intercourse is no longer possible, is centrally important.

Ginsberg et al.[7] found in a study of lower-income older adults that participants wanted to engage in sexual activities more frequently than they did, but could not often because of a lack of partners. Touching and kissing were desired, while mutual stroking, masturbation, and intercourse were less often experienced or desired. Age and health status, again, were found to be predictive of preferences for sexual activity.

INTIMACY

What becomes clear in the recent literature on sexuality and older adults is the importance of **intimacy**.[8] Sexual intimacy requires self-acceptance and risk taking. It involves purposely losing control of oneself and acquiescing to what is happening. When the result of sexual intimacy is a satisfying one, feelings of self-esteem and trust are reinforced.

Intimacy needs to be included as a component of meaningful sexuality. Women, as kin keepers, have traditionally nurtured a capacity for connection and engagement with others in all forms of intimacy. Men may have many friends, but deep and honest disclosure, so vital to intimacy, may not be a part of these friendships. Jung, in describing the years after 40, calls them the "afternoon"[9] of life and suggests that each gender come to know its polarities, the sexually opposite side of their nature: for the male, his feminine qualities; for the female, her male traits. Coming to grips with these unused and unfamiliar characteristics can involve stress and anxiety, but ultimately their emergence can lead to a freedom of expression previously unknown.[8] This "crossover" may be a key to vital aging. "Disengagement from the roles and goals of youth and from activities and ties that no longer have any personal meaning may, in fact, be necessary to make the shift to a new kind of engagement in age."[3] It can enhance sexual activity, with the woman showing more initiative but also expecting more closeness and disclosure from her partner. Couples who persevere through these growth trials can find a new depth and richness in their relationships. They will then be ready to reinvest in different ways of communicating with each other. They continue to want to genuinely touch, know, and love each other. Such renewed ties of intimacy can lead to a sense of control of life and an acceptance, rather than a fear, of aging.[10]

PHYSIOLOGIC CHANGES IN WOMEN

Undeniable changes occur in both men and women in the physiologic aspects of their sexual functioning as they age. The effects of gravity begin to be seen in both men and women as bodies begin to sag and waistlines begin to widen. The changes each gender encounters do not need to preclude sexual activity because reduced sexual hormones affect only response time and may affect the intensity of the physical response. Knowing about and understanding the effect of these changes, combined with appropriate adaptations, can actually enhance rather than deter sexual satisfaction.

Menopause, a natural consequence of getting older, is the cessation of menstruation. It is part of the climacteric, a period of time lasting from 6 to 15 years that leads up to and follows the experience of the last menstrual period. It is usually accepted as the beginning of a woman's second half of life and is a physiologic marker for changes in her sexual functioning. The average age of the last period of American women is approximately 52 years, with a range from ages 45 to 55.[11]

Much has been written in feminist texts[3,11,12] about the "medicalization" of menopause, with large portions of the medical field viewing it as a "deficiency" disease. This medicalization has intruded into the lives of younger women with the creation of a new category of disease: female sexual dysfunction, which often has the support of researchers associated with drug companies.[13] How menopause is approached and dealt with by women is significantly influenced by a combination of cultural, religious, and family experiences, as well as whether the women accept or deny the aging process.

Ironically, during the first half of the 20th century in the United States, medical intervention was seldom used for menopause because it was viewed as a natural event. Now that 50 million women are nearing menopausal age, an incredible market for manufactured hormones exists.[3] **Estrogen replacement therapy** (ERT) is recommended by physicians to treat this "deficiency disease," with its accompanying hot flashes, sweating, and vaginal dryness, and to reduce the likelihood of developing osteoporosis or heart disease. Debates regarding the necessity for ERT abound because of increased likelihood of developing uterine or breast cancer with this treatment. The final decision must be made by the individual woman based on her particular health status and unique family medical history. More natural approaches (e.g., use of homeopathic and herbal remedies, diet, and exercise) are also now preferred to help women experience the menopausal years.[11,14]

Decreasing amounts of estrogen account for many of the signs exhibited at menopause. These signs include the following:

- Vaginal changes
  - Thinning of walls
  - Decreased lubrication
  - Foreshortening of vagina
  - Delayed and reduced expansion of the vagina
- Vasomotor changes leading to hot flashes or flushes
  - Blood flows to skin causing a 4–8°F skin temperature increase
  - Sweating
  - Increased heart rate
  - Chills
  - Tingling of skin
- Less rapid and extreme vascular responses to sexual arousal
  - Waning of flush
  - Reduced increase in breast volume during arousal[14]
- Orgasm with fewer contractions
- Bladder and urethral changes
  - Increased need to urinate, particularly immediately after intercourse
  - Irritability—a variant of "honeymoon cystitis"[14]
- Diminished fatty tissue of mons
  - Labia majora become susceptible to mechanical trauma from repetitive bumping or rubbing during intercourse
- Clitoral area is more susceptible to irritation by forceful manipulation[11,12,15,16]

An obvious omission from this list of changes is a decrease in libido. Sexual desire and activity do not need to decrease during this period because "sex drive is *NOT* related to estrogen levels."[11] Libido can actually increase postmenopausally because of the elimination of pregnancy fears, decreased child care responsibilities, an increase in energy and a zest for life, and improved self-knowledge. Yet, if desire does decrease it may be the result of health problems, medications, and a lack of available partners.[17] Women age 65 and older report one or more sexual concerns, a similar number to younger women, and they also report that their partner's sexual difficulties are a significant barrier. Despite this, physicians often do not initiate a discussion about sexuality concerns with female patients, and when they do, they seldom include partners' difficulties.

PHYSIOLOGIC CHANGES IN MEN

Sexual functioning also changes for men as they age. These changes are less dramatic than those experienced by women perimenopausally. A gradual decrease in circulating testosterone after 60 years of age accounts for these changes; they do not signal a decrease in potency. Changes include the following:

- Arousal
  - Delayed and less firm erection with longer intervals to ejaculation
  - Less clear sense of impending orgasm
- Orgasm
  - Abbreviated ejaculation
  - Decreased expulsive urethral contractions
  - Decreased force of seminal fluid expulsion
  - Reduced amount of semen ejaculation; ejaculation may not occur with every intercourse
- Postorgasm
  - Rapid loss of erection
  - Longer time needed between erections
- Extragenital
  - Decreased swelling and erection of nipples
  - Absence of flush
  - Reduced elevation of testicles[11,14]

Knowing about these changes can diminish a man's fears of performance and can in fact contribute to increased sexual pleasure. Realizing the need for more prolonged and direct stimulation can lead to lengthened and more engaging lovemaking sessions, sessions that may offer a more profound sense of pleasure than when the partners were younger. The technique of "stuffing," when a partially erect penis is stuffed into the vagina and the woman tightens her vaginal muscles rhythmically to stimulate both partners, can be an effective technique.

GENDER DIFFERENCES

New meanings regarding sexuality may emerge as one ages. Despite the fact men and women develop distinctive sexual styles and gender differences persist throughout life, some older women have been affected by the current cultural expectations for sexual behavior. These cultural changes may include different sexual scripts,[18] whereby the woman can assume the lead, asking for dates or paying her share of expenses on dates. Occupational accomplishments can lead to secure jobs, increased self-esteem, role transitions (loss or change of partner), and an increase in sexual agency, including the ability to choose and have control over one's sexual life.[19]

Masturbation occurrences increased significantly over time for unmarried women, according to a nonrandomized sample of 102 respondents ages 60 to 85 in a 1985 Adams and Turner study.[19] Besides preserving sexual functioning when a partner is not available, masturbation may enhance feelings of autonomy. However, masturbation was not a favored sexual activity of the majority of those, both men and women, who engaged in it. It was viewed as a substitute sexual activity. In this same study, 85% of women and 89% of men preferred interpersonal rather than solo sexual activity if given a choice. Adams and Turner conclude their article on a hopeful note: A substantial minority of women in the study experienced an increase in the frequency of orgasm, subjective pleasure, and overall satisfaction. These changes in sexuality occurred in late middle life and beyond.[1] In the more recent Ginsberg[7] study, masturbation was not wanted by most of the participants, yet the Lindau study[5] found the masturbation rate to be higher among men (52%) than among women (25%) with a spouse or other intimate partner in the previous year.

Interviews with older adults reveal a lasting difference in how men and women view sexual activity. Duke Longitudinal Studies[20,21] have found sexual activity is more stable over time than previously thought. They found three-quarters of men in their 70s engaged in intercourse at least once a month, while more than a third of men in their early 60s and nearly 30% of men in their late 60s engaged in weekly intercourse. The majority of women were not sexually active primarily because of a paucity of partners or their male partners' decreased desire. However, the same Duke University Studies found nearly one-half of married 66- to 71-year-old women were sexually active. Nearly 30% of those closer to age 80 were sexually active. The Lindau study[5] reconfirms these findings: Even in the oldest age group, those in their 80s, 54% of sexually active adults engaged in sexual activity 2–3 times a month, with 23% once a week or more. Oral sex was more frequent among younger respondents, likely an indication of the cohort effect.

In interviews with 10 high-functioning, healthy, active, married and divorced or single women older than 60 years, Crose and Drake[22] found a decrease in incidence but a constant or increased level of sexual satisfaction from when they were younger. These women also felt that they displayed more positive sexual attitudes over time. Sexual encounters had become less pressured, pregnancy was no longer a fear, and seeking pleasure for themselves was an acceptable goal. Masturbation was increasingly used by these women to relieve sexual tension. They indicated a stimulating relationship was a prerequisite to sex. Women maintain and renew ties of intimacy (with both men and women), and this may help them to maintain a sense of control in their later lives.[3]

Prevailing public attitudes that women, after disability, are less interested in sex and that their physiologic response is affected led Nosek and colleagues[23] to survey the top concerns of women (1,150 women ages 18–65) with physical disabilities. They found these women were concerned about the following issues:

- The satisfaction of their partners
- Feeling sexually unattractive

- Others viewing them as sexually unattractive
- The physical issues of urinary or bowel accidents

They wanted to receive information about the following topics:

- Coping emotionally with the changes in sexual functioning
- Helping a partner cope emotionally with limitations on sexual activity
- Methods and techniques to achieve sexual satisfaction

Despite these findings, women were less likely to have received information about sexuality after injury. This report underscores the importance of psychosocial factors in sexual functioning.

Couples, "two people in a committed relationship which may include but is not exclusive to heterosexual married and cohabitating couples"[24p. 268] are also greatly affected when one partner becomes disabled. A majority report a decline in sexual activity frequency, a necessary change in its pattern, as well as a decline in both satisfaction and interest. Yet a desire for more satisfaction was expressed.[25] Fear, feelings of discomfort, and increased stress affecting their roles and personal boundaries are the reasons for these limitations. Those with postdisability-formed relationships report greater satisfaction (both with frequency and variety of sexual activity).[26] The longer a partner acts as a caretaker in a predisability-established relationship, the more difficult achieving intimacy can become.[27] Associations with other people and activities appear to be the strongest predictor of positive marital adjustment.[28] Education and counseling also can help.

Recognition of the importance of continuing sexuality in the lives of older adults can help people to enhance self-esteem and increase their options for intimacy. Combined with more realistic expectations about age-related changes, this recognition can assist in the development of adaptive coping strategies.

OLDER LESBIANS AND GAY MEN

Older **lesbian** and **gay** people are a diverse group—a group whose popular image is often a negative one. Their issues with sexuality are both similar to those heterosexuals confront and different. Ageism added onto homophobia increases the challenges faced by aging lesbians and gays as they deal with their changing and developing sexuality. Negative stereotypes of lonely, depressed, oversexed, unattractive, and unemotional older lesbians and gay men are myths. Friend,[29] in an article on older lesbian and gay people, reports a substantial portion of older gay men were found to be "psychologically well-adjusted, self-accepting, and adapting well to the aging process," and a majority of older lesbian women studied were found to be happy and well adjusted.

Friend, using a social construction theory, proposes that the concept of heterosexuality has shaped or constructed the homosexual identity as one of sickness. The current older lesbian and gay cohorts have had to manage heterosexism for the greater part of their lives.

They have had to reconstruct the meaning of a homosexual identity in an attempt to control their own sexuality. Cass[30] identifies the developmental stages that gays and lesbians progress through as identity, confusion, comparison, tolerance, acceptance, pride, and synthesis. Stages mastered at appropriate ages facilitate maturity, while inability to master certain stages leads to immaturity and feelings of incompetence.[31] Reconstructing their identities often involves conflicts with family and friends and active attempts to initiate social change. They may be the only group who needs to inform their family of origin about their changed group membership status—their "coming out."[32] Efforts to find a niche in society often lead to high levels of adjustment where lesbians and gays develop skills that facilitate their ability to manage the aging process. Such experience develops a "crisis competence" flexibility in gender role and a redefinition of family[29] that provide a unique perspective on other crises in their lives. The fact that they may not be able to count on family in old age has encouraged this group to plan more carefully for older age.

Lesbian women can and do experience sexual difficulties. Instead of one woman undergoing menopausal changes in the relationship, there may be two, and at the same time. One may experience a decreased interest in sex.[18] Same-gender relationships can, because of a certain closeness that comes from being the same gender, become extremely close and confining, necessitating the establishment of a healthy balance between togetherness and aloneness. Expectations, because of being the same gender, that the other will intuitively know what is wanted and needed may be unrealistic and, as with heterosexual relationships, require good communication between partners.

Pope[33] makes eight recommendations for health care practitioners in their interactions with older lesbians and gays: take a nonjudgmental approach, assess their identity development stage, develop an awareness of their cultures, develop an awareness of the societal discrimination they face, understand the importance of sex for older gay men and relationships for older lesbians, understand there will be a variety of sexual behaviors to satisfy older gays and lesbians, and develop a positive view of sexual activity in this population.

ADDRESSING SEXUAL ISSUES

Because sexuality is such a primal core of our lives, it is a necessary part of a functional evaluation throughout the life span, even in end-of-life situations.[34] It is identified as an activity of daily living and falls within the domain of practice of many health care practitioners.[35] When the issue of sexuality is viewed as another aspect of the day-to-day activities in which a client will be involved and when its psychosocial importance is understood, it needs to be included in assessment procedures. Mentioning it to clients as yet another aspect of daily life to be considered provides an opportunity for clients to talk about their functioning in this area and to pursue any desired intervention.

It is crucial for practitioners to have a clear comprehension of their own comfort level in dealing with issues of sexuality. An obvious prerequisite is an acceptance of one's own sexuality, which requires a level of maturity and a period of introspection. A helpful tool is Annon's four-level **PLISSIT model**,[36] which not only identifies the level of intervention needed by a client, but also assists the practitioner in understanding the level at which he or she can comfortably provide intervention.

Annon's model is a conceptual scheme for differentiating and treating sexual problems and concerns. His schema can help distinguish those who are likely to respond to sex education and brief sex therapy from those who need intensive psychotherapy. Each descending level requires more expertise from practitioners so the approach can be geared to their own level of competence. Knowledge of resources available within their treatment site or community is a necessary component of this approach so that referrals can be handled smoothly.

The four levels of treatment within the PLISSIT model are as follows:

- *Permission*:   The client is given permission to discuss any concerns and is reassured as a sexual being; affords an opportunity for practitioners to provide a nonjudgmental and relaxed environment in which to share their knowledge.
- *Limited information*:   Specific factual information directly relevant to the particular sexual concern is provided on a one-on-one basis; myths and misconceptions, particularly about disabilities, can be dispelled.
- *Specific suggestions*:   Strategies or alternatives are provided to change or influence the specific problem behavior; the partner needs to be involved at this level; positioning and adaptive equipment are examples.
- *Intensive therapy*:   Long-term treatment for chronic sexual problems is provided.

Health care practitioners need to proceed only to the level to which they feel comfortable and for which they feel prepared. Many will feel able to deal effectively with the first three levels. Inherent in this is preparation for the requisite referral information and knowledge about myths, various disabilities, and cultural sensitivity. What is crucial, however, is being able to calmly relay information in an accepting and nonjudgmental manner and smoothly refer to others, such as occupational therapists and psychologists, for their expertise when necessary.

For practitioners to be able to help clients deal with their sexual concerns they need to exhibit the following characteristics:

- Sensitivity
- Understanding of the effect of losses on the mind, spirit, and body
- Knowledge of the processes of diagnoses, as well as knowledge of available resources
- Respect for cultural and gender differences in sexual expression
- Familiarity with a wide number of possible strategies for intervention

They also need to be aware of the following assumptions:

- The client will bring up sexuality issues.
- Chronological age may indicate an increased or decreased libido.

- The client's sexual preference fits with practitioners' views of morality.
- The client is monogamous.
- The client shares practitioners' views on morality.

In other words, practitioners may need to make the first move and be aware of indirect attempts on the part of the client (jokes, for example) to bring up the topic.

Inappropriate client/patient sexual behavior (ISB) can interfere with client care and intervention. Definitions of ISB vary and depend on personal sensitivity to appropriateness. ISB can range from offensive jokes and flattering comments, to asking for a date and/or deliberate touching, to exposure and attempts at sexual fondling.[37] These types of behavior are common in the health care field[38–40] and occur along a continuum of mild to severe. Disinhibition from neurological conditions, longstanding sexual dysfunctions, fear of loss of sexual function, a diversion from treatment, and an attempt to gain power or control are possible causes of this behavior. ISB can be defined as sexual harassment because of its unwelcome nature, its possible interference with an individual's work performance, and the creation of a hostile, offensive work environment.[41] Ignoring the behavior may be the practitioner's response, but this accomplishes nothing. There are more effective ways to respond. Although each case must be viewed individually and contextual clues are of paramount importance, practitioners can be assertive, provide nonthreatening feedback to the client, be honest, and be clear. Discussing the issue with the client can lead to a positive therapeutic relationship.[42] Friedman recommends that practitioners do not ignore this behavior. Practitioners should not accept any behavior from a client they would not accept from anyone else. Immediate reporting of repeated behavior must occur, and an interdisciplinary behavioral plan may need to be developed, which is often appropriate for clients with dementia. Practitioners also need to respond to prevent such behavior from negatively affecting them.

With aging comes an increase in both chronic and acute physical problems and disabilities. Typical older adults have a number of chronic conditions that can affect them not only physically, but also emotionally and sexually. Some of the most prevalent chronic conditions of those 65 years and older are arthritis, hypertension, heart disease, deformity or orthopedic impairment, and diabetes.[43]

Another approach to addressing sexual issues is to look at the areas of sexual concern for those who are physically challenged, whether from a recent injury or because of chronic problems. These areas fall into four general categories:

- Self-esteem
- Body image
- Relationships
- Family[44]

Questions about continued worthiness as a man or woman can arise soon after the disability occurs or they may appear gradually as a chronic condition worsens with age.

Issues about whether one's body can be trusted or respected again are likely to coincide with questions regarding self-esteem. Anxiety about the ability to maintain or initiate new relationships, from social to intimate, also surfaces. Options for sexual relations and for continuing to fulfill family roles effectively may also need to be addressed.

Practitioners prepared with a foundation of healthy acceptance of their own sexuality and a desire to holistically treat those who are aging can effectively use their clinical knowledge and skills to help in the recovery of a client and/or in the client's ability to learn to live with one or more disabilities. Approaching sexuality from a positive viewpoint, based on what does work rather than on what the person cannot do, and from a base of open communication and intimacy can make a crucial difference.[45]

SAMPLE DIAGNOSTIC CATEGORIES

Knowledge about specific diagnostic categories likely to be associated with being older, as well as the coexistence of multiple chronic illnesses, is necessary to deal with sexuality issues effectively and sensitively. Building on psychosocial issues that have been mentioned earlier using Annon's PLISSIT model and taking into account the areas of sexual concern for those who are physically challenged can help a health care practitioner assist a client. A combination of these two approaches is used to demonstrate how sexual issues can be dealt with in the following three diagnostic categories, chosen for their prevalence in older adults.

Arthritis   Limitations imposed by arthritis and rheumatism affect more than 30% of people age 65 and older. Sore joints, range-of-motion limitations, loss of mobility, and pain with movement can impede sexual performance, yet regular sexual activity can lead to adrenal gland production of cortisone and can decrease stress and lead to less pain, discomfort, and depression.[45] The following are suggestions for older adults to deal with the problems a diagnosis of arthritis may cause:

- Rest prior to sexual activity to prevent fatigue.
- Place a pillow under limbs that are painful.
- Use aspirin prophylactically for pain before sexual activity.
- Use a hot shower or other heat source before sexual activity.
- Experiment with alternative positions, ones that do not put prolonged pressure on involved joints.
- Use alternatives to intercourse such as mutual masturbation or oral sex.
- Empty bladder before sexual activity to increase comfort.
- Exercise regularly to increase or maintain joint mobility.
- Communicate with the partner about fears.
- Use a warm waterbed.[46]

Heart Disease Heart disease can lead to anxiety about and avoidance of sexual activity. However, the energy expenditure of the average sexual act approximates walking rapidly or climbing one or two flights of stairs. Four to 5 weeks after a coronary attack an individual is usually ready to resume these activities. However, it is not uncommon for men to have sexual difficulties for up to 6 to 12 months after recovery. Fear of sudden death during sex, low endurance, and medication-induced erectile problems feed a man's anxiety. In fact, death during coitus accounts for less than 1% of sudden coronary deaths, and, of these, 70% occur during extramarital relations.[47] Women with heart disease are less likely to develop subsequent sexual problems.

Suggestions for dealing with the effects of heart disease include the following:

- Take a less active role in the sexual act.
- Learn and use relaxation techniques.
- Masturbate as an alternative.
- Take time for foreplay to allow the heart to warm up slowly.
- Avoid sexual activity when you are anxious or fatigued or when the weather is extremely hot, cold, or humid.
- Use positions that both conserve energy and are non-weight-bearing (sitting or side-lying, for example).[46]

Cerebrovascular Accidents and Stroke Cerebrovascular accidents (CVAs) lead to sensation loss, perceptual problems, loss of strength and mobility, visual problems, and/or communication problems. Suggestions for older people with this diagnosis include using touch, smell, and vision rather than speech, as well as the following:

- Experiment with comfortable positions.
- Have your partner stay within the visual field.
- Use a waterbed.
- Use a vibrator to compensate for weakness or incoordination.
- Stimulate areas that remain responsive to touch.[46]

An alternative way to present helpful possibilities is one that does not rely on diagnostic categories but rather on symptomatology. The chart in **Table 8-1** is self-explanatory.

THE INFLUENCE OF MEDICATIONS

Knowledge of how medications can affect sexual functioning is also important for effective intervention with sexuality concerns. Honest reporting of concerns to the physician is necessary. Alternative medications, ones that may eliminate or reduce any sexual problems, may be available. A list of commonly used drugs and their possible side effects is included in **Table 8-2**.

TABLE 8-1   Presenting Problems and Potential Solutions.

Presenting Problem	Possible Diagnoses	Precautions	Potential Solutions
Decreased endurance	Arthritis Cardiac disease Post CVA Parkinsons's disease	Avoid extreme temperatures, heat, cold, humidity. Avoid anxiety and fatigue. Avoid sexual activity until 1 hour after a large meal. Avoid alcohol.	Rest prior to sexual activity. Schedule sexual activity for best energy time during day. Utilize sexual positions and techniques that require less energy: • Affected partner lying on back (no energy expended to support weight on arms) • Both partners in spoon side-lying position with back of one to front of another (no overworking of muscles to support weight) • Ample direct genital foreplay Use masturbation as alternative
Pain, stiff joints, or decreased range of motion	Arthritis	Pain: Respect pain. Support painful area. Do not continue painful motion. Avoid staying in one position too long. Be well rested.	Place pillow under affected limbs. Precede sexual activity with warm bath, hot shower, or other heat source. Take aspirin prophylactically for pain prior to sexual activity. Exercise regularly to increase or maintain joint mobility. Use warm waterbed. Use relaxation techniques. Experiment with alternative positions, ones that do not put prolonged pressure on involved joints: • Rear entry supported by woman • Nonaffected partner on top Use prescribed muscle relaxants for high tone prior to sexual activity.
Contractures	Arthritis Post CVA	Avoid stress to contractures.	Use comfortable positions. Work within pain-free range of movement.
Tremors	Parkinson's disease Medication-related side effect		Use positions that incorporate weight bearing on affected limbs. Either decrease or increase movement, depending on which produces fewer tremors.

TABLE 8-1   Presenting Problems and Potential Solutions. *(continued)*

Presenting Problem	Possible Diagnoses	Precautions	Potential Solutions
Bladder/bowel dysfunction	Post CVA Spinal cord injury	Have towels nearby in advance.	Discuss fears and concerns with partner before sexual activity. Determine safest time during urinary schedule for sexual activity. Use protective covering on mattress. Man can wear condom for small amounts of urinary incontinence during sexual activity. Empty bladder before sexual activity. If on catheterization program, catheterize and empty bladder before sexual activity. Secure indwelling catheter prior to sexual activity (woman, to abdomen; man, to penis) Use extension on tubing for bedside drainage bag for more maneuverability.

Data from: Laflin, M. Sexuality and the Elderly. In CB Lewis (ed.), *Aging: The Health Care Challenge.* 3rd ed. Philadelphia: F. A. Davis; 1996:364. Leiblum, SR. Sexuality and the Midlife Woman. *Psychology of Women Quarterly,* 1990;14:495. Lewis, CB (ed.). *Aging: The Health Care Challenge.* Philadelphia: F. A. Davis; 1985:293. Montgomery, EA, Hogan, LS. *A New Beginning: Sexuality and Rehabilitation.* Boston: Spaulding Rehabilitation Hospital; 1992. Siegal, DL, et al. Menopause: Entering Our Third Age. In PB Doress, DL Siegal (eds.), *Ourselves Growing Older.* New York: Touchstone Books; 1987:116.

SEXUALITY ISSUES FOR THOSE WHO ARE INSTITUTIONALIZED

When older adults become dependent and are institutionalized, their need for intimacy and sexual expression does not disappear. Their needs for intimacy may in fact increase as they make efforts to cope within a constrained environment. They may suffer from what Ghusen[48] terms "emotional malnutrition." Nursing home residents report they support the sexual rights of their peers whether or not they personally are sexually active. Health care providers must acknowledge these needs and take steps to accommodate them as important signs of respect; this is normally done on a case-by-case basis. Some institutions have set aside one room where couples may spend time alone to pursue whatever course of intimacy they choose; other organizations help schedule time alone for couples in shared rooms when the roommate is regularly out of the room.[49] Staff are educated to be accepting of expressions of intimacy and sexuality (masturbation, hand holding,

TABLE 8-2   Drug-Induced Sexual Dysfunction.

Drug	Potential Effects
Alcohol (ethanol)	Libido enhanced at low does; does-related progressive decline due to central nervous system depressant effects; can result in failure of erection in men and reduced vaginal vasodilation and delayed orgasm in women; can also cause disinhibition, impaired judgment, and decreased ability to enjoy sexual encounter
Amphetamines	Libido enhanced at low doses; possible erectile dysfunction in men with higher doses may cause hyperexcitability, tremulousness, and anxiety
Anticonvulsants	Reduced libido; can cause drowsiness, irritability, dizziness, confusion, ataxia, and slurred speech, as well as nausea, constipation, and/or diarrhea, which may interfere with sexual activity
Antidepressants	
Tricyclics; monoamine oxidase inhibitors	Decreased libido, erectile dysfunction, impotence, delayed and/or painful ejaculation, and anorgasmia in men; decreased libido, delayed orgasm, and anorgasmia in women
Selective serotonin reuptake inhibitors	Delayed orgasm, anorgasmia (primarily with fluoxetrine)
Trazodone	Priapism, increased libido in women
Antihypertensives	
Diuretics	Decreased libido, erectile dysfunction, impotence, gynecomastia
Beta-blockers	Erectile dysfunction, decreased libido, impotence
Alpha-blockers	Erectile dysfunction, priapism
Calcium-channel blockers and methyldopa, clonidine, hydralazine	Erectile dysfunction
Barbiturates and benzodiazepines	Libido enhanced at low doses; progressive decline with higher doses due to central nervous system depressant effects
Cocaine	Erectile dysfunction, ejaculatory dysfunction, anorgasmia

Data from: Nolin, TD, Aldridge, SD. Drug-Induced Sexual Dysfunction. *Clinical Pharmacy,* 1982;1:141–147. Lee, M, Sharfi, R. More on Drug-Induced Sexual Dysfunction. *Clinical Pharmacy,* 1982;1:397. Smith, RJ, Talbert, RL. Sexual Dysfunction with Antihypertensive and Antipsychotic Agents. *Clinical Pharmacy,* 1986;5:373–384. Thompson, JF. Geriatiric Urologic Disorders. In LY Young, MA Koda-Kimble (eds.), *Applied Therapeutics: The Clinical Use of Drugs.* Vancouver, WA: Clinical Therapeutics; 1995:103–111. Troutman, WG. Drug-Induced Sexual Dysfunction. In PO Anderson, JE Knoben (eds.), *Handbook of Clinical Drug Data.* Stamford, CT: Appleton & Lange; 1997:686.

kissing, touching, petting)[21] and to know when to guide the involved people into more private areas.

Special needs may also be apparent in the community partners of those who are institutionalized. Providing time and space for intimacy when it is desired is important, as is offering counseling and understanding from the medical staff.[50]

A primary issue of concern in this area is of competence. Determining whether an older adult is capable of making a choice and not being taken advantage of is crucial. Guidelines have been proposed by Lichtenberg for use in long-term care settings.[51] They are based on the Mini Mental State Examination score of at least 14 and a subjective interview that addresses awareness of others, capacity to decline uninvited sexual contact, and realization a relationship may be time limited.[51]

Ghusen offers several strategies to enhance sexuality expression for institutionalized older adults.[48] Practitioners need to be aware of the myths and realities of sexuality, to be educated about older adults' sexual needs, to help shield residents from abuse, to reexamine their own prejudices, and to work to change policies into ones that promote a high quality of life for residents and help families not to impose their own biases on their elder family members. Finally, he recommends alternate outlets for sexual expression, ones that maintain and restore ego strength.

RESPONSIBLE SEXUAL BEHAVIOR

Age is not an excuse for failure to follow safe sex practices. Sexually transmitted diseases and HIV cases do exist in the elderly population. Statistics from the Centers for Disease Control and Prevention show that approximately 15% of the newly diagnosed cases of HIV are among Americans 50 years or older.[52] The incidence of HIV is rising faster among this age group than it is in younger age groups with a male:female ratio of approximately 9:1.[53-55]

This older group differs from those who are younger with AIDS. They show the largest proportion of cases in any adult age group attributed to heterosexual transmission;[56] other cases are ascribed to blood transfusions occurring before 1985;[57] and approximately 16% in a study of older adults became infected from IV drug use.[56] However, homosexual or bisexual behavior remains the predominant risk factor for HIV infection up to the age of 70.[57] The Centers for Disease Control and Prevention has generated data implying stability in HIV diagnoses of persons 50 and older; yet the number of older adults diagnosed with AIDS and those living with HIV is increasing. Nonspecific symptoms can frequently be overlooked because of the high level of chronic illnesses in the older population. AIDS dementia complex may be the initial manifestation of HIV infection and needs to be part of any differential diagnosis of older adults with diffuse cognitive dysfunction.[58] This type of dementia progresses more rapidly than that of Alzheimer's disease.

Educational efforts regarding safe sexual practices have been almost exclusively directed to younger cohorts, which is at least partially explained by the societal stereotype that older adults are no longer sexual. Consequently, safe sex practices are not subscribed to by this age group. At-risk persons older than 50 were only one-sixth as likely to use condoms as compared with at-risk persons in the 20- to 29-year-old group.[53] Additionally, atrophic vaginal tissue changes in older women make them particularly susceptible to lesions that may readily admit HIV.[57]

Recommendations to improve safe sex practices in this group include fostering an increased awareness on the part of health care practitioners, particularly physicians, of the need to routinely make sexual histories a part of their medical examinations.[57,58] The University of Colorado study supports the willingness of older adults to talk about sexuality in their lives. This process also involves demystifying the stereotype that older adults are sexually inactive. Health care practitioners also need to be aware of the different ways sexually transmitted diseases (STDs) may be transmitted among older adults, the appropriate modes of treatment, and a sensitivity to how safe sex information is acknowledged by clients and shared with significant others.[56] Support, in all forms, must be provided for this group, as for any age group.

SUMMARY

Acknowledging the importance sexuality plays in all of our lives and displaying a sensitivity to the personal nature of this component of our lives can help health care practitioners assist older adults to deal with sexuality issues effectively. Providing empathy and appropriate information, devising adaptations, and encouraging experimentation to find resolutions can be invaluable services to clients. Tact, discretion, and judicious use of humor are also effective tools on which health care practitioners can rely. When health care practitioners routinely discuss sexuality as another one of the activities of daily living, clients can talk about and deal with any issues in this area. Collaborative problem solving can help to empower the client to gain control over this most intimate of areas. The resulting feelings of wholeness and connectedness to another are gifts we can give.

Review Questions

1. Sexuality is not only an nine-letter word. It can best be defined by which of the following phrases?
   A. Sexual intercourse
   B. Basic to our sense of self
   C. Intimacy is a prerequisite
   D. A dynamic concept defined in a mutually satisfying way by both partners

2. Choose the statement that is *not* true: Aging
   A. Causes physiologic changes in both genders
   B. Precludes sexual activity
   C. For women has become medicalized (in its treatment of menopause)
   D. Causes a decrease in testosterone in men, but not necessarily a decrease in potency

3. Choose the *true* statement that best completes the following sentence: For women, sexuality changes in later life can include
   A. An increase in orgasm frequency, subjective pleasure, and overall satisfaction
   B. Masturbation as a favored sexual activity
   C. Increased lubrication of the vaginal walls
   D. Few vasomotor changes

4. Choose the *false* statement that best completes the following sentence: For men, sexuality changes in later life can include
   A. A rapid loss of erection
   B. A reduced amount of ejaculate
   C. An increase in potency
   D. Less dramatic changes than those experienced by premenopausal women

5. Which of the following issues do older lesbian and gay people face that heterosexuals do not encounter?
   A. Homophobia
   B. Ageism
   C. Aging bodies
   D. Negative stereotypes

6. Which of the following is *not* helpful to a practitioner in dealing with issues of sexuality?
   A. A sense of humor
   B. An understanding of his or her own comfort level with issues of sexuality
   C. A knowledge of sexuality resources
   D. Waiting for the client to bring up concerns about sexuality

7. Choose the following phrase that best describes the four areas of sexual concern for those who are physically challenged.
   A. Self-esteem, body weight, appearance, and activity level
   B. Family, relationships, body image, and self-esteem
   C. Fear, relationships, loss of libido, and self-esteem
   D. Appearance, family, ability to perform, and friendships

8. The most common diagnostic categories that may affect sexuality in older adults are:
   A. Arthritis, heart disease, and cerebrovascular accident
   B. Spinal cord injury, multiple sclerosis, and burns
   C. Diabetes, glaucoma, and tinnitis
   D. Vertigo, arthritis, emphysema, and macular degeneration

9. Utilizing sexual positions and techniques that require less energy is a method that is helpful for all people with the following diagnoses *except*
   A. Parkinson's disease
   B. Postcerebrovascular accident
   C. Glaucoma
   D. Cardiac disease
   E. Arthritis

10. Fill in the blank with the best choice. Exercising regularly, using a warm waterbed, using relaxation techniques, and experimenting with alternative positions are examples of potential solutions for the presenting problem of _____.
    A. Sensory changes
    B. Paralysis
    C. Abnormal muscle tone
    D. Pain

11. The best approach to dealing with inappropriate client/patient sexual behavior is
    A. Ignore the behavior and continue with the course of intervention
    B. Confront the client immediately and end the intervention session
    C. Speak to your supervisor at the end of the intervention session
    D. Address the problem immediately by letting the client know that that kind of behavior will not be tolerated

12. A gay or lesbian lifestyle has often better prepared these groups to deal with
    A. Domestic violence and abuse
    B. Adapting to the losses associated with aging
    C. Planning more carefully for older age
    D. Inappropriate sexual gestures

Learning Activities

1. Describe your first discoveries of sexual feelings.
2. How have your family, culture, and religion affected (a) your own sexuality? and (b) your views on the sexuality of others?
3. a. What effects has peer pressure had on your sexuality?
   b. How can cohort effects influence one's sexuality?
4. Using the PLISSIT model and considering the four areas of sexual concern, develop a plan that addresses the specific diagnosis, age, and concerns of the following clients:
   a. A woman, age 72, with a total hip replacement and arthritis who is interested in continuing sex with her partner.
   b. A 65-year-old man with congestive heart failure who is very concerned about continuing his sexual relationship with his 55-year-old wife.

   c. A 70-year-old man post right cerebrovascular accident who is experiencing both sensory changes (decreased sensation on the left side; decreased left visual field) and decreased endurance. Despite these, he wishes to maintain an intimate relationship with his wife of more than 50 years.

5. Bring in advertisements and/or jokes that depict older adults and sexuality both in positive and negative ways. Discuss their veracity and the stereotypes they defy or confirm.

REFERENCES

1. American Association of Retired Persons. *A Profile of Older Americans*. Washington, DC: American Association of Retired Persons; 1995.
2. Hettler, B. *Test Well Wellness Inventory*. Stevens Point, WI: National Wellness Institute; 1979.
3. Friedan, B. *The Fountain of Age*. New York: Simon and Schuster; 1993.
4. Starr, BD, Weiner, MB. *The Starr–Weiner Report on Sex and Sexuality in the Mature Years*. New York: Stein and Day; 1981.
5. Lindau, ST, Schumm, LP, Laumann, EO, Levinson, W, et al. A Study of Sexuality and Health Among Older Adults in the United States. *New England Journal of Medicine*, 2007;357(8): 762–766.
6. Gott, M, Hinchliff, S. How Important Is Sex in Later Life? The Views of Older People. *Social Science and Medicine*, 2003;56:1617–1628.
7. Ginsberg, TB, Pomerantz, SC, Kramer-Felley, V. Sexuality in Older Adults: Behaviours and Preferences. *Age and Ageing*, 2005;34:475–480.
8. Butler, RN, et al. Love and Sex After 60: How Physical Changes Affect Intimate Expression. A Roundtable Discussion: Part 1. *Geriatrics*, 1994;49(9):21–27.
9. Bruce, MA, Borg, B. *Frames of Reference in Psychosocial Occupational Therapy*. Thorofare, NJ: Slack; 1987:47, 196.
10. Comacho, ME, Reyes-Ortiz, CA. Sexual Dysfunction in the Elderly: Age or Disease? *International Journal of Impotence Research*, 2005; 17:S52–S56.
11. Northrup, C. *Women's Bodies, Women's Wisdom*. New York: Bantam Books; 1994.
12. Siegal, DL, et al. Menopause: Entering Our Third Age. In PB Doress, DL Siegal (eds.), *Ourselves Growing Older*. New York: Touchstone Books; 1987:116.
13. Moynihan, R. The Making of a Disease: Female Sexual Dysfunction. *British Medical Journal*, 2003;326:7379 Health Module, 45–47.
14. Weed, SS. *Menopausal Years: The Wise Woman Way*. Woodstock, NY: Ash Tree Publishing; 1992.
15. Masters, WH. Sex and Aging—Expectations and Reality. *Hospital Practice*, August 15, 1986, 175.
16. Kiernat, M. *Occupational Therapy and the Older Adult: A Clinical Manual*. Gaithersburg, MD: Aspen; 1991:39.
17. Nusbaum, MRH, Singh, AR, Pyles, AA. Sexual Healthcare Needs of Women Aged 65 and Older. *Journal of American Geriatrics Society*, 2004;52(1):117–122.
18. Leiblum, SR. Sexuality and the Midlife Woman. *Psychology of Women Quarterly*, 1990;14:495.
19. Adams, CG, Turner, BE. Reported Change in Sexuality from Young Adulthood to Old Age. *Journal of Sex Research*, 1985;21(2):126.
20. Pfeiffer, E, et al. Sexual Behavior in Middle Life. *American Journal of Psychiatry*, 1972;128(10):82.
21. Steinke, EE. Sexuality in Aging: Implications for Nursing Facility Staff. *Journal of Continuing Education in Nursing*, March/April 1997;28(2): 59–63.
22. Crose, R, Drake, LK. Older Women's Sexuality. *Clinical Gerontologist*, 1993;12(4):51.

23. Nosek, MA, et al. Sexual Functioning Among Women with Physical Disabilities. *Archives of Physical Medical Rehabilitation*, February, 1996; 77:107.
24. Esmail, S, Esmail, E, Munro, B. Sexuality and Disability: The Role of Health Care Professionals in Providing Options and Alternatives for Couples. *Sexuality and Disability*, 2001;19(4): 267–282.
25. Sadoughi, W, Leshner, M, Fine, HL. Sexual Adjustment in a Chronically Ill and Physically Disabled Population: A Pilot Study. *Archives of Physical Medicine and Rehabilitation*, 1971; 52(7):311–317.
26. Kreuter, M, Sullivan, M, Siosteen, A. Sexual Adjustment After Spinal Cord Injury (SCI) Focusing on Partner Experiences. *Paraplegia*, 1994;32:225–235.
27. Miller, L. Sex and the Brain-Injured Patient: Regaining Love, Pleasure and Intimacy. *Journal of Cognitive Rehabilitation*, 1994;12(3):12–20.
28. Urey, JR, Viar, V, Henggeler, SW. Prediction of Marital Adjustment Among Spinal Injured Persons. *Rehabilitation Nursing*, 1987;12(1): 26–27.
29. Friend, RA. Older Lesbian and Gay People: A Theory of Successful Aging. *Journal of Homosexuality*, 1991;20(3–4):99.
30. Cass, V. Homosexual Identity Formation: A Theoretical Model. *Journal of Homosexuality*, 1979;4:219–235.
31. Coleman, JC, Butcher, JN, Carson, RC. *Abnormal Psychology and Modern Lives*. 7th ed. Glenview, IL: Scott, Foresman and Company; 1984.
32. Elliot, JE. Career Development with Lesbian and Gay Clients. *Career Development Quarterly*, 1993;41(3):210–226.
33. Pope, M. Sexual Issues for Older Lesbians and Gays. *Topics in Geriatric Rehabilitation*, 1979; 12(4):53–60.
34. Stausmire, JM. Sexuality at the End of Life. *American Journal of Hospice and Palliative Care*, 2004;21(1).
35. Friedman, JD. Sexual Expression: The Forgotten Component of ADL. *OT Practice*, January 1997, 20.
36. Annon, JS. The PLISSIT Model: A Proposed Conceptual Scheme for the Behavioral Treatment of Sexual Problems. *Journal of Sex Education and Therapy I*, Spring/Summer 1976.
37. Friedman, JD. Inappropriate Patient Sexual Behavior: Part I: Understanding This Prevalent Situation. *Advance for Occupational Therapy Practitioners*, September 17, 2007, 46–47.
38. McComas, J, Hebert, C, Geacomin, C, Kaplan, D, Dulberg, C. Experiences of Students and Practicing Physical Therapists with Inappropriate Patient Sexual Behaviour. *Journal of Physical Therapy*, 1993;73:762–769.
39. Schulte, HM, Kay, J. Medical Students' Perceptions of Patient-Initiated Sexual Behavior. *Academic Medicine*, 1994;69:842–846.
40. Zook, R. Sexual Harassment in the Workplace. *American Journal of Nursing*, 2000;100(12): 24AAAA–24CCCC.
41. Equal Employment Opportunity Commission. Guidelines on Discrimination Because of Sex. *Federal Register*, November 10, 1980, 74676–74677.
42. Schneider, J, Wierakoon, P, Heard, R. Inappropriate Client Sexual Behaviour in Occupational Therapy. *Occupational Therapy International*, 1999;6(3):176–194.
43. Adams, PF, Benson, V. Current Estimates from the National Health Interview Survey. National Center for Health Statistics. *Vital Health Statistics*, 1991;10(184).
44. Fox, S. Dismissing Taboos: OTs Integrate Sexuality into "Whole Reason" Treatment Approach. *Advance for Occupational Therapists*, June 18, 1990, 13–17.
45. Joe, BE. Coming to Terms with Sexuality. *OT Week*, September 19, 1996, 13.
46. Laflin, M. Sexuality and the Elderly. In CB Lewis (ed.), *Aging: The Health Care Challenge*. 3rd ed. Philadelphia: F. A. Davis; 1996:364.
47. Lewis, CB (ed.). *Aging: The Health Care Challenge*. Philadelphia: F. A. Davis; 1985:293.
48. Ghusen, H. Sexuality in Institutionalized Patients. *Physical Medicine and Rehabilitation*, 1995;9(2): 475–486.
49. Galindo, D, Kaiser, FE. Sexual Health After 60. *Patient Care*, April 15, 1995, 25–41.
50. McCartney, JR, et al. Sexuality and the Institutionalized Elderly. *Journal of American Geriatric Society*, 1987;35:331–333.

51. Lichtenberg, PA. *A Guide to Psychological Practice in Geriatric Long-Term Care*. New York: Haworth Press; 1994.

52. National Institute on Aging. Study Sheds New Light on Intimate Lives of Older Americans. Retrieved September 5, 2007, from http://nia.nih.gov/NewsAndEvents/PressReleases/PR20070823sexlives.htm

53. Feldman, MD, et al. The Growing Risk of AIDS in Older Patients. *Patient Care*, October 30, 1994, 61–63.

54. National Institute on Aging. Sexuality in Later Life. Retrieved September 5, 2007, from http://www.niapublications.org/agepages/sexuality.asp

55. National Institute on Aging. Study Sheds New Light on Intimate Lives of Older Americans. Retrieved September 5, 2007, from http://www.nia.nih.gov/NewsAndEvents/PressReleases/PR20070823sexlives.htm

56. Stall, R, Catania, J. AIDS Risk Behaviors Among Late Middle-Aged and Elderly Americans: The National AIDS Behavioral Surveys. *Archives of Internal Medicine*, 1994;154:57–63.

57. Whipple, B, Scura, KW. The Overlooked Epidemic: HIV in Older Adults. *American Journal of Nursing*, 1996;96(2):23–28.

58. Wallace, JI, et al. HIV Infection in Older Patients: When to Suspect the Unexpected. *Geriatrics*, 1993;48(6):61–70.

ADDITIONAL READINGS

Boston Women's Health Collective: *Our Bodies, Ourselves: A New Edition for the New Era*. New York: Simon and Schuster; 2005.

Cole, E, Rothblum, E. Commentary on "Sexuality and the Midlife Woman." *Psychology of Women Quarterly*, 1990;14:509.

Cross, RJ. What Doctors and Others Need to Know: Six Facts on Human Sexuality and Aging. *SEICUS Report*, June/July 1993, 7.

Doress, PB, Siegal, DL (eds.). *Ourselves Growing Older*. New York: Simon and Schuster; 1987.

Goldstein, H, Runyon, C. An Occupational Therapy Educational Model to Increase Sensitivity About Geriatric Sexuality. *Physical and Occupational Therapy in Geriatrics*, 1993;11(2):57.

Mooradian, AD, Grieff, V. Sexuality in Older Women. *Archives of Internal Medicine*, 1990;150:1033.

Pendleton, HM, Schultz-Krohn, W (eds.). *Pedretti's Occupational Therapy: Practice Skills for Physical Dysfunction*. 6th ed. St. Louis, MO: Mosby Elsevier; 2006.

Pfeiffer, E, et al. The Natural History of Sexual Behavior in a Biologically Advantaged Group of Aged Individuals. *Journal of Gerontology*, 1969;24:193.

Schiavi, RC, et al. Sexual Satisfaction in Healthy Aging Men. *Journal of Sex and Marital Therapy*, 1994;20(1):3.

Smedley, G. Addressing Sexuality in the Elderly. *Rehabilitation Nursing*, 1991;16(1):9.

Chapter 9

LIVING OPTIONS AND THE CONTINUUM OF CARE

ANN O'SULLIVAN, OTR/L, LSW, AND
REGULA H. ROBNETT, PhD, OTR/L

Home, as Mahmud Darwish, the famous Palestinian poet wrote, is "your life and your cause bound up together. And before and after all of that, it's the essence of who you are."
Home is where we start from, but home is also where we are bound for, the place we always seek.
　　　　　　　　　　　　　　　　　　　　　　　　　　　　　　　—David Steindl-Rast

Chapter Outline

Behavioral Objectives

Upon completion of this chapter, the reader will be able to:

1. Describe housing options for people who are able to live independently, including advantages and disadvantages.
2. List group housing options and relate these to older adults' needs.
3. Define assisted living.
4. Describe how home health care and rehabilitation fit into the health care continuum.
5. Discuss past and current perceptions of long-term care.
6. List factors associated with long-term care needs.
7. Discuss how health care professionals can help facilitate a supportive environment for older clients.
8. Discuss factors that contribute to older adult health and well-being in any setting.
9. Identify the importance of family caregivers for older adults, and discuss contributions and needs of this group and their role in providing long-term care.

Key Terms

Activities of daily living	Long-term care
Adaptation	Long-term care insurance
Adult day services	Medicaid
Agency on Aging	Medicare
Aging in place	Moving in together
Assisted living	Naturally occurring retirement community
Board and care facilities	Nursing facilities
Cohousing	Physiatrists
Congregate housing	Rehabilitation
Continuing care retirement community	Residential care
Empowerment	Reverse mortgage
Family caregiver	Shared homes
Home health care	Single-room occupancy units
Hospice	Skilled care
Independence	Universal design
Instrumental activities of daily living (IADLs)	

The living environment is intimately related to health care. Physically and cognitively able older adults may continue to live independently in their own homes, while those with physical and/or cognitive disabilities may need assistance or a more supportive environment. This chapter explores the continuum of options for older people, looking at different living environments, along with their limitations and advantages, and relating these options to the health care requirements of older adults. This chapter also covers the basic tenets of environmental adaptation. Adapting activities or the environment can be an important component of an individual's safety and independence in all settings.

THE HOUSING AND HEALTH CONNECTION

INDEPENDENCE

There are many factors that can influence choices, and, indeed, the living situation can influence one's overall abilities and quality of life. **Figure 9-1** illustrates the complexity of the living environment and its health connection. For example, physical abilities certainly have an impact on where one lives. If you use a wheelchair, the optimal living situation does not involve a three-story home with numerous staircases. On the other hand, going up and down stairs several times a day actually can help a person maintain endurance and vital physical skills. Another example involves the activities of daily living; by completing tasks such as self-care (safely within the supportive environment), one is able to maintain these skills longer. If we expect decline because we have reached a certain age, we may be more likely to experience that decline (see Chapter 4), and this decline certainly impacts where we can live. This chapter explores some of these living environment continuum variables.

In a study researching the link between health and housing, MacDonald and associates[1] found that the desire for independence was extremely strong among the older adults who participated in their study. However, **independence** was interpreted in a number of

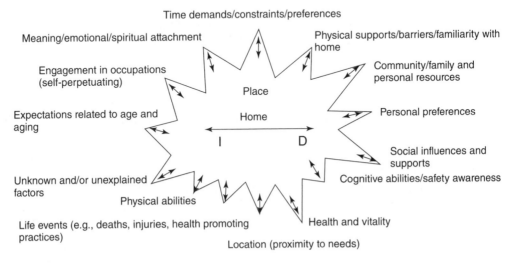

FIGURE 9-1 The housing continuum ranges from completely independent living (I) to totally dependent living (D).

different ways. While some viewed it as living comfortably without needing regular assistance from anyone else, others viewed independence as living in one's own apartment or home rather than a nursing home and as the ability to make one's own decisions. Certain participants viewed independence as not being a burden to their family, while others viewed being independent as being able to manage with just the help of their families, not outside resources. Independence was on a relative scale, not an all-or-nothing construct, at least to this group of senior citizens.

As health care practitioners, our job is to promote the level of independence sought by older people. We must first seek to understand the meaning of independence to the person and respect his or her particular viewpoint, even if it differs from our own. Then those of us who assist people in gaining and maintaining their independence (e.g., therapists, nurses) must use all our creative and scientific resources to promote the kind of life the older adult is seeking.

EMPOWERMENT

Empowerment is closely related to independence, or perhaps more aptly stated, freedom. It relates not only to people's ability, but also to the right to make choices affecting their own lives. Decisions made by a competent person of any age should garner our respect, as stated earlier, even if these choices do not fit in with our own comprehension of what is right for the person.

Participants in the study by MacDonald and colleagues[1] clearly stated that they sought control over, and thereby wanted to make choices about, their own lives, particularly in three areas:

1. The type of environment in which they live (housing in general)
2. Where they would go if they needed additional care (continuum of care)
3. Control over their day-to-day lives (reflecting their personal view of independence)

Health care professionals need to keep the idea of empowerment at the forefront when working with and for older people, respecting and encouraging choices whenever possible. We may need to remind those who have forgotten that choices exist; it is their right and privilege to guide the course of their daily lives.

Along with making choices does come a certain amount of responsibility. At the very least, each person should be given the choice of whether or not to accept this level of responsibility. Indeed many of the problems of aging may be directly related to what theorists call the "environmentally induced loss of control."[2] Respecting freedom of choice supports people to "gain mastery over their lives."[2] On a community or national level, the results can be dramatic. People come together through support groups, coalitions, organizations, and associations to reach common goals by working collectively. These goals can be as diverse as improving housing conditions and access to health care to lowering the crime rate. Old age is not a stage when one must simply become a victim of fate, but rather a time when older adults can offer years of valuable past experience and current free time to significantly improve the quality of their own and others' lives. As an example, many localities nationwide have formed "triads" to bring law enforcement, older adults, and the community together to promote senior safety and to reduce unwarranted fear of crime. Groups are organized at the grassroots level, with support at the national level, and conduct organized programs and activities, such as distributing emergency cell phones, offering daily phone check-in programs, and providing community education relating to safety.[3]

ENGAGEMENT IN PERSONALLY MEANINGFUL ACTIVITIES

Involvement in enjoyable and productive activity is paramount to productive aging.[4] Longevity is associated with being active,[5] and successful aging includes maintaining physical activity and pursuing cognitive challenges.[6] Continued participation involves reassessing one's needs and desires. Older people may need to refocus to remain engaged when life changes, such as retirement or the death of a spouse, occur. The choice of purposeful activity may need to be altered to accommodate changing strengths and abilities.

Nevertheless, as health care practitioners, we can promote an optimal level of participation through our own particular health care provider roles. A significant lack of interest in day-to-day activities or life in general may indicate clinical depression (see Chapter 4). Encourage the older person to seek assistance from a physician if this seems to be the case. At other times the person may need assistance in finding meaningful activities or hobbies. A referral to a recreational or occupational therapist may be appropriate if the person can no longer participate in or enjoy past occupations (including hobbies, home management, and work activities).

Many communities offer opportunities for older adults to volunteer using the skills they have developed over a lifetime. The Retired and Senior Volunteer Program (RSVP) is an example of a national program that matches volunteers with community needs. Local **Agencies on Aging** can be a resource for learning how older adults can connect with opportunities for service. Agencies can be found through the Eldercare Locator website (www.eldercare.gov) maintained by the Administration on Aging.

An important consideration in fostering the involvement of older adults is to engage them in the choice and planning of the activity as well. Although encouragement and enthusiasm for participation may be appreciated, individuals should never be forced to attend an event, and neither should anyone's activity preferences be assumed without consulting with that person.

SOCIAL AND EMOTIONAL SUPPORT

All these realms—independence, empowerment, social support, and purposeful activities—are hardly distinct from one another. By focusing on one, other areas may also improve. Numerous studies have linked the concept of social support and interaction to better health. The social support theory purports that those who are lacking adequate social support systems are more susceptible to disease because of a decrease in functioning of the body's immune system. During tense times, the love and support of other people can decrease a person's stress level and may also help to increase a person's sense of control.[2]

Marriage is correlated with a higher level of life satisfaction in older people, but one spouse, more often the woman, is nearly always left alone after the death of the other. Widows and widowers may need to find a replacement social support system after the death of their spouse. In two separate studies, Hong and colleagues[7] found that life satisfaction was positively correlated with the frequency of participation in group activities and high level of interaction with friends. Perhaps it is evident that close human connections are crucial in attaining and maintaining wellness for most people of all ages. People do not generally thrive in isolation. Yet as people get older, if their senses become impaired and they are less mobile, isolation becomes a greater risk. Older adults may not want to be a burden on close friends or family, or they may feel uncomfortable if they can no longer hear conversations as well or walk as quickly or as far. For whatever reason, social withdrawal can occur. This, in turn, may lead to further decline both socially and physically.

Health care professionals should attempt to intervene and stop this downward spiral. Not only can we lend a listening ear, but also we can encourage human interaction (and animal interactions as well, if desired), either directly by setting up and becoming involved in programs or by making appropriate referrals to those who can (e.g., activity directors, social workers, nurses, recreational therapists), and by supporting efforts to create communities that are accessible to all. At least one study has found that older people value emotional support and that they feel it is important to feel "cared about" rather than just "cared for."[8]

Intergenerational programs, which bring together older adults and younger people, have gained popularity in recent years. Many school systems, universities, senior centers, and community agencies create opportunities for children and older adults to learn about each others' experiences and gain an appreciation for each others' wisdom. Some programs (such as Foster Grandparents) have been developed to promote volunteer opportunities for older adults to connect and work with children and young adults. Some programs offer a small stipend for low-income seniors. While the youth gain valued friendships and guidance about making decisions, the older adults benefit from the social involvement and the chance to use their skills and share their experience. Both groups improve their awareness of issues facing the other generation. The community also benefits through the utilization of dormant resources.

FAMILY EXPECTATIONS AND CULTURE

A family's ethnic and religious background can influence the way it approaches aging and caregiving. Different cultures have different expectations about how a person is treated as

BOX 9-1 MY CHILDREN ARE COMING TODAY.

My children are coming today.
They mean well, but they worry.
They think I should have a railing in the hall.
A telephone in the kitchen.
They want someone to come in when I take a bath.
They don't really like my living alone.
Help me be grateful for their concern.
And help them to understand that I have to do what I can.
They're right when they say there are risks.
I might fall. I might leave the stove on.
But there is no challenge, no possibility of triumph, no real aliveness without risk.
When they were young and climbed trees and rode bicycles and went away to camp,
I was terrified. But I let them go.
Because to hold them would have hurt them.
Now our roles are reversed. Help them see.
Keep me from being grim or stubborn about it, but don't let them smother me.

Anonymous

Source: Reprinted with permission from *Aging Arkansas.* Arkansas Aging Foundation, Little Rock, AR, September, 1995, p 8.

he or she ages, how much and what types of assistance are provided by family, or where/ with whom an older person will live (see **Box 9-1**). As health care providers, it is our responsibility to be aware of and respect these cultural factors, and to provide care that is consistent and compatible with older adults' and families' beliefs. It is important to note that, although rates of caregiving vary somewhat by ethnicity,[9] **family caregivers** provide similar types of care and experience similar stresses regardless of ethnic background.[9] Professionals should avoid making assumptions about the division of caregiving duties within a family. Clarifying the amount and types of care, the caregiver's expectations of assistance from other family members, the actual extent of assistance provided by family members, and the family's comfort with the caregiving arrangement will help in realistically assessing the situation.[10]

AGING IN PLACE

Aging in place is a person's ability to continue to live in his or her home safely, as independently as possible, and comfortably, regardless of age, income, or ability level. It means living in a familiar environment and being able to participate in family and other community activities.[11] Several factors can contribute to an individual's ability to continue to do this.

ACCESSIBILITY

Participation is difficult or impossible if activities take place in an environment that is not easily accessible. A supportive environment fosters comfort, safety, and ease of navigation and movement. Although the ideas presented here are not difficult to grasp, the process of adapting a home to fit the requirements of a particular individual with special needs usually requires technical skills and clinical reasoning. For a full home safety evaluation, a physician should refer the client to an occupational and/or physical therapist.

Environmental design that fits the needs of older people basically falls into two categories:

- Building new, accommodating structures
- Adapting existing structures

The typical newly built home is not designed with aging in mind, even though each of us is headed in that direction. With multiple living levels, narrow doorways, and inaccessible spaces (especially for those who use wheelchairs), existing homes may not be very suitable for aging in place.

UNIVERSAL DESIGN

Universal design is the design of products and environments to be usable by all people, to the greatest extent possible, without the need for **adaptation** or specialized design. The intent of universal design is to simplify life for everyone by making products, communications, and the built environment more usable by as many people as possible at little or no extra cost. Universal design benefits people of all ages and abilities.[12]

A good example of universal design is lever door handles. While they are easier for a person with arthritis or upper extremity weakness to use, they are also easier for anyone carrying groceries or wearing mittens.

Other design features that support people with a range of abilities include the following:

- Bright lighting (people older than age 60 require twice the amount of illumination needed by a 20-year-old).[13]
- Either single-story construction or living areas easily accessed by ramp, stair glide, or elevator.
- Anti-slip floor finishes.
- Doorways wide enough to allow a wheelchair or walker to pass through easily.
- Easy to reach switches and outlets.
- Bathroom grab bars.
- Levers on faucets.

ADAPTATION AND COMPENSATION

Most people wish to remain in their own homes for as long as possible. This presents a problem when the home can no longer offer a safe and comfortable living space. A full home evaluation is usually warranted to determine whether changes can be made. At times, the proposed accommodations will involve extensive remodeling such as building a bathroom on the first floor or tearing down walls to increase accessibility. Entry steps may need to be replaced by a ramp to allow for wheelchair access. Ramps are not safe unless they are built at least to Americans with Disabilities Act (ADA) specifications, which are available at local independent living centers or on the Internet (the grade should not exceed 1 inch of height per foot of length). Doorways may need to be widened to accommodate a wheelchair, and kitchens may need to be remodeled to allow continued use. Chair lifts may need to be added to existing stairways (**Figure 9-2**).

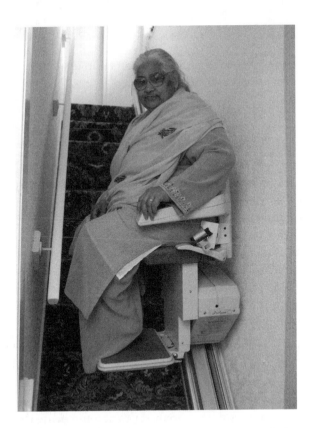

FIGURE 9-2 Stairlifts can be helpful but, of course, should only be used if needed as stairclimbing is great exercise. (© John Birdsall/age fotostock)

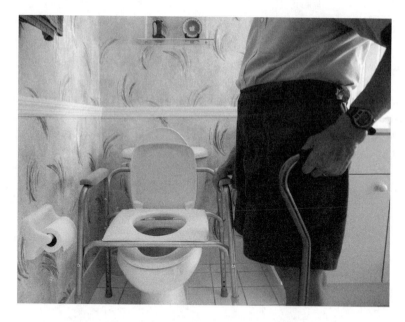

FIGURE 9-3 Many fairly easy adaptations can be made in a home to increase the resi-dent's safety. (© *Mark Gabrenya/Dreamstime.com*)

Many changes are less drastic and therefore more acceptable and more affordable to home owners. These changes may include the following:

- Adding raised toilet seats and grab bars in the bathroom (**Figure 9-3**)
- Tacking down or eliminating scatter rugs
- Improving lighting levels
- Using shower seats or bath transfer benches
- Eliminating clutter and excess furniture
- Checking smoke alarms
- Resetting the water heater to a lower temperature (not exceeding 120°F)
- Removing door thresholds
- Moving commonly used items into easily reached spaces

Not all older people need to make all these changes to be safe, although these accom-modations are unlikely to cause harm to anyone. Many other minor adjustments in the home, or small equipment purchases, may also be helpful. A physical or occupational therapist can offer guidance in making decisions regarding home safety (**Figure 9-4**).

In addition to altering the environment to accommodate the changing needs of the aging adult, the person may also learn compensatory strategies to remain as safe as pos-sible in the home. As protection from possible injury, a rehabilitation specialist, such as

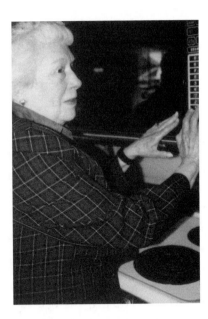

FIGURE 9-4 Marge, who is legally blind, has made simple adaptions to her microwave so she can continue to use it. (*Courtesy of Marge's family*)

an occupational or physical therapist, may help an older person learn to do the following:

- Transfer into and out of the tub or shower safely
- Use a walker or cane to compensate for decreased balance or strength
- Use safer techniques when using kitchen appliances
- Use different, more effective techniques for completing their daily activities
- Use joint protection and energy conservation techniques
- Compensate for changes such as decreased eyesight, decreased memory, or decreased hearing (see Chapters 4 and 5)

This is just a small sample of accommodations and compensatory strategies that can be used on an individual basis as needed. Through these techniques and others, many people are able to remain in their environments of choice more safely and for a longer time.

INDEPENDENT LIVING

Many older adults prefer to maintain living arrangements in their lifetime homes, even when these homes may present environmental barriers, activity challenges, or may contribute to financial hardships. These homes are often the ones in which they raised their children; the homes may offer more space than is now needed, require outdoor maintenance, such as snow shoveling or lawn mowing, or necessitate the use of stairs. The reasons for staying in these homes can be very compelling. A few possibilities are listed here:

- Older people may feel that by giving up their home, they are giving up their freedom and independence.
- They may feel emotionally attached to a home that holds years of cherished memories.
- They may like the neighborhood and not want to leave friends.
- They may want to maintain a large house for when family and friends visit.
- Some people fear that if they indicate a need for any additional support or assistance, they will be placed in a nursing facility.
- Many people, of all ages, either do not like or are even fearful of change.

As health care professionals, we must respect competent older peoples' right to make their own decisions, which may include a wish to remain in their own homes, even if we do not agree. This can be difficult for families and friends to accept. Older people with disabilities overwhelmingly prefer to receive long-term care in their own home or a community setting.[14] Studies have shown that the delivery of home or community-based long-term care services is a cost-effective alternative to nursing homes and is what most Americans would prefer.[15] Well-meaning family members may insist that the older adult leave the familiar home, but this kind of interference may be more detrimental than helpful.

Garrett speaks to this difficulty when he describes an elderly woman, Violet, who was forced to leave her home with steep stairs, several cats over whom she regularly tripped, an outdoor toilet, and a gas stove.[16] Her children insisted that she move to a modern apartment that they believed would be much safer. However, because of Violet's hearing impairment and her lack of familiarity with the new surroundings and the way things worked in the apartment, she became isolated and depressed. Garrett contends that, although safety is crucial, the home environment should be of the person's choosing if at all possible. He states that home improvements to increase safety may be a preferred alternative to moving out of the home.

Unfortunately, the lack of adequate income may preclude some older people, especially women, from staying in their homes even if they want to and are capable of doing so. The Profile of Older Americans: 2005 indicates that 9.8% of older adults were below the poverty level in 2004.[17] Older women had a higher poverty rate (12.0%) than did older men (7.0%) in 2004.[17] In 2003, 42% of older householders spent more than one-fourth of their income on housing costs,[17] and consequently about a third of the nation's elderly citizens reported not having enough money left over for essentials like food, clothing, and health care.[18]

The **reverse mortgage** program is one option that has made it possible for many older people (especially women at or below the poverty level) to afford to stay in their own long-term homes. Through this program, borrowers use their home as collateral, and the bank sets up either an annuity or a line of credit to be used as needed until the home is sold or the loan repaid. This allows those with inadequate monthly income, but with substantial home equity, to continue to reside in their own homes. When the older person decides to sell, or he or she dies, the bank recovers its investment.[19]

Naturally occurring retirement community (NORC) is a demographic term to describe a neighborhood or building in which a large segment of the residents are older adults. In general, they are not purpose-built senior housing or retirement communities and were neither designed nor intended to meet the particular health and social services wants and needs of older adults. Most commonly, they are simply neighborhoods where community residents have either aged in place, having lived in their homes over several decades, or they are the result of significant migrations of older adults into the same area.[20] Several of these NORCs have received federal and private grants to offer supportive services to residents, promote independence, create a sense of community, and meet unmet needs. The overarching goal is to help older adults remain in their homes of choice and experience a high quality of life.[21] In St. Louis, the Jewish Federation partnered with Washington University to research the needs of older adults in the identified NORC. This led to regular educational (wellness) programming, social activities, resident councils, and information exchange. A transportation program was initiated to help with grocery shopping. When it was learned that the residents really wanted transportation to cultural events instead (because family and friends were helping with groceries), it evolved into a popular day trip program. Ongoing funding through the National Center on Aging is supporting development of the use of resident volunteers to continue identifying needs and making services available.[22]

LIVING OPTIONS FOR OLDER PEOPLE

Although reasons for staying in one's familiar home may be compelling, for some older adults, the decision to move may be the necessary or preferred option. People may decide to move for reasons such as limited finances, social isolation, desire to be closer to family or friends, wanting fewer home management responsibilities, experiencing a loss of functional ability, and/or seeking a more moderate climate. There are many living options for older adults. This section highlights a range of them, including those for people who are independent, and across the continuum for those who need assistance with **activities of daily living** (ADLs).

LIVING WITH FAMILY

Many families consider the option of **moving in together**. Family members might move into the older adult's home, the older adult might move into a family member's home, or an in-law apartment might be made available. These arrangements work very well for some families, and not as well for others. Unfortunately, if the situation is not satisfying for everyone, it can be difficult to make changes without emotional upset. Before making this type of move, everyone involved might benefit from considering the following questions:

- Has the relationship been open and honest?
- How have past conflicts been resolved?
- Is there enough room in the home for everyone to have privacy?
- Can the home be made appropriately accessible for everyone?
- How much assistance is needed and what is realistically available?
- How will expenses be divided?
- Are all household members' needs being considered?
- What will be the division of labor?
- Can everyone set appropriate limits?
- If the situation does not work, what are the alternatives?

HOMELESSNESS

Although the proportion of older persons in the total homeless population has declined, the number of homeless older adults (age 50 and older) has grown. This escalation is likely to continue as increasing numbers of people reach older adulthood and the demand for affordable housing continues to outstrip supply.[23] Older homeless persons are of special concern because of their vulnerability to victimization both in shelters and on the streets, their frailty caused by compromised mental and physical health, and the limited resources available to them through traditional service systems for older adults.[23] Factors contributing to an older person becoming homeless may include deinstitutionalization, poverty (especially among elderly women), and the lack of affordable housing. People may become homeless for the first time after the death of a spouse, child, or friend who had been caring for them or providing financial support.[23]

SINGLE-ROOM OCCUPANCY

Since 1988, the federal government has been supporting the development of **single-room occupancy** (SRO) **units**, partially funding rehabilitation of existing structures to create subsidized housing for individuals with very low incomes. These single-room units are usually found in cities and offer shared bathroom and kitchen facilities. They are considered by some to be a substandard housing type. However, these single rooms do offer a low-cost independent living alternative, especially for those who have little money and weak family ties, and they have served as a positive alternative to homelessness.[24]

SUBSIDIZED SENIOR HOUSING

The federal government and state programs offer affordable senior housing in many areas. Rent is generally based on a percentage of a person's income. In 2008, there were more than 300,000 units in the United States, but for every unit, there were 10 eligible older adults on waiting lists for it (average waiting time is 13.4 months).[25] For those who are able to access this option, it can offer security, user-friendly design, affordability, and a sense of community.

COHOUSING

Cohousing is a type of collaborative housing in which residents actively participate in the design and operation of their own neighborhoods.[26] Whereas NORCs develop where people are already living, cohousing is an intentional community, with private homes and common facilities, consensus decision making, shared responsibilities, and mutual assistance. The idea originated in Denmark and began appearing in the United States in the early 1980s. In recent years, there has been interest in cohousing specifically as an option for older adults, adding elements of universal design, caregiver support, and other features to promote the ability of residents to age in place.

SHARED HOMES

Shared homes can be an alternative to moving in with family. In this arrangement, people might share expenses or exchange services for rent. For instance, a homebound homeowner might have someone do house and yard work in exchange for free lodging.[27] Adults might opt to share a home to reduce expenses (such as heating), to share chores, and for companionship.

CONGREGATE HOUSING

Congregate housing encompasses a multitude of different options, including independent living units, adult congregate living facilities, rental retirement housing, and senior retirement centers. These units, which are sometimes subsidized by state and federal government programs, are difficult to describe comprehensively because they can vary so much from one another. Generally, they do not offer personal assistance or health services, although residents may be able to access home care services through an outside agency. These units may resemble any other apartments, with private bathrooms and kitchen facilities, and with safety features to support independent function. In addition, they usually offer group dining, housekeeping, and socialization opportunities.

LONG-TERM CARE

Long-term care is an array of long-term services and supports used by people who need assistance to function in their daily lives. It can include personal care, rehabilitation, social services, assistive technology, health care, home modifications, care coordination, assisted transportation, and more. Services may be needed on a regular or intermittent basis over a period of several months, years, or for the rest of a lifetime. Services may be delivered in individual homes, in assisted living or supportive housing, in adult day centers, or in nursing facilities or other institutional settings. The need for long-term care is usually measured by assessing limitations in an individual's capacity to perform or manage tasks of daily living, including self-care and household tasks.[14] It is important to note that 80% of individuals age 75 and older have no functional limitations requiring assistance from another person.[28]

FAMILY CAREGIVERS

Most people who need long-term care (nearly 79%) actually live at home or in community settings, not in institutions.[29] They depend exclusively on their family and friends for help. The vast majority (78%) of adults in the United States who receive care at home get all their care from family caregivers (unpaid family and friends). Another 14% receive some combination of family care and paid help; only 8% rely on formal (paid) care alone.[30] Family caregivers will likely continue to be the largest source of long-term care services in the United States; in fact, by 2050, we will likely have 37 million of them.[31]

PAYING FOR LONG-TERM CARE

Nearly 40% of long-term care spending is paid for by private funds. Medicare pays for 19%, Medicaid, which covers health care costs for individuals with limited financial resources, pays 49%.[25]

In 2004, almost all (96%) noninstitutionalized persons age 65 and older in the United States were covered by **Medicare**. Medicare covers mostly acute care services and requires beneficiaries to pay part of the cost, leaving about half of health care spending to be covered by other sources.[17] Medicare Part A, which most people get when they turn 65, covers hospitalization, rehabilitation, home health care, and hospice. Medicare Part B, for which an additional premium is paid, covers physician visits and durable medical equipment. Medicare Advantage Plans (formerly known as Part C) function as health maintenance organizations (HMOs), providing managed care benefits. Medicare Part D plans cover prescription medications. Medicare, however, does not pay for nonskilled nursing facility care or for ongoing personal care or housekeeping assistance at home.

Medicaid covers health care costs for individuals with limited financial resources. It is jointly funded by the federal government and each state. Federal regulations specify what can be covered and how states administer their programs, and states determine how their individual programs will cover and pay for services. It is important to be familiar with the regulations in the state in which the individual resides because these vary from state to state. Medicaid may cover skilled care in the home, some assisted living care, and some nursing home care for eligible individuals. Medicaid was covering the costs of the care for almost 58% of Medicare beneficiaries residing in nursing homes in 2001.[17] To rebalance state spending for institutional services and home and community-based services (HCBS), all states, at varying rates, have been changing the way that Medicaid long-term care services are delivered and financed to allocate a higher proportion of dollars to HCBS.[32]

As people survive longer, the need for care is also increasing, and paying for that care becomes a concern. Many people are purchasing **long-term care insurance** as a way to pay for services they may need in the future while protecting their financial assets (e.g., in 2005, an estimated 7 million policies were in place[33]). Depending on the individual policy purchased, long-term care insurance may cover personal care and homemaking assistance in the home, assisted living, nursing facility care, or other services.

OPTIONS FOR SERVICES AND CARE

HOME HEALTH CARE

Services provided at home, known as **home health care**, have existed for well over 125 years. It's purpose is to provide skilled care in the home (**skilled care** is a term used to describe services requiring a high level of skill, which can only be provided by credentialed professionals, to ensure safe and effective care).

Approximately 7.6 million individuals currently receive care from 83,000 home care agencies because of acute illness, long-term health conditions, permanent disability, or terminal illness. In 2007, annual expenditures for home health care were projected to be $57.6 billion.[34] There are currently more than 9,200 Medicare-certified (meaning that they meet certain guidelines and are able to bill Medicare for skilled services) home care providers in the United States, offering therapies (including occupational, physical, and respiratory therapies, and speech-language pathology services), home health aide services, social work intervention, and sometimes psychological and nutritional counseling, in addition to nursing care services.

As the population ages, this number is expected to rise. Because of the expansion of the 85-and-over cohort as well as the capability of technological advances to save lives we previously would have lost, we can expect growth in the need for home care. Technological development is also allowing an array of new services to be provided in the home, from dialysis to blood pressure monitoring and reporting. Payers are requiring providers to collect and report data on the outcomes of the care they provide. Payment systems through Medicare and other programs are intended to encourage efficient and effective care, and support accountability for treatment. In addition, studies have shown that the delivery of home- or community-based long-term care services is a cost-effective alternative to nursing homes and is what most Americans would prefer.[35] This combination of factors suggests that we can expect continued growth and a larger number of options in this area of service delivery.

REHABILITATION

Rehabilitation is the process of helping someone regain the highest possible level of functioning after an injury or illness. Rehabilitation specialists, including **physiatrists** (who are physicians specializing in rehabilitation), nurses, and therapists, work with patients or clients in home, community, and residential facility settings, as well as in the hospital. Rehabilitation services are provided at different levels of intensity. In an acute rehabilitation setting, where a patient can stay for days or a few weeks, the patients generally receive 3 or more hours of skilled therapy per day, at least 5 days per week. Through medical management and therapy, they are expected to make significant gains in a reasonable and expected period of time. Therapists, rehabilitation nurses, and physiatrists are experts in judging whether or not this is likely to occur.

For example, after a stroke, or cerebrovascular accident (CVA), patients often can make good progress in regaining the strength, balance, and motor control to do the tasks they want or need to do. If they make excellent and quick gains, they may return home directly from the rehabilitation hospital. However, if their gains are slower or not as significant, they may need alternative placement (e.g., assisted living or nursing facility) prior to or instead of going home. Or if their level of endurance cannot withstand an acute level of rehabilitation, they may receive a lower intensity of therapy services in a skilled nursing facility (SNF).

Through rehabilitation, which includes exercise, education, and training/retraining in activities of daily living (ADLs), **instrumental activities of daily living** (IADLs; e.g., home management tasks), mobility, communication, and other functional tasks as needed, many people have been able to return to their former level of independence. This is accomplished through the restoration of function and/or through the use of compensatory measures to make up for lost skills. Adaptation of the environment may also be needed, and was described earlier in this chapter.

ADULT DAY SERVICES

Adult day services are community-based group programs with specialized plans of care designed to meet the daytime needs of individuals with functional and/or cognitive impairments. Because they offer structured care in a protective setting, these services can help people with disabilities live at home, while allowing caregivers time to work or rest. Participants have opportunities for social engagement, activities, and meals, in a environment that offers staff availability when needed. Although some states, long-term care insurance policies, and veterans' programs can help with funding, most adult services are paid for privately.[36]

RESIDENTIAL CARE

Residential care facilities can have multiple labels, including adult residential facilities, adult group homes, domiciliary homes, personal care homes, family care, adult foster care, rest homes, board and care homes, and assisted living facilities. All have the common theme of bridging the gap between independent living and 24-hour-per-day nursing care.[37] States have different definitions and degrees of licensing and regulation for the various types of facilities. The Assisted Living Federation of America defines **assisted living** as a long-term residence option that provides resident-centered care in a residential setting. It is designed for those who need extra help in their day-to-day lives but who do not require 24-hour per day skilled nursing care.[38] Residents rent apartments and receive needed assistance with ADLs and IADLs as part of their monthly rental fee. The amount of assistance available varies between facilities and regions. Most states regulate these facilities. This model of housing seeks to allow independent decision making, while promoting the safety of all residents. The apartments are "homelike" and environmentally accessible. Residents are encouraged to bring personal furnishings and continue community involvement.

Community or shared space is also a feature of assisted living facilities. Dining rooms, laundry areas, libraries, and activity/physical fitness areas are located to promote social interactions.[39] Although an initial move is necessary to establish themselves at an assisted living facility, many older people find relocating is well worth the consequent security it brings. Although residents are encouraged to maintain an optimal level of functioning, they also can trust that if health issues do arise, they will receive the needed care in their new home for as long as possible.

In 2004, there were approximately 36,000 assisted living residences in the United States, housing more than 900,000 people.[40] Facility sizes vary greatly, as do fees charged and services provided. Residences typically provide 24-hour supervision, three meals per day in a group dining room, personal care, social activities, housekeeping, and arrangements for transportation.

Many assisted living providers offer services to people with a range of care needs. Some facilities offer specialized units for people with dementia to ensure both their safety and their engagement in meaningful activities. Other facilities may opt not to accept residents with significant cognitive compromise, if the facility is not set up to accommodate safety concerns such as wandering.

Board and care facilities are also considered to be in this residential care spectrum, but they differ from many assisted living centers in that they tend to be located in traditional, large single-family homes. These homes typically provide meals, transportation, other services, and "protective oversight" as needed. A board and care home has generally one to six beds, which may be located in either private or shared bedrooms.[41]

Nursing facilities house only a relatively small percentage (4.5%) of the total 65 and older population, but the percentage increases dramatically with age, ranging from 1.1% for persons 65–74 years to 4.7% for persons 75–84 years and 18.2% for persons 85 and older.[17] Nonetheless, an impression persists among some older adults and the general public that nursing home care is an inevitable, and undesirable, part of growing older. A 2007 survey of more than 800 older adults and adult children revealed that people were more fearful of losing their independence (26%) or moving into a nursing home (13%) than they were about dying (3%). Adult children's concerns about their parents' well-being if they had to leave their homes centered on the older adults' sadness at loss of independence (89%), fear of leaving their homes (70%), the risk of mistreatment (82%), and potential unhappiness in a facility (79%).[42]

Nursing facility care may be needed by those people who have disabilities interfering with their self-care skills. Because of their physical or cognitive impairments, others must assist them in completing their daily tasks. If the need for assistance is greater than what is available through family caregivers and/or professional providers in other settings, a move to a nursing facility may be the option of choice for safety and comfort.

Nursing facilities provide round-the-clock care through the use of paid caregivers, primarily nurses and aides. In the past, people generally entered a nursing home to live out their final days. In recent years, the concept of nursing facility care is changing, and the services provided are increasingly focused on rehabilitation. Older people are often admitted to the facility for a short stay to improve their functioning enough so that they are able to transfer to a less restrictive environment.

In addition, some providers are rethinking how the facility supports its residents. One approach currently gaining visibility is the Eden Alternative. This nonprofit organization provides education and resources to help long-term care organizations change their culture and environments from being facilities for the frail to being habitats for human beings. Their focus is on ensuring meaning, variety, warmth, and autonomy in these settings. The philosophy includes encouraging resident autonomy, creating opportunities for meaningful activities, including caring for other living things, and enhancing spontaneity and variety throughout the day.[43]

CONTINUING CARE RETIREMENT COMMUNITIES

Health care for life can be obtained at **continuing care retirement communities** (CCRCs), which have existed for more than a century, but which have just recently gained popularity in the United States. These facilities are specifically designed to provide lifetime care within one community, so residents often move there while still independent and then change residences within the community if medical and/or personal care services are needed.[41] To join, the person generally pays an entrance fee and a monthly fee, and in return gets a home and certain services (specific to that CCRC).[44] These homes are arranged in a community and may be free-standing houses, condominiums, or apartments and include residential treatment facilities. The services may be optional for the resident and may range from no outside services at all to comprehensive health care services as needed. Services available may include housecleaning, meals, recreational programs, transportation, grounds upkeep, laundry service, individual medication management, respite care, rehabilitation, nursing services, health promotion programs, recreational programs, assistance with personal care, and social services.

HOSPICE CARE

Supportive and palliative care provided to people at the end of life is part of the **hospice** movement. The focus is on comfort and quality of life, rather than curative treatments. Although the concept of hospice care dates to ancient times, the first hospice in the United States was started in 1974. Medicare added a hospice benefit in 1983. Services may be provided in a client's home (including assisted living and nursing facilities), hospital, or a separate hospice facility. Services include medical, emotional, and spiritual care for terminally ill people and their families. Under the Medicare hospice benefit, eligibility includes a prognosis of 6 months or less, "if the disease runs its normal course." Beneficiaries receive a wider range of covered services and supports than would be available under traditional Medicare Part A.[45]

Hospice care, although well known for those with cancer, can be appropriate for people with many other medical diagnoses, including end-stage cardiac or pulmonary issues, renal failure, dementia, and neurological degenerative conditions. Although it is available through the last expected 6 months of life (and beyond, if a person survives longer), many patients are on the benefit less than a week, which may indicate a reluctance on the part of patients, families, or medical personnel to address a terminal prognosis.[45] Trends indicate that as more patients and families are educated about its possible benefits, hospice may become a more attractive alternative in the last days of life.[45]

OVERSIGHT

Oversight of long-term care is performed by a number of entities. Medicare audits and surveys providers who participate in the Medicare program to ensure that they are in compliance with all state and federal requirements. States also survey licensed facilities. Agencies and facilities opting for additional accreditation, such as provided by The Joint Commission (TJC) or the Community Health Accreditation Program (CHAP), are subject to additional requirements related to care provided. The Long Term Care Ombudsman Program, which is part of the Administration on Aging, works with long-term care providers and consumers to improve quality and resolve issues.[46]

SUMMARY

An adequate or desired living situation can provide the foundation for maintaining quality of life for older adults. Although safety is paramount, perhaps an equally important consideration is respecting choices made by competent older adults and supporting their quality of life in the environments of their choosing. Such a home, described by Garrett,[2] "fulfills many needs: it is a place of shelter and security, inspires a sense of belonging and mastery, and allows the person to be him or herself, reinforcing (by the presence of significant personal items) their life and identity."

Older people have a variety of opportunities to live in such a home, whether it is a house, apartment, SRO, CCRC, assisted living facility, or nursing facility. The home should be as pleasing to the individual, as affordable, and as accessible as possible. Along with safe and enjoyable surroundings, older people also need social support systems (provided by their families or beyond) and opportunities to participate in personally meaningful activities and contribute to their communities, for these are the tools to promote healthy aging.

Review Questions

1. Most older people would prefer to live _____ if widowed.
   A. Alone
   B. With their children
   C. In their own home
   D. In an SRO

2. Universal design
   A. Supports aging in place
   B. Can be used only with new construction
   C. Requires single-story construction
   D. Is helpful only to people with disabilities

3. All the following characteristics describe SROs except
   A. Private bathrooms
   B. One room
   C. Limited kitchen facilities
   D. Low cost

4. Which one of the following services is not available at CCRCs?
   A. A continuum of long-term care as long as needed
   B. Assistance with personal care
   C. Rehabilitation services
   D. Hospital services

5. _____ is/are an option for short-term rehabilitation care before moving to another setting.
   A. Single-room occupancies
   B. Skilled nursing facilities
   C. Subsidized housing
   D. Residential care facilities

6. Home health care is expanding for all the following reasons *except* which one?
    A. Most people prefer to recuperate at home
    B. Expansion in the number of available home health workers
    C. Technological advances
    D. The aging population

7. Rehabilitation
    A. Can only take place in the hospital
    B. Involves at least 4 hours of therapy per day
    C. Doctors are called physiatrists
    D. Therapists are called physiatrists

8. Hospice
    A. Is only for people in the last few days of life
    B. Is only for people with terminal cancer
    C. Is only for people with 6 months or less life expectancy
    D. Is staffed only by volunteers

9. Assisted living facility care would be appropriate for someone who
    A. Needs complete assistance with all activities of daily living
    B. Is completely independent in his or her personal care
    C. Requires some assistance with ADLs and IADLs now
    D. Needs a short rehabilitation stay

10. What may be the most important aspect of life quality for older adults?
    A. Having choices respected and supported
    B. Living with family
    C. Having lots of friends
    D. Maintaining former lifestyle

Learning Activities

1. Without referring back to the chapter, individually list the five most important things for you when considering your own environment when you are older. Compare your answers with the group. What can you learn from the answers of others?

2. Brainstorm about different ways that older people can improve their quality of life. Be creative. Remember in brainstorming there are no wrong answers. Can you, as health care professionals, assist in the improvement process? How?

3. Spend some time designing your future retirement community. You can list features or draw them out. Be specific. Share the designs among the group.

REFERENCES

1. MacDonald, M, et al. Research Considerations: The Link Between Housing and Health in the Elderly. *Journal of Gerontological Nursing*, 1994; 20:5–10.

2. Minkler, M. Community Organizing Among the Elderly Poor in the United States: A Case Study. *International Journal of Health Services*, 1992; 22:303–316.

3. National Association of Triads. The Makeup of Triad. Retrieved July 2, 2008, from http://www.nationaltriad.org/tools/Triad-at-a-Glance.pdf

4. Kerschner, H, Pegues, JA. Productive Aging: A Quality of Life Agenda. *Journal of the American Dietetic Association*, 1998;98(12):1445–1448.

5. Terracciano, A, et al. Personality Predictors of Longevity: Activity, Emotional Stability, and Conscientiousness. *Psychosomatic Medicine*, 2008; 70(6):621–627.

6. Phillips, EM, Davidoff, D. Normal and Successful Aging: What Happens to Function as We Age. *Primary Psychiatry*, 2004;11(1):35–38, 47.

7. Hong, LK, Duff, RW. Widows in Retirement Communities: The Social Context of Subjective Well-Being. *The Gerontologist*, 1994;34:347.

8. Cox, J. It's a Lifeline. *Elderly Care*, 1996; 8:13–15.

9. National Alliance for Caregiving and AARP. Caregiving in the US. Bethesda, MD: National Alliance for Caregiving; 2004.

10. Yarry, S, Stevens, EK, McCallum, TJ. Cultural Influences on Spousal Caregiving. *Generations, American Society on Aging*, Fall 2007;31(3):24–30. Retrieved February 14, 2009, from http://www.asaging.org/publications/dbase/GEN/Gen.31_3.Yarry.pdf

11. National Aging in Place Council. Aging in Place Glossary of Terms. Retrieved July 9, 2008, from http://www.naipc.org/AGuidetoAginginPlace/GlossaryofTerms/tabid/103/Default.aspx

12. Center for Universal Design, North Carolina State University. About Universal Design. Retrieved July 16, 2008, from http://www.design.ncsu.edu/cud/about_ud/about_ud.htm

13. Cannava, E. "Gerodesign": Safe and Comfortable Living Spaces for Older Adults. *Geriatrics*, 1994;49:45–49.

14. Houser, A. Long-Term Care Fact Sheet. AARP. 2007. Retrieved July 4, 2008, from http://www.aarp.org/research/longtermcare/trends/fs27r_ltc.html

15. Kassner, E. *Medicaid and Long-Term Services and Supports for Older People: Fact Sheet*. Washington, DC: AARP Public Policy Institute; 2005.

16. Garrett, G. But Does It Feel Like Home? Accommodation Needs on Later Life. *Professional Nurse*, January 1992;7:254–257.

17. Administration on Aging, U.S. Department of Health and Human Services. *A Profile of Older Americans: 2005*. Washington, DC: U.S. Department of Health and Human Services; 2005.

18. Gilderbloom, JI, Mullins, RL. Elderly Housing Needs: An Examination of the American Housing Survey. *International Journal of Aging and Human Development*, 1995;40:57–72.

19. Stucki, B. *Use Your Home to Stay at Home*. Washington, DC: National Council on the Aging; 2005.

20. United Jewish Communities, All About NORCs. Retrieved July 7, 2008, from http://www.norcs.com/index.aspx?page=1.

21. Ormond, BA, et al. *Supportive Services Programs in Naturally Occurring Retirement Communities*. Washington, DC: U.S. Department of Health and Human Services; 2004.

22. Opp, A. Productively Aging: St. Louis's Naturally Occurring Retirement Community. American Occupational Therapy Association. Retrieved July 10, 2008 from http://www.aota.org/news/centennial/40313/aging/40617.aspx

23. Rosenbeck, R, Bassuk, E, Salomon, A. Special Populations of Homeless Americans. Retrieved July 4, 2008, from http://aspe.hhs.gov/progsys/homeless/symposium/2-Spclpop.htm

24. U.S. Department of Housing and Urban Development. Single Room Occupancy Program (SRO). Retrieved July 3, 2008, from http://www.hud.gov/offices/cpd/homeless/programs/sro

25. American Association of Homes and Services for the Aging. Aging Services: The Facts. Retrieved June 19, 2008, from http://www.aahsa.org/article.aspx?id=74

26. The Cohousing Association of the United States. What Is Cohousing? Retrieved July 7, 2008, from http://www.cohousing.org/what_is_cohousing

27. U.S. Office of Personnel Management. *The Handbook of Elder Care Resources for the Federal Workplace*. Retrieved July 7, 2008, from http://www.opm.gov/Employment_and_Benefits/WorkLife/OfficialDocuments/HandbooksGuides/ElderCareResources/index.asp

28. Gist, J, et al. The State of 50+ America. Public Policy Institute, AARP. Retrieved June 30, 2008, from http://www.aarp.org/research/longtermcare/trends/fifty_plus_2007.html

29. Agency for Healthcare Research and Quality. *Long-Term Care Users Range in Age and Most Do Not Live in Nursing Homes: Research Alert*. Rockville, MD: AHRQ; 2000.

30. Thompson, L. *Long-Term Care: Support for Family Caregivers*. Washington, DC: Long-Term Financing Project, Georgetown University Press; 2004.

31. U.S. Department of Health and Human Services, Assistant Secretary for Planning and Evaluation. *The Future Supply of Long-Term Care Workers in Relation to the Aging Baby Boom Generation*. Report to Congress. Washington, DC: U.S. Department of Health and Human Services; 2003.

32. Fox-Grage, W, Coleman, B, Freiman, M. Rebalancing: Ensuring Greater Access to Home and Community-Based Services. AARP. Retrieved July 4, 2008, from http://www.aarp.org/research/housing-mobility/homecare/fs132_hcbs.html

33. Kassner, E. Long-Term Care Insurance. AARP. Retrieved July 4, 2008, from http://www.aarp.org/research/health/privinsurance/fs7r_ltc.html

34. National Association for Home Care and Hospice. Basic Statistics About Home Care. Retrieved July 4, 2008, from http://www.nahc.org/04HC_stats.pdf

35. Wakabayashi, C, Donato, KM. *The Consequences of Caregiving for Economic Well-Being in Women's Later Life*. Presented at the annual meeting of the American Sociological Association, San Francisco; 2004.

36. Pandya, S. Adult Day Services. AARP. Retrieved July 4, 2008, from http://www.aarp.org/research/housing-mobility/homecare/aresearch-import-839.html

37. Golant, SM. *Housing America's Elderly: Many Possibilities/Few Choices*. Newbury Park, CA: Sage; 1992;7:229–246.

38. Assisted Living Federation of America. What Is Assisted Living? Retrieved July 4, 2008, from http://www.alfa.org

39. Just, G, et al. Assisted Living: Challenges for Nursing Practice. *Geriatric Nursing*, 1995;16: 165–168.

40. National Center for Assisted Living. Assisted Living Facility Profile. Retrieved June 19, 2008, from http://www.ncal.org/about/facility.cfm.

41. Family Caregiver Alliance. *Fact Sheet: Residential Care Options*. Retrieved June 30, 2008, from http://www.caregiver.org/caregiver/jsp/content_node.jsp?nodeid=1742

42. Prince, D, Butler, D. *Final Report: Aging in Place in America*. Clarity and the EAR Foundation. Retrieved July 8, 2008, from www.clarityproducts.com/research/Clarity_Aging_in_Place_2007.pdf

43. The Eden Alternative. Retrieved June 30, 2008, from http://www.edenalt.org

44. AARP. Continuing Care Retirement Communities. Retrieved July 8, 2008, from http://www.aarp.org/families/housing_choices/other_options/a2004-02-26-retirementcommunity.html

45. Hospice Association of America. Hospice Facts and Statistics. Retrieved July 4, 2008, from http://www.nahc.org/HAA/

46. National Long Term Care Ombudsman Resource Center. What Does an Ombudsman Do? Retrieved July 9, 2008, from http://www.ltcombudsman.org/ombpublic/49_151_855.cfm

LEGAL AND FINANCIAL ISSUES RELATED TO HEALTH CARE FOR OLDER PEOPLE

TIMOTHY M. VOGEL, Esq.

Chapter Outline

Behavioral Objectives

Upon completion of this chapter, the reader will be able to:

1. Understand the value of personal autonomy in a patient's legal, medical, care, and financial decision making.
2. Describe the differences between mental competency and legal capacity.
3. Appreciate the need for sound legal decision making.
4. Describe surrogate health care decision making, when it is appropriate, and what is involved.
5. List the differences between voluntary and involuntary decision making.
6. Define the terminology related to a durable financial power of attorney, power of attorney, end-of-life care declaration, and trusts.
7. List the terms a power of attorney (POA) document must satisfy to be considered valid.
8. Understand the standard of legal capacity needed for an individual to sign various legal documents.
9. Describe the flexibility and limitations of voluntary decision making.
10. Describe when it is necessary to petition a probate court to appoint a guardian and conservator for a person.
11. List how the rights of a person are protected with the appointment of a guardian or conservator.
12. Describe what is involved with being a witness to a legal document.
13. Describe the three primary ways to pass property after death and what is involved in a will contest.
14. List the questions that would help empower your clients and their families to recognize and select quality long-term care services.
15. Describe the services of a geriatric care manager.
16. Describe the limits of Medicare and Medicaid for long-term care services.
17. List the five factors to consider when deciding on a long-term care insurance policy.
18. Describe what to consider in developing a plan to fund long-term care services.

Key Terms

Abuse

Advance directive

Agent

Alleged incapacitated person

Attorney for the alleged incapacitated
   person

Attorney-in-fact

Beneficiary

Capacity

Community spouse resource allowance

Competency

Conservator

Corporate trustee

Durable

Durable financial power of attorney

Elder law attorneys

End-of-life care declaration

Fiduciary

Financial exploitation

Geriatric care managers

Grantor

Guardian

Guardian ad litem

Health law attorneys

Incapacity

Intestacy statute

Involuntary civil commitment

Irrevocable trust

Last will and testament

Living will

Long-term care insurance

Long-term care plan

Medicaid

Medicaid exempt assets

Medical statement of incapacity

Medicare

Medicare Advantage programs

Medicare supplemental insurance (Medigap)

Neglect

Oral health care directive

Ownership designation

Patient Self-Determination Act

Personal autonomy

Pooled trusts

Power of attorney

Power of attorney for health care

Principal

Processing the estate through probate court

Reverse mortgage

Revocable living trust

Settlor

Special needs trust

Successor agent

Surviving joint owner

Supplemental care trust

Testamentary trust

Trust

Trustee

Uncompensated asset transfer

Uniform Health Care Decisions Act

Visitor

Written health care directive

Elder law attorneys commonly advise and represent older persons and their families on medical and long-term care planning, as well as in crisis situations. Likewise **health law attorneys** counsel health care professionals on a variety of health care delivery, regulatory, and professional conduct issues.

This chapter offers advice for health care professionals on legal and financial issues from the elder law perspective: What are solid planning steps for individuals to make and communicate health care decisions? How are disputes among family members regarding health care decisions resolved? How is payment for medical and long-term care best obtained?

Every society has issues of law, money, health care, and decision making. However, this chapter focuses on these issues as they relate to the delivery of medical and health care services for older people in the United States. It explains a variety of legal and financial issues that patients, their families, and health care professionals commonly face.

The application of this practical advice depends to some degree on your particular health care position, the hospital, facility or agency where you work, as well as the state or local law. It is crucial to know the protocol of your hospital, facility, or agency in a particular situation. By building awareness of the situations described in this chapter, you can prepare yourself in advance to respond, based on your particular health care institution. With whom should you talk? Where do you report incidents? Where do you refer patients who have questions or need advice about health care decisions or payment for medical and health care services? What is the institution's procedure to comply with your state law that may mandate you to report cases of older adults who have suffered **abuse**, **neglect**, or **financial exploitation**? The answers to these questions can be found in the following pages.

HEALTH CARE DECISION MAKING

Our society and culture place a high value on **personal autonomy**—the ability of an adult to make decisions for oneself and control one's life. Personal autonomy is often the basis for medical, health care, legal, financial, and personal decision making. Personal autonomy is commonly explained to patients and clients with the phrase: No one will make better decisions for you than you will make for yourself.

However, illness and accidents may leave a person unable to understand what is involved in a particular decision or unable to make and communicate desires. This condition, known as **incapacity**, may arise in medical, health care, residential, financial, and/or legal situations. At one time or another, each of these areas presents circumstances requiring decisions to be made when an individual becomes incapacitated and unable to make decisions or communicate decisions.

Competency is a measure of an individual's mental process, which can be measured by a physician, psychiatrist, or psychologist, commonly through a mental status exam. **Capacity** is the application of an individual's competency to a set legal standard, such as the person's ability to make a decision or sign a legal document. Examples of such decisions and documents include making a medical decision, deciding to give property to a loved one, making a gift, signing a legal document such as a power of attorney, last will and testament, contract, deed, trust, tax return, or application for coverage or benefits under insurance or Medicaid.

As an aspect of personal autonomy, an adult is presumed to have the capacity to make legal, financial, medical, and care decisions. Incapacity is often expressed as the inability of an individual, because of a physical or mental condition, to make reasonable decisions about self or property. Thus, this chapter refers to a person's capacity or incapacity to make decisions, and not to the individual's competency.

THE NEED FOR SOUND LEGAL DECISION-MAKING AUTHORITY

A number of problems are likely, if legal decision-making authority is not established for the incapacitated person who cannot make or communicate decisions. Medical decisions, including end-of-life care decisions, cannot be made. Financial accounts and property cannot be managed for the incapacitated person or for the support of the spouse and dependents. The capable spouse, family member, or other trusted individual must secure authority to make legal, financial, and health care decisions for the infirm individual in the event of incapacity. Each partner of a married couple has the ability to make decisions for her- or himself. Thus, generally a spouse has no legal right to make legal, financial, or medical decisions for the other spouse. One option is for the infirm individual to voluntarily sign a health care directive (sometimes known as a power of attorney for health care or health care proxy).

Another option exists in states that have a law such as the **Uniform Health Care Decisions Act** (UHCDA). The UHCDA surrogate health care decision section addresses the situation when a patient is incapacitated, unable to make or communicate a health care decision, and has no signed health care directive or a court-appointed guardian. In these states, physicians and other health care providers may recognize the authority of a surrogate health care decision maker for the patient. The surrogate health care decision maker may be the spouse, other family member, or close friend. The surrogate decision maker is authorized to make general health care decisions if the patient has been determined by the primary physician to lack capacity and no power of attorney agent or guardian exists. The surrogate is also authorized to withhold or withdraw life-sustaining treatment for a patient.

However, when there is a dispute between family members, or if the physician or health care provider questions the authority of the surrogate, the surrogate's authority may be insufficient. In such situations it still may be necessary to petition probate court to appoint a guardian with health care decision-making authority.

Another option exists in the area of financial decisions. Commonly, both the incapacitated person and the capable spouse are named as joint owners of bank or investment accounts. As a joint owner, the able spouse has authority to have full access to the account. However, conducting transactions involving jointly owned real estate and some joint investments may be difficult when the signatures of both joint owners are required. If there is no **durable financial power of attorney** (DFPOA) for the incapacitated spouse, the other spouse may have to resort to petitioning the probate court to appoint a conservator.

In almost all cases, it will be necessary to establish decision-making authority for an incapacitated person. The next section concerns voluntary decision-making arrangements. The following section discusses establishing involuntary decision making by petitioning the probate court to appoint a guardian and/or conservator.

VOLUNTARY APPROACHES TO DECISION MAKING

Voluntary decision-making authority is available to establish an appropriate range of decision-making authority involving legal, financial, and health care decisions. Voluntary decision making is usually superior to petitioning the probate court to appoint a guardian and conservator. Legal documents for voluntary decision making are almost always quicker, more flexible, more confidential, and less expensive than going to probate court. It is almost always best for a person to select someone to make decisions for him or her in the event of incapacity. The alternative is to rely on family or close friends (who may or may not have honorable intentions), local adult protective services agencies, or a judge to select who will make medical and financial, personal and sensitive decisions for the incapacitated person.

The voluntary approach to establishing decision-making authority involves a person who is willing and able to voluntarily sign a legal document. These legal documents are commonly known as **advance directives**. This term explains its meaning: In *advance* of something happening to the individual, he or she signs a written *directive* stating who should make decisions for him or her in the event of incapacity. Depending on the state, advance directive documents may be called a general power of attorney, durable financial power of attorney, health care directive, health care proxy, living will, or end-of-life care declaration. This person who has legal authority and responsibility to make decisions for another is called a **fiduciary**. In most states, the fiduciary appointed by the probate court to make personal, medical, care, educational, and residential decisions is called the **guardian**. The person appointed to make money, investment, and property decisions is called the **conservator**. Sometimes one person is appointed to be both guardian and conservator for the incapacitated person. In other cases, one person is appointed the guardian and another person is appointed the conservator.

In most circumstances, it is recommended that a person should execute a durable financial power of attorney (DFPOA) and a **power of attorney for health care** (POAHC), or the equivalent document used in the state. Although the terminology may vary from state to state, it is useful to review the general terminology of power of attorney (POA) documents:

- **Power of attorney** (POA) is the legal document setting out the legal authority of the agent to act for the principal.
- The **principal** is the person who signs the document.
- The **agent** is the person whom the principal authorizes to make decisions. In some states, this person may also be called the **attorney-in-fact**.
- At least one **successor agent** should be named to make decisions if the primary agent becomes unable or unwilling to act as agent. In that event, there may not be an agent available to act for the principal, and thus it may become necessary to petition the probate court to appoint a guardian and conservator.
- **Durable** means that the power of attorney document remains valid after the principal becomes incapacitated.

A power of attorney (POA) document must satisfy certain terms to be valid:

- The POA must name the principal and the agent, and if possible a successor agent or agents. Even the best crafted DFPOA or POAHC becomes useless if the named agent becomes incapacitated or dies without the document providing for a successor agent.

- Both the DFPOA and POAHC should be *durable*. This term means that the POA document remains valid if the principal should become incapacitated.
- Some states require the POA to contain specific language, such as authorizing the agent to use the principal's funds to make gifts. Such gifting authority is necessary to avoid any problems. The capable spouse may need the DFPOA to transfer the infirm spouse's joint home ownership. The couple's assets may need to be restructured to meet Medicaid requirements.
- Further, some states require the POA to include statutory warning language to the principal and the agent. Without such language, the POA will be invalid or lack authority in crucial areas.

Signing requirements for POA documents vary among the states. Some states require that the principal's signature be notarized. Other states require that there must be two witnesses to the principal signing the document. It is appropriately cautious to have two witnesses and a notary sign each POA document.

LEGAL STANDARDS FOR DECISION-MAKING CAPACITY

The legal standard regarding sufficient capacity to make a decision or sign a legal document usually depends on state law and sometimes on federal law. In general, to make a decision or sign a legal document, the individual must understand the action to be taken or the decision to be made and must intend to or want to sign the document. For example, to sign a contract, the individual need not understand every term of the document. What the person must know is that the document is a contract to do something (such as to buy or sell a house for a certain price at a specific time), and that the person wants to undertake the action described in the contract.

The legal standard to execute a will is that the person must want to sign the will, know what property he or she owns, and can name his or her relatives who likely would inherit his or her estate. Many persons with early Alzheimer's disease or another form of dementia may still have sufficient legal capacity to sign a contract or a will.

Depending on the type of legal document, one or two witnesses and possibly a notary may be required to be present when the person signs the document. That the person has the legal capacity to sign the document is determined at the time the document is signed. The function of a witness is to acknowledge that the person knew what he or she was doing and voluntarily signed the document. If it is established that the person had legal capacity to sign the document, the document remains valid even if the individual later suffers an accident or illness that leaves him or her incapacitated.

It is the lawyer's duty to determine whether the person has sufficient capacity to sign the document. A physician, psychiatrist, or psychologist may test the individual's mental competency. However, the lawyer knows the particular legal standard and what the law requires for the person to sign the particular legal document.

BEING A WITNESS TO A LEGAL DOCUMENT OR A WILL

Sometimes nurses, social workers, or other health care professionals working in a hospital or facility are asked to witness the signing of legal documents. First, you should know the institution's policy on staff witnessing legal documents. Sometimes witnessing a legal document takes more time than anticipated. If you are asked to be a witness at the signing of a document, your responsibility is to observe the individual's actions during the process. Note what he or she may say about the document and his or her willingness to sign the document. Most states require two witnesses at the signing of a will. The responsibilities of a witness are not difficult. A witness must be present when the person signs the will. To the best of the witness's knowledge, the witness must be able to state that the person was of the legal age to sign a will (usually 18), seemed to be of sound mind, and was under no pressure to sign the will.

A health care professional may become involved in a family dispute about a patient signing a will. If you feel the patient does not know what he or she is doing, or is being forced to sign the will, you should refuse to witness the signing of the will. On the other hand, if you feel the patient knows the situation and wants to sign the will, as a witness you are helping the patient create a legally enforceable written record of his or her wishes.

HEALTH CARE DECISIONS

Certainly, it is preferred for patients to be able to communicate directly to the physician or health care provider as to what care they want to receive or refuse. Such an **oral health care directive** takes precedence over the individual's **written health care directive** or POAHC. However, if the individual lacks the ability to make or communicate these crucial health care decisions, the POAHC is an essential written health care directive. Unless specifically limited, the health care decision-making authority of the agent is both broad and general.

If the principal has the ability to make and communicate health care decisions to the physician or other health care provider, the principal's health care decision in the immediate time will take control. This is true even if the principal has signed a written health care directive or if the health care agent objects to the principal's health care decision. Depending on facts of the situation, there may be a challenge of the principal's capacity to make health care decisions.

General POA terminology is usually used in a written health care directive. The principal signs a written health care directive, commonly called a power of attorney for health care. In the POAHC, the principal appoints an agent and successor agents to make health care decisions if the principal becomes incapacitated. A well-drafted POAHC includes an authorization to release information for all information under the HIPAA

(Health Insurance Portability and Accountability Act) federal medical privacy law so that the agent has full access to HIPAA-protected health care information. In states with the Uniform Health Care Decisions Act, in the POAHC, end-of-life health care decisions, formerly referred to as a living will, should be included.

Individuals should have the opportunity to sign an **end-of-life care declaration**, formerly known as a **living will**, stating the degree of medical intervention each person wishes to receive during a terminal condition. The end-of-life care declaration is commonly included within the POAHC. Under the federal **Patient Self-Determination Act**, hospitals and medical facilities receiving federal funding must make available to patients on admission health care directive and end-of-life care declaration forms.

The law establishing surrogate health care decision authority is described earlier. You should determine whether your state has a surrogate health care decision-making law. Remember that the authority for a surrogate to make health care decisions exists only if the principal is not currently able to make or communicate health care decisions and there exists no valid written health care directive, such as a POAHC.

THE FLEXIBILITY AND LIMITATIONS OF VOLUNTARY DECISION MAKING

It is almost always best for a person to make voluntary decision-making arrangements by signing the DFPOA or a POAHC equivalent in the person's state. Consulting a lawyer—such as an elder law attorney who is familiar with the state law about voluntary decision-making arrangements and POA documents—will generally be quicker and less costly than petitioning the probate court to appoint a guardian and conservator. The lawyer can tailor the terms of the POA documents to meet the principal's needs with regard to the type of health care treatments and interventions the principal wants to receive or reject in the event of incapacity, the specific language concerning the sale or transfer of property in the specific state of residence, questions related to eligibility and applying for Medicaid, provisions the principal wants to make for a disabled spouse or child, and whom the principal wants included or excluded from decision making should the principal become incapacitated.

When the principal signs a POA document, the principal keeps the authority to amend or revoke the document as long as the principal has legal capacity to take such action. Also, he or she retains the ability to make a full range of legal, financial, medical, and health care decisions on his or her own without the permission of or without even consulting the agent, even if those decisions may be against the best interests of the principal. If the principal has the capacity to sign a POAHC, the principal will continue to have the capacity to make health care decisions until some intervening accident or illness renders the principal incapacitated. For example, Mrs. Jones has signed a POAHC appointing her daughter Mary as her health care agent. Mrs. Jones has early stage dementia, but usually she still can make her wishes known. Mary believes her mother would receive better care if she moves from the home where she has lived for years to an assisted living facility with a respected dementia care unit. Mary uses her authority under her mother's POAHC to sign the assisted living facility admissions documents.

Mary moves her mother into the facility, but Mrs. Jones misses her home very much. In several days, Mrs. Jones goes to the facility social worker and states that she is moving back home today. Mrs. Jones is still able to make her own decisions, and Mary cannot stop her based on her decision-making authority in the POAHC. As described in the section on involuntary decision making, only a probate court order appointing a guardian and conservator would be legally binding and thus would need to be respected by Mrs. Jones, Mary, and the facility.

Mary and the facility social worker certainly can make an effort to convince Mrs. Jones that she will receive the best care in the assisted living facility. Mary may also hire a geriatric care manager to help create a good care system for her mother at home. If Mrs. Jones continues to refuse to cooperate, Mary may consider seeing a lawyer to petition the probate court to appoint Mary as her mother's guardian and conservator. Mary must decide whether or not her mother has a physical or mental condition that prevents her from making reasonable decisions about herself or her property. Going to probate court may be a long and expensive process. There is also the risk that Mrs. Jones will fight Mary's petition to the probate court or that the probate court may appoint someone else, rather than Mary, as Mrs. Jones's guardian and conservator. This case demonstrates the problems that may arise in the case of making decisions about best care.

FAMILY DISPUTE RESOLUTION

Medical, health care, and long-term care situations can create great stress involving the patient/resident, family members, and other close persons. Some of these situations involve tensions or anxiety about health care decisions. Others involve concern about the facility or residence where the person will be transferred. Money, property, wills, estate plans, and how to pay for care are all topics that can cause controversies and tensions within families. Sometimes one or several family members will directly challenge the authority of the POA agent. Other times, the agent is either unable or unwilling to make decisions for the principal.

Reviewing the facts and options as comprehensively as possible with the individual and family members can be crucial in resolving these dilemmas. Social workers may be helpful in resolving familial disputes of this nature. In many areas of the country, mediators experienced in resolving these issues are available as well.

Although there is a significant value in discussion and consensus decision making, sometimes individuals and families are unable to resolve medical and care disputes. Some of these disputes may end up being discussed by the hospital or facility ethics committees. As described in the next section, in some cases someone may have to petition probate court, have all concerned individuals tell their stories to the judge, and have the judge decide. If the patient/resident is able to make and communicate decisions, the judge may help him or her to understand the medical and care situation and options. Once the appropriate decision maker has been identified, the health care professional should provide information on the issues and options so that the decision maker can make the most thoughtful decisions for the individual.

INVOLUNTARY DECISION MAKING

The involuntary approach is necessary when the individual does not have the ability to make or communicate decisions voluntarily. Because the person is not able to state who should help him or her make decisions, if necessary, a request on behalf of the person must be filed in a court—in most states, the probate court—to appoint a decision maker for the person. This involuntary approach usually results in the probate court appointing a person to make personal and financial decisions for the incapacitated person.

Utilizing the involuntary decision-making process may be necessary in several circumstances. For example, if the individual never has signed a DFPOA or POAHC and now lacks capacity to execute those documents; or the signed documents are not legally valid or legally sufficient for the situation; or a family dispute arises about the decision maker or decisions made. In those instances, it may be necessary to petition the probate court to appoint a guardian and conservator. Whereas petitioning probate court may be necessary in some circumstances, well-drafted POA documents tailored to meet the needs of the principal, spouse, and family members are more flexible, quicker, and less expensive.

State laws, such as the Uniform Health Care Decisions Act, have established a system for physicians and health care providers to recognize the decision-making authority of surrogate health care decision makers. Such laws have reduced the need for health care facilities to petition the probate court for emergency medical decision-making authority when the incapacitated patient does not have a POAHC. However, the surrogate decision-making process will not work in all situations. It is sometimes still necessary to petition probate court for appointment of a guardian to make health care decisions.

When appointed by the probate court, the guardian makes personal decisions for the incapacitated person, usually in the realm of medical, care, and residential issues. The conservator makes decisions regarding the protected person's money and property. For a guardian or conservator to be appointed, the individual must have a physical or mental condition such that he or she lacks the ability to make or communicate reasonable decisions regarding personal, medical, property, or financial matters.

State laws may offer some protections for the rights of the **alleged incapacitated person** (AIP)—the person who allegedly has impaired decision-making abilities but upon whom the probate court has yet to decide. Depending on state law, the probate court may require a **medical statement of incapacity** signed by a physician or licensed psychologist to document the existence of the physical or mental condition and its functional limitations on the allegedly incapacitated person. The probate court also may appoint a

visitor—usually a nurse or social worker—to report to the court after visiting the individual, the proposed guardian or conservator, and the individual's proposed residence. The probate court may also appoint an **attorney for the alleged incapacitated person** or a **guardian ad litem**.

An attorney for an allegedly incapacitated person has the duty to legally represent the allegedly incapacitated person and articulate the individual's position on the case to the probate court. For example, the attorney may report that the individual is capable of making decisions, or that the individual agrees to the appointment of a guardian or conservator but wishes a certain person appointed with specifically limited powers.

A guardian ad litem has the responsibility to interview the allegedly incapacitated person and investigate the situation. The guardian ad litem advises the probate court as to what actions are in the allegedly incapacitated person's best interests, even if the person objects to that course of action.

INVOLUNTARY CIVIL COMMITMENT FOR THOSE WHO ARE A DANGER TO THEMSELVES OR OTHERS

Whereas in most states the appointment of a guardian or conservator is usually handled by the probate court, some states have laws assigning **involuntary civil commitment** cases to another court rather than probate court. You should learn how your state handles involuntary civil commitment cases.

In most states, if a person suffers from a mental condition or psychosis such that he or she is deemed a danger to himself or herself or to others, the police or some other person can petition the appropriate court to order the person to be confined, usually to a mental hospital or facility. Each state law differs as to the person's rights in an involuntary civil commitment, such as how long the person can be held without a hearing, whether the person will be appointed a lawyer, and when there will be a second hearing to determine if the person continues to be a risk and should be held longer. After a person has been through involuntary civil commitment, it may be necessary for a family member or adult protective services to petition the probate court to appoint a guardian and conservator, if the person remains incapacitated and if someone must be appointed to make personal, medical, or financial decisions for the person.

ESTATE PLANNING AND TRUSTS: HOW PROPERTY IS PASSED TO AND MANAGED FOR THE BENEFIT OF OTHERS

Health care professionals may be present during the time in a patient's life when medical, care, legal, and financial issues are decided or disputed. Another important aspect of decision making is how to pass property after death and who will benefit. There are three primary ways that property is passed after death.

OWNERSHIP DESIGNATION

Ownership designation is when the individual establishes joint ownership of property or lists beneficiaries' names, usually on life insurance policies or retirement accounts. This happens while the person is alive and has the capacity to select those who should receive the property after the person dies. Most important, if property passes to the **surviving joint owner** or **beneficiary**, that property will pass regardless of what is stated in the person's last will and testament. Sometimes, a health care professional will be asked to witness a deed establishing joint ownership or a beneficiary designation form.

PROCESSING THE ESTATE THROUGH PROBATE COURT

Administering an estate through court—in most states called probate court—is what most people identify as the primary way to pass property after death. It is not necessary to **process an estate through probate court** when all of the deceased's property is passed to the surviving joint owner or beneficiary.

After death, when property remains in the sole name of the deceased individual, it is usually necessary to process the estate through probate court to transfer property to the intended persons. State probate laws and procedures establish this process. During their lifetime, people can sign a **last will and testament** (LWT, or will). In this document, they state who will receive the property they own at death that does not pass by joint ownership or beneficiary designation. In the LWT, the person can also name who will administer the estate. Traditionally, the person who administers the estate is called the executor, but in many state the person is now called the personal representative.

If the deceased did not have a valid LWT at time of death, or if no valid will can be found, the estate property will pass according to the state's **intestacy statute**. The intestacy statute states how property should pass. If the deceased left no indication of how the property should pass after death, then the state intestacy statute lists the order of inheritance. Intestacy statutes vary among states, but a common intestacy statute inheritance pattern among persons who survive the deceased is spouse and children, parents, siblings, aunts and uncles, nieces and nephews, cousins, and on through other relatives. Only if the deceased leaves no valid ownership designation, no valid will, or no living relative listed in the intestacy statute will the property pass to the state.

There are protections for the surviving spouse, dependent children, and creditors when an estate is processed through probate court. Most states have laws requiring the surviving spouse and dependent children receive a certain portion of the estate if they have been left out of the will. Creditors must be paid before distributions are made from the estate. If a house with a mortgage is in an estate, the mortgage must be paid before other creditors are paid or estate distributions are made.

Some states have streamlined estate administration procedures allowing an estate to be processed through probate court in several months at low cost. The probate court appoints the personal representative. That person then pays the estate bills, distributes the estate property according to the will or the intestacy statute, and notifies the court when the estate is closed. In other states, the court is involved in all stages of estate administration and must review and approve finances before the estate can be closed.

TRUSTS

A properly written and functioning trust may effectively pass all property after death. Key trust terminology helps explain how trusts work:

- The **trust** is the document that establishes the rules by which property will be managed for the benefit of another.
- The **grantor** (also known as the **settlor**) is the person who signs the trust document and establishes the trust.
- The **trustee** is the person who administers the trust by following the rules in the trust. The trust commonly names an initial trustee and successor trustees for when the initial trustee is no longer able to administer the trust. Most trustees are individuals, but a bank or corporation can be named as a **corporate trustee**.
- The beneficiary is the person to whom the trustee distributes money, property, or services. The trustee also can pay for services, such as home health care, directly to the provider for the benefit of the beneficiary. The trust commonly names an immediate beneficiary and future beneficiaries.
- A common trust form is a **revocable living trust** (RLT). In most states, in an RLT, the grantor can be the initial trustee and the initial beneficiary. Prior to death the grantor can revoke or amend the RLT. In states where the procedure to process an estate through probate court is lengthy and expensive, many persons set up an RLT to avoid that probate process.
- A trust whose terms are included within a last will and testament is called a **testamentary trust**. A testamentary trust functions only if its operation is required by the terms of the will and the facts at the time of death. For example, a will may have a testamentary trust to provide education and support for grandchildren under the age of 25. If all the grandchildren are older than 25 when the grandparent dies, this testamentary trust will not come into operation.
- An **irrevocable trust** cannot be changed after the grantor signs it. In most cases, when property is transferred to an irrevocable trust, the property cannot be returned to the grantor. Although irrevocable trusts can be useful for tax purposes, in most cases they will not shelter property from consideration in determining Medicaid eligibility.

CHALLENGES TO ESTATE PLANNING DECISIONS

Challenges to the validity of a will after death of a testator may be common in movies, books, and theater, but in real life they are rare and seldom successful. Although the law of will contests vary among states, there are several common grounds to challenge or contest the validity of a will.

In many states, if a will was signed before two witnesses and a notary, there is a legal presumption that the testator properly signed the will. Anyone challenging the will would have to present strong evidence of improper conduct at the will signing, such as the testator not knowing the document was a will or someone forging the testator's signature. Courts strictly demand clear and convincing evidence to invalidate a will. Courts discourage will contests to keep persons who feel they were unfairly treated in a will from clogging up the court with unsupported will contests.

Most will challenges are for undue influence. A common example is that of 92-year-old Mr. Smith who had a will evenly dividing his estate between his children. The home care agency assigned an attractive young woman, Jane Jones, as his personal care attendant. Within 3 weeks, Mr. Smith signed a new will leaving all of his estate to Jane Jones. For the children to challenge this will, they would have to prove that Mr. Smith depended on Ms. Jones, and that she encouraged him to change his will for her benefit.

Thus, if a health care professional acts as a witness for a patient signing a will, there is a very small chance after the testator's death that the witness will become involved in a court case challenging the validity of the will. Also, if the patient's will leaves a portion of the estate to the hospital, health care facility, or any health care professional involved with the patient, the health care professional should avoid any conflict and refuse to witness the will.

SPECIAL NEEDS TRUSTS, SUPPLEMENTAL CARE TRUSTS, AND POOLED TRUSTS

Certain trusts are carefully structured so that a Medicaid recipient can receive benefits from the trust without losing Medicaid eligibility. These trusts should be carefully prepared to strictly comply with federal and state Medicaid law. An experienced elder law attorney familiar with these types of trusts and the state Medicaid program should be consulted to prepare such a trust.

When Congress authorized these trusts, it recognized the usefulness of these trusts to older and disabled individuals. The purpose of these trusts is to provide goods and services to improve the trust beneficiary's quality of life while still allowing the beneficiary to remain eligible for Medicaid. Thus, Medicaid covers the beneficiary's medical and primary care expenses, such as nursing home costs. The trustee can use the trust funds to improve the quality of the beneficiary's life through non-Medicaid covered goods and services such as special therapy, companionship, training, education, transportation, recreation, and travel. In the right circumstances, your patient might greatly benefit from one of these trusts.

- **Special needs trust**. In this situation, an example is a grandparent who wants to leave money to improve the quality of life of a grandchild who is developmentally disabled and lives in a group home. The trustee is permitted to make trust distributions as long as these do not violate the rules of any government programs with financial eligibility rules, such as Medicaid or Supplementary Security Income (SSI). The trustee cannot give any cash to the beneficiary. The grandparent can set up the special needs trust by signing it during the grandparent's lifetime or including it as a testamentary trust in the grandparent's will. Upon the death of the grandchild, any remaining funds in the trust will be distributed according to trust terms, most likely to other family members the grandparent selected.

When a parent needs Medicaid and has a child receiving disability benefits, it is possible to set up a version of the special needs trust. Medicaid exempts the transfer by the parent to a child who is receiving Social Security disability benefits, even if the child is an adult. The parent can set up a special needs trust that will not violate the child's Medicaid and SSI eligibility. At the child's death, any money left in the trust is distributed according to the child's last will and testament or, if the child does not have a will, according to the intestacy statute.

- **Supplemental care trust**. In 1993, Congress authorized a type of trust allowing Medicaid recipients under age 65 to transfer funds—usually from an inheritance or a personal injury settlement—without being penalized for an asset penalty. Like a special needs trust, the trustee is permitted to make trust distributions as long as these do not violate Medicaid rules and do not distribute cash to the beneficiary. The trust must be set up by the individual's parent, guardian, or a court. At the death of the individual, any remaining funds must first reimburse the state for the Medicaid the person received.
- **Pooled trusts**. In 1993, Congress authorized pooled trusts for Medicaid recipients. In a pooled trust, an individual sets up an account in a larger trust fund administered for disabled persons. The person is permitted to make this transfer without any Medicaid transfer penalty. The pooled trust management committee can make distributions for the benefit of the disabled person, but cannot distribute cash directly to the individual. A pooled trust is a great benefit for disabled individuals who have smaller amounts of money. Upon the individual's death, the terms of the pooled trust agreement determine how much of the remaining account funds must be used to repay Medicaid and how much will be left to benefit the pooled trust and its other beneficiaries.

MAINTAINING CARE FOR THE INDIVIDUAL'S WELL-BEING

Chapter 9 describes the range of long-term care services. This chapter focuses on how the older person is able to access and fund the appropriate care services necessary for the individual's well-being.

From the perspective of an elder law attorney, long-term care planning begins with a simple goal for the client: access to quality care. This is an essential human need in every circumstance. Long-term care planning is crucial because long-term care is the most expensive direct health care expense for which older Americans have personal liability. This focus on quality care concerns the full range of services provided by a variety of delivery systems funded through a number of private and public sources. In the broadest sense, *long-term care* is a term that covers many levels of care ranging from subacute hospital care, skilled nursing care, rehabilitation care, general nursing facility care, assisted living facility care, and a variety of home health care and community-based services.

Quality of care issues arise all along this spectrum—including family caregivers, parents residing with family members, respite care, home health care agencies, multilevel facilities, assisted living facilities, residential care facilities, boarding homes, continuing care retirement communities, adult family care homes, general nursing homes, skilled nursing facilities, rehabilitation facilities, subacute care facilities, and hospice care.

As recently as the early 1990s, the common long-term care options were limited to family help at home, usually by a wife or daughter, in-patient hospital care for acute conditions, and nursing home care when the patient could not stay at home. No longer does this linear progression accurately reflect the long-term care environment of the 21st century.

Empowering your patients and their families to recognize and select quality long-term care services involves educating the individual and the family. Many needs must be assessed. What kind and how much care or assistance does the patient need? Where is the best place for these services to be received? What payment options are available? How does the family view the situation? Here are questions to ask when considering the quality of long-term care services for a particular patient:

- How would you like to be treated in a similar situation?
- Are the patient's needs being met?
- Is the care provided harming or causing the patient to deteriorate?
- What do the caregiver and the family need?
- Where can those services best be obtained?
- What is working best, and what can be improved?
- What does the patient need that is not being provided?
- How can the family enable and help the service provider to recognize and address the patient's needs?

Geriatric care managers (GCMs) can play an important role in helping the older client and the family access quality care. These are independently employed professionals who are commonly licensed as nurses or social workers. They can review an individual's needs for home health care, assisted living, or nursing home care and help identify resources in the community to provide that care. They may also be able to provide supervision for the recommended care. They are able to provide care information to family members and assist them in making care decisions.

A GCM can be an important complement to a hospital or nursing home care coordinator, discharge planner, or social worker. A GCM has the experience to identify the patient's care options upon which the elder law attorney can focus funding possibilities. The GCM can help the family evaluate the patient's care needs and identify available quality long-term care services. The care manager can also advocate for the patient who is caught in the "patient shuffle" as he or she is moved from a hospital, to skilled care, to a nursing facility, to home, to a hospital, to an assisted living facility, to home, and so on. A geriatric care manager might help to minimize the risks, including a significant risk of mortality, for those patients caught in this shuffle.

SUPPORTING THE INDIVIDUAL'S AND THE FAMILY'S ECONOMIC SECURITY

In long-term care planning, it is important to consider the economic security of the spouse at home as well as the patient's other family support obligations for dependents. Eligibility for Medicaid nursing home services includes calculations to protect assets and income for the community spouse and dependent children. It is crucial to secure a payment source for the patient's care services, whenever the patient and family are budgeting for long-term care expenses.

Long-term care planning is more complex where there is a second or multiple marriages. The children may say, "It is fine that mother found a new husband after dad died. However, now he is getting Alzheimer's disease and all of the money my father worked so hard to save is going to pay for his nursing home care." Medicaid rules treat all couples the same whether they have been married for 5 or 55 years.

An increasing number of older couples, primarily heterosexual, are choosing not to marry. Commonly, these unmarried couples need help planning to provide economic security for the partner left at home. When one partner applies for Medicaid, the Medicaid rules do not consider the assets of the other partner. However, the other partner also does not benefit from the Medicaid rule that exempts transfers between married spouses. When one member of an unmarried couple needs long-term care, it is best to consult an attorney experienced in this area.

Although many men work hard to provide caregiver services to a loved one, the majority of caregivers are wives or daughters. Everyone involved in long-term care planning should consider the issues caregivers face and not ignore their needs. Some families are motivated by this reality. They will plan for a loved one possibly needing long-term care services to avoid the women in the family having their lives disrupted by extended caregiver responsibilities. In other families, the women will need to or choose to surrender their careers, their independence, and their own health to care for a family member.

A caregiver who is strained to the point of collapse, of course, greatly complicates the situation. Quality long-term care services can ease the situation. Long-term care consumer support groups, such as the Alzheimer's Association, also can provide essential support, education, and empowerment for the caregiver and the family. Sharing experiences can strengthen the caregiver, leading to positive effects for the patient, the family, and better opportunities for obtaining quality long-term care services.

LACK OF A PAYMENT SOURCE

Many individuals who do not have health care insurance are adults between the ages of 18 and 65. The cost of providing medical care continues to rise during adulthood peaking in old age. Many states have expanded Medicaid coverage for children under 18. Frequently, most adults older than 65 are covered by Medicare or retiree health insurance. When a patient does not have a source of payment for hospital, medical, therapy, or long-term care services can be great stress placed on the patient and his or her family. (See **Table 10-1** for a summary of the average care costs for individuals of various ages.)

Health care payment problems may become the source of family disputes. You need to know the resources available, or to whom the family should turn, in the event that patients do not have health insurance, Medicare, or Medicaid. A social worker at your health care facility can help the beleaguered family sort out these issues and make referrals to others who can help the family as well.

ABUSE, NEGLECT, AND FINANCIAL EXPLOITATION

Financial exploitation of older adults does exist. When an older patient needs nursing home care or other long-term care services, many families do not understand Medicaid, especially its asset transfer rules. In such situations, some families adopt the attitude that it is better for them to take the older person's money or property because otherwise it will just go to pay for nursing home care. Financial pressure and caretaker stress in some instances can lead to physical abuse and neglect of the older individual.

You should know your profession's and your health care institution's protocol when you suspect physical abuse, caregiver or individual self-neglect, and financial exploitation. You may be mandated to report such cases to the Adult Protective Services agency in your

TABLE 10-1 Average Annual Cost per Consumer for Health Care.

Age	Cost in Dollars 1995	Cost in Dollars 2005 (2004–2006)
≤25	$465	$705
35–44	$1,609	$2,284
65–74	$2,617	$4,379
>75	$2,683	$4,282
Average (all ages)	$1,732	$2,664

Sources: U.S. Census Bureau. *Statistical Abstract of the United States, 1997.* 17th ed. Washington, DC: U.S. Department of Commerce; 1997: 119. U.S. Census Bureau. Average Annual Expenditures per Consumer Unit for Health Care, 2004–2006 (Table 133). Retrieved March 1, 2009, from http://www.census.gov/compendia/statab/cats/health_nutrition.html.

state. Law enforcement officials are improving in their response and investigation of financial exploitation. In some cases, an elder law attorney should be consulted about recovery of property and legal damages.

PLANNING FOR MEDICAL AND LONG-TERM CARE FINANCING

Health care professionals encounter patients and their families who need to understand both individual care needs and how to fund that care. Most health care professionals are not trained to advise patients and families on the eligibility and coverage details of Medicare; medical, supplemental, and long-term care insurance; and Medicaid. However, if health care professionals have an overview of long-term care funding options, they can help clients and families manage care option decisions, as well as understand which professionals, including elder law attorneys, to consult.

KNOW AVAILABLE RESOURCES

Health care professionals know paying for health and long-term care is frequently a source of great stress and disputes for patients/residents and their families. Cases of financial exploitation may arise out of the fear that all the individual's money and property will go to pay for medical and long-term care expenses. Therefore, health care professionals need to know the resources available in their organization and in the community. They need to educate individuals and their families using objective and up-to-date information on medical and long-term care payment options. Referrals to experts in these realms are usually appropriate. In recent years, federal and state Medicaid laws and rules have become stricter. Individuals and family members need to know how they can operate lawfully given their current medical, long-term care, and financial situation. Elder law attorneys are a good source of information to help individuals learn how to best utilize what is available to them to make good decisions and to find, procure, and pay for quality care.

LIMITS OF MEDICARE FOR LONG-TERM CARE SERVICES

Medicare is a national health care insurance policy for most people age 65 and older, and many people with long-term disabilities. Most older Americans are covered by Medicare Part A for hospital care and Part B for outpatient physician services. Because Medicare has deductibles and copayments, most Medicare recipients also purchase **Medicare supplemental insurance**, known as **Medigap**. Most Medigap insurance policies are offered with a number of federally regulated care and price options. A patient's Medigap policy needs to supplement the Medicare-provided skilled and rehabilitation care services adequately. Medicare provides a limited period of skilled nursing and rehabilitation care, commonly covering 20 to 100 days of posthospital care. This Medicare benefit is an important bridge to non-Medicare-covered long-term care services through home health care, assisted living, or general nursing home care. The Medicare program does not cover long-term custodial care (e.g., in a nursing home).

An increasing number of older and disabled persons are not covered by traditional Medicare. Federal, state, and municipal retirees may have non-Medicare health insurance or Medicare with a different type of Medicare supplemental insurance. Some employers offer retirees a different type of Medicare supplemental insurance. More people have converted from traditional Medicare to **Medicare Advantage programs**, which incorporate the supplemental insurance coverage into their primary premium and provide coverage on a health maintenance organization (HMO) model.

With all nontraditional Medicare options, the patient and family members need to get advice from a knowledgeable source—inside or outside the facility—who understands what is included in the individual's health care coverage and how that differs from the traditional Medicare/Medigap coverage. Several nontraditional Medicare options are more restrictive in their coverage of skilled and rehabilitation care. Thus, a patient who needs rehabilitation after a stroke or broken hip may be forced to apply for Medicaid earlier than usual to get rehabilitation coverage.

FUNDING LONG-TERM CARE

When an individual needs long-term care services—most commonly assisted living or nursing home care—there are several payment options. The person or family may pay privately through a combination of income, financial resources, home equity, and property. Long-term care is relatively expensive. Although costs vary widely among parts of the United States, *monthly* private pay rates for assisted living facilities range from $2,500 to $6,000 per month, and nursing home care can range from $3,500 to more than $12,000. (See **Table 10-2** for information on nursing home expenditures by year.)

Long-term care insurance is the only readily available insurance that covers such services. Long-term care insurance may be useful in combination with the individual's other financial resources. However, long-term care insurance is not an option available just as needed; it is the best option if purchased well in advance of need.

Another funding option for long-term care is qualifying for the federal–state **Medicaid** program administered by a state agency. Medicaid is a program for low-income people or those whose care costs exceed their income. It was not intended to pay for long-term care for large numbers of persons.

Individuals must pay for long-term care services from their own funds or long-term care insurance until they meet the Medicaid eligibility requirements. In recent years, federal and state laws and rules have limited Medicaid eligibility, severely penalized short-term asset transfers, and increased estate collections for Medicaid services received by persons after age 55. Given the individual and family situation, patients may be well served to consult an elder law attorney and a financial planner to establish a plan on how they will pay for long-term care services. These professionals can help the individual and

TABLE 10-2. Nursing Home Expenditures 1980–2006 in Billions of Dollars.

Year	Cost
1980	17.6
1985	30.7
1990	50.9
1995	77.9
2000	90
2006	115

Sources: U.S. Census Bureau. *Statistical Abstract of the United States, 1997.* 17th ed. Washington, DC: U.S. Department of Commerce; 1997: 112. U.S. Department of Health and Human Services, Centers for Medicare and Medicaid Services. Nursing Home Expenditures 2007. Retrieved March 1, 2009, from http://cms.hhs.gov/NationalHealthExpendData/downloads/highlights.pdf.

the family plan how to use their available financial resources to fund their long-term care costs, with or without applying for Medicaid, while also supporting the person's spouse.

Although in many cases private payment for long-term care services is not an option, in other cases it is an option worth investigating. This is especially true in the few states that have established Medicaid-funded assisted living programs. In those states, assisted living facilities may or may not participate in the Medicaid assisted living program. Sometimes assisted living facilities may require the resident to pay privately for a number of months before the person can apply for the Medicaid assisted living program. Thus, it may be necessary for an individual to develop a strategy to be able to private pay for a number of months before applying for the Medicaid assisted living program.

BASIC MEDICAID ELIGIBILITY

Federal Medicaid law is passed by Congress. When a state administers Medicaid, the state selects various program and regulatory options within the federal Medicaid framework. What is true of the Medicaid in one state may not be true of how another state runs its Medicaid program.

In general, there are three primary eligibility requirements for Medicaid nursing home coverage:

- For Medicaid nursing home care, the individual must classify as needing nursing facility (NF) level care. Some states have made this into a gatekeeping process whose purpose is to strictly limit persons who qualify for Medicaid nursing home assistance. This strict review has kept many patients from qualifying for Medicaid NF services, even if they would be financially eligible otherwise.

- The individual's assets must be reduced below the Medicaid limits. **Medicaid exempt assets** include the individual's home, personal and household items, and prepaid funeral and burial expenses. Medicaid has a general $2,000 exemption for cash, financial accounts, and other nonexempt assets, although some states have increased that amount. When one spouse is receiving Medicaid NF care, in addition to other Medicaid exempt assets, the community spouse can exempt the **community spouse resource allowance** (CSRA). The maximum CSRA in 2008 is $104,400, although some states set a lower CSRA. The CSRA is crucial to the financial protection of the community spouse. If all of the family's savings are consumed on one spouse's nursing home care, the other spouse may spend years or even decades in poverty.
- The individual must not be ineligible for Medicaid because of an **uncompensated asset transfer** (otherwise known as a gift) made during the lookback period—which is now 36 months prior to Medicaid application and which will lengthen to 60 months by February 2011. Asset transfers have become much stricter in recent years. Medicaid exempts some asset transfers, and some asset transfers can be reversed. However, the individual must document and explain all asset gifts during the lookback period. A nonexempt asset transfer may cause a person to be ineligible for Medicaid and subsequently not have the funds needed to pay for crucial long-term care. To provide a payment source for the facility, as well as to protect the individual and the spouse, if there is any possibility that the person made a Medicaid disqualifying asset transfer, the individual should be advised to promptly consult an elder law attorney experienced in Medicaid law and procedure.

FUNDING CARE WITHOUT MEDICAID

For some patients, Medicaid may not be available for the type of care that they need because of their income or assets or because of assets that they have gifted during the asset transfer lookback period. Because of increasing budget pressures, Medicaid is being cut back. What if there was no Medicaid to help older and disabled persons pay for assisted living or nursing home care? More likely, what if the legal and financial costs of qualifying for Medicaid become so burdensome as to become unacceptable? With increasing restrictions in Medicaid financial eligibility, level-of-care reviews, asset transfer penalties, as well as increasing Medicaid estate collections, these are relevant questions.

In these situations, patients and their families need advice from an elder law attorney to develop legal and financial planning strategies to finance long-term care services. The clients keep asking, "How do we find, get, and pay for good care?" What is needed is a variety of strategies for older persons and their families to finance long-term care expenses when government programs are no longer available, or acceptable, to them. The following approaches may help many more families than anticipated to finance long-term care without resorting to Medicaid:

1. *Focus on good care.* When lawyers and financial professionals advise patients and their family, the focus should be on excellent care for the older person. Saving money is important, as well as passing wealth to children. However, planning is best accomplished when good care becomes the leading value.
2. *Work with a team of professionals who understand how to plan for and finance long-term care.* Elder law attorneys working with geriatric care managers, accountants, financial advisers, long-term care insurance professionals, and reverse mortgage specialists can form a team to assemble key elements of the long-term care plan.
3. *Understand the five sources of long-term care funding.* Federal Medicaid and its administration in every state will likely continue to change significantly over time. Medicaid may become so restrictive that it will no longer be a practical way for most people to fund long-term care. That leaves five primary non-Medicaid sources of value to fund long-term care:
   a. Fixed income—Social Security and pensions
   b. Investments—savings, retirement funds, stocks, bonds
   c. Real estate equity—most commonly the home, sometimes the family cottage or rental real estate
   d. Insurance benefits—long-term care insurance (LTCI), as well as Medicare's limited long-term care coverage
   e. Funds from the children—from income or investments
   Under the current Medicaid system, the person's home is an exempt asset, and there is no legal obligation for the children to support their parents. However, if government long-term care funding is not available or an acceptable option, the older person and/or the family need to determine where the money will come from to pay for long-term care.
4. *Use income first for long-term care expenses.* Long-term care financial planning should begin by constructing an income and expense budget to support the older adult who needs care, as well as the spouse/partner (if there is one) and the family home. For daily living expenses and long-term care costs, it is best to use income sources prior to making withdrawals from savings or investments. This income-first approach may make large long-term care expenses more affordable.
5. *Make the most of investments.* Even in current financial markets, for many older persons, investment earnings and asset appreciation remain the best path over time to improve their financial situation. A qualified financial adviser who is aware of the person's potential long-term care needs can be of assistance. The investment adviser must help analyze the individual's or couple's risk tolerance, as well as the appropriate balance of income and equity growth to fit with their current and future long-term care needs.
6. *Make small investments to maintain the highest possible level of personal independence.* Many older people remain at home with little support or assistance until their condition deteriorates and expensive nursing home care is the only appropriate placement.

It is preferable to make small investments earlier on to maintain the individual's highest possible level of independence. Such expenditures in independence include in-home or outpatient rehabilitation services; home companion help with housekeeping, meal preparation, home maintenance (including adaptive equipment), and transportation; adult day care; respite care; and bookkeeping and bill paying services. A geriatric care manager can construct a plan to utilize these timely investments.

7. *Use the value of the home.* Understandably, many persons are emotionally attached to the homes they have worked hard to own and maintain. Many older clients underestimate the significance of the value of their home, which is commonly their most valuable asset. This home value may offer a way to finance their future care as well as to maintain their security. Their home is where they will likely receive early level home health care. The functional usefulness of the home should be judged in terms of the care, mobility, and transportation needs of both spouses, as well as the maintenance and tax costs associated with the property. A **reverse mortgage** may be the best way to fund essential care. Another approach is for the children to purchase the home from the parents at the current fair market value, and thereby gain the benefit of its future appreciation while helping out the parent(s).

8. *Appreciate the value of combined housing.* Many families are considering the option of housing that combines older and younger generations. It may be possible to build an addition on the parent's home, the child's home, or sell both homes and purchase a new home to accommodate the needs of younger and older family members alike. Such combined housing may allow families to provide quality care for an older individual for a number of months or years without resorting to expensive full-time facility care. Families should discuss in advance issues that could lead to disputes, such as dividing expenses, chores, space, and belongings. (See Chapter 9 for more details.)

9. *Purchase long-term care insurance when appropriate.* The scope and level of benefits of **long-term care insurance** (LTCI) must be suitable for the person's financial circumstances. It is essential to research the options. If LTCI is determined to be an option, consulting a long-term care insurance professional can help the older person or the family to determine appropriate policy components and premium costs, as well as to identify a financially stable insurance carrier. (See the section titled "Important LTCI Policy Provisions" later in this chapter.)

10. *Increase tax deductions to reduce tax liability.* If there is one, the silver lining to long-term care expenses is the federal tax deduction. An accountant should be consulted to maximize the individual's long-term care income tax deductions and how these offset income. Reducing tax liability provides more funds for necessary care expenditures.

11. *Provide family funding so that appreciating property may pass on to family members.* Adult children may look at their parents' care needs and financial situation and then search for ways they can financially contribute to their parents' assisted living or nursing home expenses. When the children provide immediate funds to their parents,

the children may gain significant future financial benefits. If the children purchase residential, recreational, or commercial real estate from their parents, the immediate funds will provide crucial immediate care for the parents. The children are likely to gain future appreciation in the property value. Upon death, the parents might also be able to pass an IRA or other qualified retirement fund to the children with significant deferred tax benefits.

12. *A long-term care plan can stabilize the situation and preserve realistic options.* Timing is everything. It is important to educate older persons and their families to take action prior to when a long-term care crisis hits. A well-laid-out **long-term care plan** anticipates many (if not all) long-term care situations and recommends realistic options. The plan can be adjusted for a mix of funding by the parents and the children. A successful long-term care plan must balance ongoing developments, the client's income and assets, the spouse or partner, the family and step relations, government long-term care strategies and funding, and the performance of the economy.

Often this is a complex mix. For years, elder law attorneys and their clients have talked about how to preserve the family assets in the context of achieving financial eligibility for nursing home assistance. The scope of planning needs to be broadened to focus on how older and disabled persons will be able to find, get, and pay for good care.

IMPORTANT LONG-TERM CARE INSURANCE (LTCI) POLICY PROVISIONS

Following are key LTCI terms. A LTCI professional should be able to discuss these points in an informed, low-pressure manner.

- *Daily benefit rate.* This is calculated in dollars per day available for nursing home coverage. Some clients will insure for the full cost of nursing home care, while others will insure for only a portion. Nursing home costs will continue to increase because the Medicaid system underpays nursing homes, and therefore private pay nursing home rates are likely to increase much faster than general inflation. Most policies have different daily benefit rates for assisted living and home health care benefits. To keep the person home as long as possible, it may be best to select a high home health care rate.

- *Benefits paid on an indemnity or reimbursement schedule.* Indemnity benefits pay on a daily schedule for each day one receives a covered long-term care service. Reimbursement benefits pay for actual costs incurred up to a daily maximum.

- *Elimination period.* The elimination period is stated in terms of days—30, 60, 90, 180, or 365—that the insured person receives covered long-term care services before LTCI benefits start. Beware of policies that greatly extend the elimination period for home health benefits. This may happen when one receives health care services only a few days per week, and the policy only credits toward the elimination period days of actual service received as opposed to calendar days.

- *Length of benefit period.* The benefit period may be 12, 24, 36, 48 months, or lifetime. Of course, the longer the benefit, the greater level of security for the LTCI beneficiary.
- *Benefit triggers.* The insured person must demonstrate certain functional problems before benefits can be paid. LTCI benefits are triggered by the onset of the individual's inability to perform activities of daily living (ADLs) or other cognitive deficit. A policy's benefit triggers must be thoroughly reviewed to estimate the likelihood that the policy will pay meaningful benefits.
- *Difference between qualified and nonqualified polices for tax purposes.* This is essential since the passage of the Health Insurance Portability and Accountability Act of 1996 (HIPAA). The policy's tax-qualified status determines the level of tax deductibility of premiums paid, as well as the tax exemption when policy benefits are paid. A qualified insurance agent can explain the tax-qualified status of the policy.
- *Inflation protection.* Inflation protection provides increased daily benefits over time. Because long-term care costs most likely will increase faster than general inflation, understanding and selecting the policy's inflation protection are important.
- *Home health coverage and assisted living coverage.* Adequate coverage in these areas is essential coverage when the insured person wants to stay at home or stay out of a long-term care facility. Make sure home health care and assisted living are covered at a realistic daily benefit with a reasonable elimination period.
- *Financial soundness of the company.* Current economic conditions make it especially important to be confident in the future viability of the company as well as in the stability of future premiums.
- *Possible future premium increases.* A low premium price now may mean that the company will drastically increase premiums for all policyholders in the future when substantial claims are made on the policies. The premium should be in line with the competition for similar policy coverage.
- *Pooled benefit provisions.* Some policies create a pool of benefits from which the insured may draw to cover an increased number of days of home health, assisted living, or nursing home care over the life of the policy. Other policies offer increased total benefits if spouses buy LTCI coverage together.
- *Life insurance benefits.* Some companies offer hybrid policies combining long-term care benefits with a life insurance benefit. These may be available in certain combinations to the insured while alive and the named beneficiaries after the insured's death. Make sure the hybrid policy makes more financial sense than separate LTCI and life insurance policies.

SUMMARY

This chapter introduces a variety of legal, financial, and care issues from the perspective of an elder law attorney. Although this material is designed to provide authoritative information regarding the subject matter covered, it is offered with the understanding that it does not constitute individual legal advice. The specific individual circumstances facing your clients, residents, or family members will dictate the appropriate legal and financial advice for the situation.

Health care professionals need to understand the range of care and payment options facing clients and their families. They need to know what type of professional can assist their patients and family members; for example, an attorney skilled in elder law, qualified financial planner, long-term care insurance agent, reverse mortgage specialist, gerontological social worker, or geriatric care manager. The key is to help the client and/or family understand the options, determine the care needed and the available resources to pay for that care, while protecting the spouse or partner if there is one. The goal should be optimal, cost-effective care.

The opinions expressed in this chapter are entirely based on the opinion of the author, who has more than 20 years of experience in elder law. Further information can be obtained by consulting an elder law attorney or other professional expert in your area.

Review Questions

1. *Capacity* refers to
   A. One's willingness to make health care decisions
   B. One's ability to plan for the future
   C. One's competency to make a legal decision
   D. One's degree of intelligence

2. An advance directive
   A. Is not legally binding
   B. May also be called a health care proxy
   C. Is issued by the primary care physician
   D. Relates only to end-of-life care

3. A person who has legal authority and responsibility to make decisions for another is called a(n)
   A. Fiduciary
   B. Attorney
   C. Principal
   D. Caregiver

4. An older person asks you to be a witness to signing his will. Which of the following does *not* concern you?
   A. Your institution's policy on staff witnessing legal documents
   B. That the person voluntarily wants to sign the will
   C. Observing the individual's actions during the process
   D. That the person understands all the details of the contract

5. For a competent patient, which of the following is true?
   A. An oral health care directive takes precedence over the individual's written health care directive.
   B. A written health care directive takes precedence over the individual's oral health care directive.
   C. A POAHC takes precedence over the individual's oral or written health care directive.
   D. The physician's directives take precedence over the individual's oral health care directive.

6. The _____ makes personal decisions for the incapacitated person in the realm of medical issues, and the _____ makes decisions regarding the protected person's money.
   A. Principal, conservator
   B. Conservator, guardian
   C. Guardian, fiduciary
   D. Guardian, conservator

7. Who of the following listed usually has the role of guardian ad litem?
   A. An attorney named by the probate court
   B. An attorney named by the incapacitated person
   C. A family member named by the probate court
   D. A family member named by the incapacitated person

8. A geriatric care manager does each of the following *except*
   A. Identify available quality long-term care services
   B. Help the family evaluate the available services
   C. Help the family review the legal issues in long-term care
   D. Review the needs of the incapacitated person

9. A trust generally
   A. Establishes the rules by which property will be managed
   B. Gives details about one's end-of-life care wishes
   C. Is irrevocable once it is signed
   D. Is necessary to pay for long-term care

10. The Medicare program pays for all of the following *except*
    A. Hospital stays
    B. Custodial care
    C. Outpatient visits
    D. Home health care

11. Mr. Davis needs long-term care. He is unable to take care of himself and can no longer live with his wife because she is too frail to help him, although she can still take care of herself. He has a house worth approximately $200,000 and about $50,000 in a savings account. In the past year, he gave his daughter $50,000 to purchase a house for herself. Mr. Davis's family thinks he should be eligible for Medicaid because his monthly income is low. What is the primary reason he may not qualify?
    A. He can still complete basic grooming tasks.
    B. He has a house worth too much money.
    C. He has too much money in the bank.
    D. He recently transferred assets to his daughter.

12. Which of the following is *not* considered an essential source of funding for long-term care?
    A. Social Security income
    B. Investments
    C. Medicare
    D. Medicaid

Learning Activities

1. Conduct a debate on paying for long-term care in the United States. Why is this such a timely issue? What are potential solutions? Try to reach consensus on some issues with the entire group.

2. Discuss the issues surrounding advanced directives, including personal choices, compliance, and the consequences of noncompliance. Write a simplified advance directive for yourself. Share these with a partner or the group. Do you know the wishes of your older family members?

3. Revisit the case of Mrs. Jones in the section "The Flexibility and Limitations of Voluntary Decision Making" (pp. 293–294). Discuss the legal, social, psychological, and possibly, the biological implications of this case. Although we know how the law views Mrs. Jones's rights, can you put yourself in Mrs. Jones's shoes? How about her daughter's?

4. For a semester project, explore health care programs for older adults in other countries such as Canada, Finland, Russia, Iraq, Brazil, Australia, China, and Nigeria. Answer questions such as follows: How are older adults cared for in this country? How do these health care programs compare with our own? What could we learn from this country's system?

Chapter 11

HEALTH CARE PROVIDERS WORKING WITH OLDER ADULTS

REGULA H. ROBNETT, PhD, OTR/L, AND WALTER C. CHOP, MS, RRT

We hope that prevention and health promotion, rather than care for illness, will prevail.
—Dr. Mimi Fields, Pew Commission

Chapter Outline

Behavioral Objectives

Upon completion of this chapter, the reader will be able to:

1. Describe the overall goal of health care in the final decades of life.
2. List the possible members of a health care team.
3. Describe multidisciplinary, transdisciplinary, and interdisciplinary health care teams.
4. Briefly describe each of the following health care professions:
   - Case manager
   - Dietician
   - Emergency medical services
   - Nursing
   - Occupational therapy
   - Physical therapy

- Radiography
- Respiratory care
- Social work
- Speech-language pathology/audiology
- Therapeutic recreation

5. Describe the commonalities of health care professionals working with older people.
6. Discuss the ethical issues that relate to providing health care for older adults.

Key Terms

Aphasia	Minimum data set
Apraxia	Multidisciplinary team
Audiology	Occupational therapy
Case management	Physical therapy
Dysarthria	Radiography
Dysphasia	Radiologic technologists
Elder abuse	Registered dietician
Emergency medical services	Respiratory care practitioner
Emergency medical technician	Social work
Evidence-based practice	Speech-language pathologist
Gerontological nursing	Therapeutic recreation specialist
Interdisciplinary team	Transdisciplinary team

The purpose of this chapter is to review briefly the framework of health care for older people and to discuss some of the commonalities among the health professionals who work with this population. It is designed to give you an overview of the different professions providing health care services for older adults. Most sections describing different professions were written by an expert in that field. The disciplines are described alphabetically to avoid giving the impression that one profession in any way provides a more essential service than any other. All are valuable members of the health care team; each one provides a vital link in the continuum of care.

Because health care is most often provided in the context of a health care team, a summary of different kinds of health teams is also provided. Not all the professionals described are represented in every health care team. A team is formed to coordinate health care services for a particular patient or client and will only include the client, his or her significant others, and members of a team who directly provide the services needed for that person. Neither are all professionals who interact with the older person described; the list would be overwhelming.

Finally, the chapter offers an overview of different types of intervention and a few of the ethical issues that relate to working with those in late life.

THE PURPOSE OF HEALTH CARE

Health care is provided to keep people as healthy and functional as possible. Those who are aging successfully tend to be active members of their families and the community, sometimes in spite of physical limitations. Good health care may be able to forestall death, but perhaps a more important role is to improve the quality of life while the person is still alive. Prevention of disease or injury, as we all know, is better than attempting to cure the disease or to fix the injury. This disarmingly simple idea, however, is not a simple one to bring to fruition. Too many of life's pleasures, especially when enjoyed with no constraints, do not promote optimal health. For example, those addicted to alcohol or tobacco may get an immediate feeling of pleasure through their use, but years of unhealthy practices can take a toll on the body. Nonetheless, generally people should not be blamed for their ill health. Blaming yields no good results.

Fortunately, the body can have enormous power to heal itself, and even modest changes in lifestyle can have positive consequences on one's health. The theory of behavioral change espoused by Prochaska and DiClemente can be used with older people as well as with younger people.[1] Most health care professionals have a stake in gently moving their patients, clients, older family members, and friends (and often even themselves) toward better health. Small concrete steps seem to work best. For a detailed overview of the transtheoretical model of behavioral change see Velicer, Prochaska, Fava, Norman, and Redding.[2] Besides cutting back or quitting smoking and alcohol abuse, other changes that can positively improve health and prevent disease fall in the realms of diet, stress, health screenings, and exercise. The positive impacts of making changes in these areas are well known.

HEALTH CARE TEAMS

Health care often is provided most effectively in the framework of a team. The team consists of at least the health care provider and the patient or client, whose life is directly affected by the care given. Often, more than one professional and other patient support persons (such as family members and friends) are team players as well. Providers can include any of the following persons:

- Physicians and their assistants
- Nurses and their assistants
- Occupational, physical, respiratory, and speech therapists (assistants and aides as well)
- Case managers
- Psychologists and psychiatrists
- Nutritionists or dieticians
- Laboratory/medical technicians
- Medical equipment vendors

- Therapeutic recreation specialists
- Social workers

The three basic types of teams in today's health care arena are the following:

- Multidisciplinary
- Interdisciplinary
- Transdisciplinary

Each provides a different perspective on the roles of the providers and how they should interact with one another. Each provider in a **multidisciplinary team** has his or her own role, which is carried out without interference. For example, the physical therapist will work on gait training, the nurse on medication management, and the dietician on caloric intake. They then share any pertinent information about the patient and events that have occurred on a need-to-know basis or during a scheduled team meeting.

In an **interdisciplinary team**, patient goals are shared by members of the team; each provider works with the patient to promote the overriding (team) goals of health care intervention. The goal may be broad, such as returning the patient to an independent living situation. Within this overarching goal, each provider then has related, more discipline-specific goals for the patient intended to reach the anticipated outcome. (For example, the occupational therapist might have goals related to activities of daily living [ADLs], while the speech therapist might have communication goals.) The interdisciplinary team is often viewed as the ideal to strive for in providing services. Although it promotes the sharing of all pertinent information, it does not cross role boundaries during the health care intervention process.

In a **transdisciplinary team**, members also share their expertise with one another, and their individualized disciplinary roles are not always clear-cut. Available resources are used to their maximal potential, and carryover from one discipline to another is common. The therapists and nurses work together to support one another's goals for the patient (and may even seem to be doing one another's job).

More likely than not, as a health care professional, you will become a member of a health care team. As a team member, you will need to take on certain responsibilities, including speaking up in the group and advocating for the welfare of the client or patient. To be effective, team members need to have good communication skills, respect for other members, confidence in their own professional skills, and a commitment to the team process. The assumptions of the team process include a belief in both interdependency and the superiority of group versus individual problem solving.

HEALTH CARE PROFESSIONALS

Following is a list of health care professionals profiled in this chapter:

- Case manager
- Dietician (registered dietician [RD])

- Emergency medical services provider
- Nursing professionals
- Occupational therapy practitioner (OTR or COTA)
- Physical therapist (PT) and physical therapist assistant (PTA)
- Radiographer
- Respiratory care practitioner (RCP)
- Social worker
- Speech-language pathologist (SLP)
- Therapeutic recreation specialist (TRS)

CASE MANAGEMENT

A case manager often works as part of a health care team to ensure effective coordination of services. **Case management** is seen as a tool to promote cost-effective outcomes, and the concept is not new, having been introduced in the 1960s with the workers' compensation and rehabilitation legislation. According to the Case Management Society of America (CSMA), *case management* is a "collaborative process of assessment, planning, facilitation and advocacy for options and services to meet an individual's health needs."[3] Case management is not a separate profession; various professionals can become certified by the Commission for Case Manager Certification (CCMC) to ensure efficacious health care service use. Case managers often have training in nursing, but may come from other clinical health care disciplines such as medical social work or rehabilitation. Because of their ability to work collaboratively, their knowledge of resources in the health care arena (including funding sources), and their ability to monitor and evaluate health care services, case managers often play a primary role in many health care teams working with older adults. Case management involves troubleshooting and problem solving, patient advocacy, and determining realistic outcomes of service provision. Case managers work with older adults primarily in general hospitals, long-term care facilities, home health care, and rehabilitation centers.

For more information, contact the Case Management Society of America, 6301 Ranch Drive, Little Rock, AR 72223.

Web address: www.cmsa.org/ContactUs/tabid/217/Default.aspx

DIETICIAN

Louise D. Whitney

Clinical dieticians are a vital part of the medical team in hospitals, nursing homes, health maintenance organizations, and other health care facilities. They work with doctors, nurses, and therapists to help speed patients' recovery and lay the groundwork for long-term health care. Dieticians also work in public and home health agencies, day care centers, health and recreation clubs, and government-funded programs that feed and counsel older adults. Whenever proper nutrition could help improve someone's quality of life, they reach out to the public to teach, monitor, and advise.

Dieticians have many opportunities to work with older people in improving their nutritional well-being in a variety of settings. The **registered dietician** (RD) might visit older patients in long-term care facilities, during routine doctor's office visits, in health department settings, and in other community health and education programs. Medicare covers medical nutrition therapy (MNT) provided by a registered dietician.[4]

Crucial to the work that dieticians do in improving nutrition in older adults is the personal interview. Vital information about the patient's health history and socioeconomic background is gathered during this conversation. If the patient is not in a position to discuss this information directly with the dietician, communication with the medical team might assist the RD in developing a nutrition care plan.

Dieticians also come in contact with older adults in community health education settings. These might include informal workshops where the RD gives advice for preparing meals for one, shopping and meal planning on a limited income, and how to meet the changing nutrition needs that accompany aging.

For more information, contact the American Dietetic Association (ADA), 120 South Riverside Plaza, Suite 2000, Chicago, IL 60606-6995.

Phone: 800-877-1600

Web address: www.eatright.org/cps/rde/xchg/ada/hs.xsl/home_4682_ENU_HTML.htm

EMERGENCY MEDICAL SERVICES

Robert Hawkes

Emergency medical services (EMS) respond to accidents and illnesses outside of the hospital. Most of these emergency responses are initiated when the patient, caregiver, or bystander calls 9-1-1. EMS providers are trained basic **emergency medical technicians** (EMTs), intermediates, and paramedics. They need to be kind, objective, and extremely observant. The EMS provider helps the patient relax, while at the same time providing immediate medical care and noting important environmental and physical conditions. They perform a patient assessment, provide basic and advanced life support, and complete needed interventions prior to arriving at the emergency department. Local EMS agencies may be integrated within a fire department, be part of a hospital-based ambulance system, or be a private ambulance company that has contracted with a community to provide services. EMS providers treat patients of all ages and with various medical problems. EMS professionals are an extremely important link in the health care system, especially for older adults.

When EMS personnel respond, they may be the only people to see the patient in his or her own environment, and those observations can be extremely important in assessing and treating the patient. These observations are recorded and passed on to the physician and nurses at the hospital. Assessing the patient's living conditions can provide insight into the patient's activities of daily living (ADLs).

When approaching the home, the EMS provider makes several observations to aid in the assessment and treatment of the patient. Is the house being maintained? Are all the windows intact or are some broken? Are there light bulbs in all the sockets and do they work? Is the walkway shoveled from a snow storm or the lawn mowed? Are there old papers piled up on the porch or mail in the box?

When EMS providers are in the house, they pay attention to the temperature. Even if the room is warm enough for younger people, it still may be too cool for the patient. In older adults, chronic exposure to even mildly cooler temperatures can lead to serious medical problems. In the summer, does the patient have access to air conditioning? High energy costs may cause the patient to decide whether to heat or cool the home or to fill prescriptions.

EMS providers often look in the cupboards or the refrigerator for medications. This is a good opportunity for them to determine whether nutritional needs are being met by quickly checking to see what food is available. Is there a variety of fresh foods? Does the food appear to be old or moldy? Nutritional problems in older adults can be a cause of certain medical problems and can contribute to others (see Chapter 7).

Another important factor noted by EMS providers is whether or not the patient is still active and socializing. Clinical depression is common and often missed in this age group (see Chapter 4). Neighbors or family may report that the patient's lifestyle has changed recently or that he or she no longer goes out. A physical problem could have limited his or her activity level, leading to isolation, loneliness, or a feeling of helplessness.

Every year, thousands of older Americans are abused in their own homes, in relatives' homes, and even in facilities responsible for their care. The victim of **elder abuse** may be a person who is being harmed physically or emotionally by a neglectful or overwhelmed caregiver or being preyed upon financially. Once again, the EMS provider may be the first person in the house who is able to see the signs of abuse. The provider can look for obvious signs as well as subtle indications of abuse. Some of the signs might include inadequate clothing, broken eyeglasses, medical devices that do not work, numerous bruises, untreated cuts or injuries, or signs that medications are being administered incorrectly or being withheld. A medical history inconsistent with observed injuries is also a potential sign of abuse or neglect. In most states, EMS providers are mandated reporters and must report cases of suspected abuse and neglect to their state's Department of Adult Protective Services.

Providers are taught to rely on the patient's pain response when performing an assessment. However, some older patients have a diminished pain response secondary to a variety of physiologic changes. As a result, it is easy to miss a serious injury because the patient does not complain of pain. The EMS provider must also consider the mechanism of injury or the nature of the illness. When evaluating vital signs, the EMS provider tries to consider what is normal for a particular patient, not only the average ranges used in traditional medicine.

Findings of any medical or social problems should be documented and reported to the hospital and included on the ambulance run report. Although important for any patient, this may be even more critical for the geriatric patient to attain the appropriate follow-up care. Preconceived notions or ideas about aging and behaviors associated with the older population can alter the way a person is treated. In the field of EMS, the attitude of the caregiver can literally make the difference between life and death for a sick or injured older person.

For more information, contact the National Association of Emergency Medical Technicians (www.naemt.org) or the National Registry of Emergency Medical Technicians (www.nremt.org).

GERONTOLOGICAL NURSING

Nancy E. Smith

The health care system is in a state of continuous change. These changes affect all aspects of health care delivery, including nursing, which remains a highly respected profession as it evolves to meet current health care needs. Not only do nurses provide direct patient care, but they also plan and manage care for individuals, families, and communities. Nurse practice acts define nursing in terms of diagnosing and treating human responses to actual or potential health care problems. This framework requires nurses to possess greater knowledge and technical skills in caring for patients than ever before.

Gerontological nursing practice reflects these changes in health care and in nursing. The most significant demographic impact on health care is the greatly expanding aging population. Although nurses have always cared for older people, gerontological nursing as a specialty practice is relatively recent. The American Nurses Association (ANA) created Standards of Practice for Gerontological Nursing in 1976. A major revision of the scope and standards of gerontological nursing practice occurred in 1994 and again in 2001. This document provides a framework for nurses involved in the care of older adults. **Table 11-1** provides a brief description of standards developed by and for gerontological nurses.

Few health care settings do not include older people. Generally speaking, most health care settings also include nurses working in various capacities. Nurses are involved in direct elder care in hospitals, long-term care centers, and home care. Nurses frequently work with older patients in respite programs, geropsychiatric programs, assisted living and congregate housing centers, and adult daycare programs.

TABLE 11-1   ANA Standards of Clinical Gerontological Nursing Care.

Standard I. Assessment

The gerontological nurse collects patient health data.

Standard II. Diagnosis

The gerontological nurse analyzes the assessment data in determining diagnoses.

Standard III. Outcome Identification

The gerontological nurse identifies expected outcomes individualized to the older adult.

Standard IV. Planning

The gerontological nurse develops a plan of care that prescribes interventions to attain expected outcomes.

Standard V. Implementation

The gerontological nurse implements the interventions identified in the plan of care.

Standard VI. Evaluation

The gerontological nurse evaluates the older adult's progress toward attainment of expected outcomes.

Source: American Nurses Association. *Scope and Standards of Gerontological Nursing Practice.* 2nd ed. Washington, DC: American Nurses Association; 2001. Reprinted with permission, © 2001 Nursesbooks.org.

Many older adults enjoy a high level of health, in part as a result of health promotion activities conducted by nurses and other health care professionals. Health protection behaviors are also taught so that older individuals are able to direct their behaviors at decreasing the risk for a specific disease.[5] As people get older, a higher proportion of the population will be affected by acute and chronic physical and mental illnesses. This requires nurses to have a high level of knowledge and technical competence when caring for older patients. Nurses work closely with other health care professionals to provide appropriate and comprehensive care to geriatric patients.

Gerontological nurses are strong advocates for older adults and recognize the unique needs of the older population. A registered nurse who works daily with older people can be recognized as an expert in this area of patient care. It is possible for registered nurses (RNs) to be certified as gerontological nurses through the American Nurses Association (ANA). In addition, master of science in nursing programs prepare nurses to be gerontological clinical nurse specialists or ANA-certified gerontological nurse practitioners. Nurses also engage in research about the physical and psychosocial needs of older people. As Rempusheski has written:

Gerontological nursing encompasses the definitions of gerontology . . . , geriatrics . . . , geriatric nursing (care of an elder during wellness and illness, including promotion and maintenance of health, prevention of illness and disability, care of the ill leading to restoration, rehabilitation, or a peaceful death), and geriatric nursing research (systematic study of nursing action and theory in relation to elder care and responses by elders to care received).[6p.4]

Gerontological nursing has a challenging future. Community planning for care of older people will require multidisciplinary and interdisciplinary approaches. Nurses will continue to provide and plan for care, manage patient care, and engage in health promotion/health protection activities for older adults. They will work with other health care professionals to meet the needs of the aging population.

For more information, contact the American Nurses Association, 8518 Georgia Avenue, Suite 400, Silver Spring, MD 20910-3492.

Phone: 800-274-4ANA (Ext. 4262)
Web address: www.nursingworld.org

OCCUPATIONAL THERAPY

Regula H. Robnett

Occupational therapy (OT) is perhaps the least understood of the health professions. One hears the name "occupational therapist" and conjures up an image of someone who will help one to find a job. To many people the word *occupation* means simply "work." More than a few older people have stated to their occupational therapy practitioner that they did not need OT services because they were already retired. It takes a bit of explaining to convince the person that the inclusive view of occupation encompasses much more than paid employment.

One's occupations include all purposeful and meaningful activities done through the course of a day or waking period, and sleep too, as this is also essential to our well-being. Our occupations are divided into the realms of work or productive activities, activities of daily living (ADLs; such as bathing, dressing, grooming, and sexual expression), instrumental activities of daily living (IADLs; such as home management, caring for others, and money management), play and leisure activities (such as sports and hobbies), and social participation.[7] Occupational therapy practitioners work with people of all ages to help them in gaining or regaining function in those tasks important to them. Occupational therapy is client-centered in that the client's goals must be considered and respected as part of the habilitation or rehabilitation process. If the person is unable to express his or her goals, then the family or guardian is consulted to make sure the client's wishes are respected to the highest degree possible.

Occupational therapy practitioners believe that engaging in purposeful activities is a worthwhile endeavor in helping to improve functional performance. They are experts in task analysis; that is, they are able to break down almost any activity into its component parts to understand what skills a person needs to be successful at it. For example, even a seemingly simple task like putting on a shirt is quite complex when all the specific skills a person needs to be able to put the shirt on correctly are considered. Adults usually complete dressing tasks without expending much conscious effort. However, to complete the task of putting on a shirt in the usual way, one needs adequate range of motion and strength of the shoulders, elbows, wrists, and fingers; intact vision; proprioception (body awareness); fine and gross motor coordination; and cognition (for sequencing, choosing the proper clothing, etc.).

Strokes (cerebrovascular accidents), and other age-related ailments, tend to cause impairments in one or more of the individual component skills older people need to complete their "occupations" successfully. The occupational therapist determines what the person's strengths and areas of improvement are through an interview and evaluation process. Clinicians use the results of the assessments, as well as a variety of theories from both within and beyond the profession to guide their interventions. They use their expertise to help the person complete the tasks he or she needs and wants to be able to do.

The occupational therapy practitioner may work with older people to restore function with the ultimate goal being a return to former level of functioning. Although full return (of function) may not always be possible, the goal usually is to come as close as possible, as well as to ensure safety. For example, after a stroke, the occupational therapy practitioner may help the person to use his weaker arm more effectively, if possible, by stimulating or facilitating the muscles, guiding the arm, reminding the person to use the affected arm, and encouraging and assisting him to practice meaningful functional tasks.

The occupational therapy practitioner may need to work on helping the person adapt to a lower skill level through compensation and/or adaptation. This can involve the therapist grading (or changing) the task or the way of doing the task so that the person can be successful. For example, in donning a shirt, it may be easier for the person to wear an oversized T-shirt than it would be to wear a fitted button-down shirt. Or the person may change the orientation of the shirt so that it is easier to put on, and in occupational therapy she could practice this task. The occupational therapy practitioner may also adapt the environment to make it safer or more accommodating for the person. For example, safety for certain individuals can be increased by removing obstacles or hazards around the home or by adding grab bars. This approach of milieu enhancement can also be helpful for those with dementia or psychiatric illnesses, again through task analyses and a thorough evaluation of the person and the environment in which she lives or plans to live.

Occupational therapy practitioners may work with the client or patient to come up with creative solutions, sometimes through the use of adaptive equipment, either purchased or fabricated. For example, a universal cuff may be useful for feeding tasks for those with ineffectual grasp of one or both hands, and a sock-aid can be indispensable for those who cannot reach down to put on their socks.

Occupational therapy is a holistic profession, seeking to help the person not only physically, but cognitively and emotionally as well. OT practitioners use a therapeutic approach emphasizing prevention and protection (e.g., educating people about how to maintain or improve functioning or to protect themselves from potential harm). They are usually members of a health care team. OT practitioners work with older people in the community as well. For example, they may complete driving evaluations and improve driving performance, low vision therapy, community mobility, home safety evaluations, and lifestyle redesign.[8,9]

Occupational therapy practitioners may obtain degrees at the associate level (certified occupational therapy assistants [COTAs/OTAs]) or at the master's or doctoral level (occupational therapist, registered [OTRs]). They are regulated in every state (through licensure, certification, or trademark laws) and are required to take a national certification examination before practicing. Occupational therapists with enough experience and knowledge can apply for board certification (through the American Occupational Therapy Association, AOTA), as experts in specialty areas such as gerontology and physical rehabilitation or specialty certification in low vision or driving and community mobility. Common sites for occupational therapy practitioners working with older people include long-term care facilities, acute care and rehabilitation hospitals, home health care agencies, assisted living centers, outpatient centers, and in the community.

For more information, contact the American Occupational Therapy Association, Inc., 4720 Montgomery Lane, Bethesda, MD 20824.

Phone: 301-652-2682
Web address: www.aota.org/contactus/contact.asp

PHYSICAL THERAPY

Joyce L. MacKinnon and Linda W. Simonsen

Physical therapists (PTs) are health care professionals who have completed an entry level master's or doctorate degree program approved by the Commission on Accreditation in Physical Therapy Education (CAPTE). They have passed a national examination and are licensed by the state in which they practice. They are supported by physical therapist assistants (PTAs) who have been educated at CAPTE-approved, 2-year college-level programs. Physical therapist assistants have passed a national examination and are licensed in the states requiring licensure.

Physical therapy occurs either by or under the direction of a physical therapist. Physical therapists provide services to patients/clients who have impairments, functional limitations, disabilities, or changes in physical function and health status as a result of injury, disease, or other causes. They interact and practice in collaboration with a variety of professionals and can provide prevention and wellness services, including screening and health promotion. PTs also engage in consultation, administration, education, and research.[10]

Physical therapists and physical therapist assistants work with older adults in a variety of settings, including home, community, hospital, rehabilitation, and long-term care facilities. Some therapists have been credentialed by the American Physical Therapy Association (APTA) as certified clinical specialists in geriatrics through a rigorous testing and review process. However, whatever the background and credentials of those therapists who work with our country's aging population, they share the common focus of maintaining or improving that population's quality of life.

Many of the physiologic changes related to normal biological aging can be slowed by exercise. Specialized exercise techniques and programs developed by physical therapists can serve to improve muscle strength, flexibility, bone health, cardiovascular and respiratory response, and tolerance to activity.[11] For instance, a common age-related change is a decline in bone mass, which can ultimately cause the pathologic condition known as osteoporosis. Physical therapists can help prevent or retard osteoporosis by prescribing an exercise program of weight-bearing and resistive exercises, postural training and back extension exercises, and flexibility activities. They can also treat patients who develop this condition by providing pain relief, general conditioning activities, and back extension and abdominal strengthening exercises. In addition, exercise has been shown to provide social and psychological benefits affecting the quality of life and the sense of well-being in older adults.[12]

Although falls are not part of the normal aging process, they are relatively common among older adults. More than one-third of adults age 65 and older fall each year in the United States.[13,14] Falls are not only the leading cause of injury death in this population, but are also the most common cause of nonfatal injuries and hospital admissions for trauma.[15] Physical therapists serve a pivotal role in the implementation of rehabilitation strategies aimed at reducing fall risk in all settings. After completing a balance assessment using multiple standardized tests and measures, the physical therapist will select specific interventions designed to reduce fall risk. These might include therapeutic exercise, vestibular rehabilitation, balance and gait training, and flexibility and strength training. In conjunction with other health care professionals, the issue of polypharmacy (taking three or more medications) is addressed and the therapist will educate the older adult in psychosocial and environmental strategies for fall prevention.

Physical therapists and assistants also provide care to older adults who are experiencing functional decline secondary to a disease process or injury. The physical therapist assesses the musculoskeletal, neuromuscular, cardiopulmonary, and integumentary systems and, based on these findings, determines how system deficits affect the patient's functional activity. For instance, does the patient have enough strength, motion, and endurance to bathe and dress? Can he or she perform light housekeeping tasks and go up and down stairs? Does the patient require adaptive devices such as a cane or a walker to assist with mobility? Can the patient get out of the house, go to the bus stop, get on the bus, go to the grocery store, shop, and return home? The physical therapist and assistant will interact with other health care professionals and the patient's family to develop and meet patient-centered goals so as to encourage optimum patient functioning.

For more information about physical therapy, contact the American Physical Therapy Association, 1111 N. Fairfax Street, Alexandria, VA 22314-1488.

Phone: 800-999-2782
Web address: www.apta.org

RADIOGRAPHY

Sally Doe

Radiography is the health profession that involves imaging various anatomic regions of the body for diagnostic purposes, generally utilizing radiation (X-rays) as the source of energy. **Radiologic technologists** must use a variety of types of equipment and imaging systems depending on the complexity of the anatomic region or organs. Radiographic procedures vary from those relatively commonplace, such as radiographs of the chests or extremities, to those technologically very sophisticated, such as angiography. Diagnosis through a radiographic procedure is often one of the first areas of investigation on the patient's behalf. Consequently, radiographers often see very ill and traumatized patients as well as perform radiographs during surgery. Radiographers must, therefore, be able to adapt procedural standards and equipment limitations to the needs of a patient.

In addition to possessing excellent patient care skills and having empathy and compassion for patients, radiographers must consider several important aspects for the geriatric patient. X-ray tables are, by necessity, hard, and some radiographic procedures require the patient to remain lying on the table for perhaps as long as 1 hour. Radiographers make use of special cushioning devices designed for the X-ray table to minimize patient discomfort and must pay particular attention to the physical warmth of the patient during his or her time of relative immobilization. Excellent communication skills are of particular importance in terms of completely explaining not only the procedure to the patient but also in giving clear and concise instructions to enlist the patient's cooperation.

Other imaging modalities closely aligned with radiography include computed tomography (CT scanning), magnetic resonance imaging (MRI), sonography (formerly ultrasound), and nuclear medicine. Computed tomography and nuclear medicine utilize radiation as the source of energy for imaging, whereas magnetic resonance imaging utilizes a very strong magnetic field, and sonography utilizes sound waves. Regardless of the type of energy used, imaging requires specific orientation of the part being examined to the image receptor and requires a period of immobilization for the patient. Consequently, radiographers are ever mindful of the patient's condition and comfort.

Radiographers may obtain degrees at the associate, bachelor's, or master's level. They are licensed in the majority of states. The American Registry of Radiologic Technologists offers a national certification examination to those who have the educational qualifications. Employment sites include hospitals, outpatient facilities, physicians' offices, and home health care agencies.

For more information, contact the American Society of Radiologic Technologists, 15000 Central Avenue, S.B., Albuquerque, NM 87123.

Phone: 505-298-4500
Web address: https://www.asrt.org/

RESPIRATORY CARE

Walter Chop

Respiratory care practitioners (RCPs) work with patients of all ages; however, it is older adults who occupy the majority of their time. The need for RCPs will continue to rise with the concurrent increase in the older segment of the population.

One of the most common symptoms associated with cardiopulmonary disease is dyspnea (difficulty breathing). An estimated 45% of those older than the age of 70 exhibit dyspnea on exertion, while 65% of men and 48% of women in this age bracket have a cardiopulmonary disorder.[16] RCPs administer aerosolized medications to relieve symptoms of cardiopulmonary disease. They also monitor life support systems in intensive care units and function as vital members of the hospital cardiac arrest team. In addition to this, they perform diagnostic pulmonary function testing and arterial blood gas measurements. They also assist physicians during bronchoscopic examination of the lungs. Aerosol and humidity therapy, oxygen administration, hyperinflation therapy, chest physiotherapy, breathing retraining, and patient education are also integral parts of an RCP's duties.

Although healthy older individuals can usually compensate for age-related changes to the pulmonary system, they do, however, remain vulnerable to environmental insults such as air pollution and second-hand smoke. Older persons are also at increased risk of developing pneumonia, especially if they are residents of long-term care facilities. RCPs are in the front line treating these conditions with medication, hyperinflation therapy, aerosol and humidity therapy, oxygen, and, if need be, mechanical ventilation.

As the trend to discharge patients from acute care facilities as quickly as possible continues, both long-term care and home care will experience continued growth. RCPs work in both these settings providing and monitoring oxygen delivery and life support systems. Respiratory therapists also work in physicians' offices and sleep labs. Assessment and evaluation of the patient from a cardiopulmonary perspective are also performed by respiratory therapists in both the hospital and outpatient setting. Pulmonary rehabilitation and asthma education programs are often coordinated by an RCP.

RCPs are required to become licensed in all but two states. This helps ensure patient protection as well as establish standards for the safe practice of respiratory care. For more information on a career in respiratory care, contact the respiratory care department in your local hospital, career counselors at a school or college in your area, or the American Association for Respiratory Care, 9425 N. MacArthur Blvd., Ste. 100, Irving, TX 75063.

Phone: 972-243-2272
Web address: www.aarc.org

SOCIAL WORK

Betsey Gray

The National Association of Social Workers (NASW) defines **social work** as "the professional activity of helping individuals, groups or communities enhance or restore their capacity for social functioning and creating societal conditions favorable to this goal."[17] Social workers are particularly sensitive to the social, cultural, biological, and psychological factors that affect a person's life. They perform many functions and are often asked to act as evaluators, facilitators, advocates, community organizers, and program planners. A code of ethics for the profession emphasizes the importance of treating people with dignity and respect. Social workers view themselves as agents of change and are seen as a voice for the oppressed in our society.

In response to society's increasing awareness of older adults as a heterogeneous group with special and diverse needs, social work practice with older adults has emerged as a new and valuable specialty within the profession. Social workers with an interest and expertise in working with older populations are becoming more common in settings that provide services to this age group, including hospitals, mental health centers, residential settings, home health care/hospice agencies, and community programs.

The primary responsibility of a hospital or medical social worker is to work with the older patient in determining a plan following discharge from the hospital. This involves doing a thorough assessment of the needs of the patient, speaking with family members, and locating resources in the community. The social worker collaborates with the other professionals involved in the patient's care and at times acts as an advocate in ensuring that the patient's wishes are followed. It is important for the social worker to be familiar with community resources as well as federal and state programs potentially available to the person.

A number of mental health centers have now developed specialized units for treating older people with mental health issues. Depression and anxiety resulting from loss and isolation, dementia, substance abuse, and elder abuse are some of the problems a social worker might encounter in an older person seeking services. The social worker trained in working with older adults begins with a comprehensive biopsychosocial spiritual assessment, being sensitive to all factors that may be contributing to the problem. He or she is particularly attentive to the supports the person has and areas where these may be able to be increased. Working collaboratively with the client, a treatment plan is developed that often involves other professional services and resources in the community. The social worker can act as the case manager in accessing these resources and monitoring the delivery of services and can also provide individual, group, and family counseling, if appropriate. Integral to all the work the social worker does is the importance of treating the client with dignity and respect and acknowledging his or her right to self-determination.

For older people in residential settings such as a nursing home or assisted living facility, the social worker plays a key role. Most often the social worker is the first person to meet with the residents and their family members. It is the responsibility of the social worker to explain the procedure for admission and answer questions about advance directives, Medicare, and Medicaid. The social worker is also a member of the interdisciplinary team that completes the initial assessment of the residents. Being cognizant of the losses people experience when leaving their homes, the social worker offers support and empathy as the residents begin to adjust to their new surroundings.

Residential settings vary with regard to the social work services offered to their residents. Many are beginning to see the need for supportive services and will ask the social worker to facilitate groups for the residents. Individual counseling can also be offered to a resident when needed. In addition, groups to aid family members may be provided for the resident's family. Last, social workers lead in-service trainings for staff on various subjects relative to the work they do.

With the emergence of managed care, people are being discharged from hospitals much sooner and often return to their homes with a need for ongoing services. Through an interdisciplinary team approach, a home health care agency provides those medical and related health care interventions that allow the older adult to remain at home for as long as possible. Social workers are a fairly recent addition to the service providers available through home health care agencies. When a member of the team determines that social work services are needed, a social worker will make a home visit and complete a psychosocial assessment. The social worker will meet with the patient and family members and together work on a plan to address the problems presented. Typical problems may include financial issues, adjustment to a terminal or other severe illness, living arrangements, and family relationships. As in other settings, the social worker needs to have a working knowledge of community resources and the way to access services.

Social workers, because of their training, are often found helping communities and groups develop new programs to assist older adults. NASW is very involved in the legislative process at state and national levels. All social workers are encouraged to be politically active so as to have a strong voice in decisions being made that affect the people they are serving. As our population continues to age and legislation focuses on the older population, the voice of the social worker will be heard on many different levels in our society.

For more information, contact the National Association of Social Workers, 750 First Street, NE, Suite 700, Washington, DC 20002-4241.

Phone: 202-408-8600
Web address: www.socialworkers.org

SPEECH-LANGUAGE PATHOLOGIST

Kimberly Hillman Bassett

Speech-language pathologists (SLPs) are health care professionals who specialize in communication and deglutition (swallowing). These clinicians hold either a master's or doctoral degree in speech pathology, speech, language and hearing science, or an allied discipline and have extensive training in both normal and disordered aspects of language, articulation, fluency, voice, cognition, hearing, anatomy and physiology of the head and neck, and swallowing. Given this broad knowledge base, speech-language pathologists are well poised to care for older adults, a population known to experience a high prevalence of speech, language, and swallowing impairments related not only to acute or chronic disease processes, but to normal aging progression as well. In fact, in and of themselves, these senescent changes can significantly hinder effective communication such that they interfere with an older person's independence and quality of life, thereby underscoring the importance of the resources speech-language pathologists offer.

Audiology is the study of normal and disordered hearing and related disorders. It is closely related to speech-language pathology. Audiologists who work with the geriatric population identify those individuals who would benefit from amplification, evaluate the benefit of amplification, dispense hearing aids and other assistive listening devices, and may assist in the differential diagnosis of vestibular disorders such as dizziness or tinnitus. In addition to fitting and orienting older individuals to an amplification device, audiologists may also implement therapy addressing auditory and visual communication, provide active listening training, and provide counseling. Another role of the audiologist is to monitor older individuals for the effect of ototoxic or vestibulotoxic prescription drug use, as well as prior noise exposure. Audiologists hold either a master's or doctoral degree in audiology. Beginning January 1, 2012, a doctoral degree will be the entry-level educational requirement for the practice of audiology.

The role of the speech pathologist with the geriatric population is to identify those individuals at risk for communication and swallowing impairments; complete a thorough evaluation encompassing all aspects of communication and swallowing; develop an individualized treatment plan specific to the individuals' deficits; provide patient, family, and caregiver education; and serve as an advocate for the communication and swallowing needs of the individual. Although many older adults benefit from traditional speech-language pathology services, also known as speech therapy, it is imperative that the treating speech-language pathologist be aware of unique, age-related issues that can directly influence effective delivery of treatment. For example, financial restrictions; environmental considerations; changes in emotional, mobility, and sensory status; social isolation; and decline in memory all require that the clinician make ongoing modifications in the treatment plan to ensure that goals are functional and accommodate the older individual's communication and swallowing routines. The speech-language pathologist also collaborates with other members of the health care team, including physical and occupational therapists, social workers, nursing staff, dieticians, and physicians. Moreover, robust relationships with health care professionals across all settings are critical to providing both holistic and patient-centered services to older people. Speech-language pathologists work with older adults in a wide variety of locales, including acute care hospitals, rehabilitation hospitals, long-term care facilities, assisted living facilities, outpatient clinics, private practices, and in individual homes.

With aging comes an increased susceptibility to neurologic disorders such as a cerebrovascular accident (CVA, or stroke), Parkinson's disease, and Alzheimer's disease. Each of these disorders can result in impairments of both communication and swallowing skills. Additionally, hearing loss and associated auditory processing deficits are common in older people and can result in frustration and withdrawal from social contacts. The speech-language pathologist plays a distinct part in each of these examples, providing both restorative and maintenance services that improve, enhance, or preserve the older individual's ability to express him- or herself, hear and understand others, and take in enough food and fluids to maintain nutritional and hydration status.

In the case of stroke, the type and extent of resulting communication and swallowing deficits are directly related to the size and location of the insult. Older individuals who sustain a stroke may present with language impairments (**aphasia**), speech impairments (**apraxia** or **dysarthria**), and/or swallowing impairments (**dysphagia**). Aphasia often affects all aspects of language, including both reading and writing. Early in the recovery from a stroke, the speech-language pathologist may concentrate on swallowing issues because these can lead to aspiration and subsequent pulmonary complications if not assessed and treated soon after the stroke occurs. Subsequent diagnostics involve determining not only the impaired areas of communication, but also identifying areas of strength upon which to build treatment strategies.

Parkinson's disease is a disorder of movement and, as such, commonly interferes with both speech production and swallowing skills. Older adults with Parkinson's disease typically present with a dysarthria characterized by monopitch, monoloudness, reduced loudness overall, and short rushes of speech production. Swallowing symptoms related to Parkinson's disease include repetitive tongue pumping and a delayed swallow, among others. In addition, cognitive deficits may develop as the disease progresses. Given the degenerative nature of Parkinson's disease, the speech-language pathologist must appropriately sequence interventions, addressing current problems at the right time while anticipating future issues. Knowledge of disease progression is similarly essential to providing effective patient and family education regarding what to expect, as well as advocating for the needs of the individual as the disease advances.

Deterioration of memory and other cognitive functions is the hallmark of Alzheimer's disease and other dementias. The associated communication symptoms are directly related to this decline and are characterized by a decrease in the affected older individual's ability to understand or use linguistic information. Behavioral issues such as hallucinations or paranoia may also arise from the neuropathology of dementia and can further impede effective communication. The role of the speech-language pathologist with this population is to provide both direct and indirect treatment, enhancing spared communication systems while compensating for the disordered ones. Caregiver education is a fundamental ingredient to any intervention for dementia because it optimizes the older adult's communication function across all stages of the dementia as it progresses. Other indirect techniques include advocating for environmental modifications to make the living situation more "home-like" and development of routines.

Finally, the speech-language pathologist's expertise in swallowing and communication often places this practitioner in a situation where end-of-life issues are addressed. In such cases, the goals of speech-language pathology services are facilitative rather than restorative, and thereby are geared toward enhancing the overall quality of life as the individual nears the end of life. For instance, a speech-language pathologist may make recommendations about swallowing strategies that will allow the older individual to eat and drink as long as possible. Another example is the development of an alternative communication system to allow the older individual to indicate wants and needs effectively. The expected outcome of speech-language interventions in end-of-life care is not to improve skills, but rather to facilitate intact abilities such that the individual is able to interact with family and friends and enjoy food and fluids if so desired. It is critical in end-of-life situations to respect the patient's and family's wishes as well as any social or cultural influences that may exist.

Growing gerontological research in conjunction with the upsurge of the geriatric population will serve to continually expand opportunities for speech-language pathologists to work with older people. The American Speech-Language Hearing Association (ASHA) has already addressed the growing need for expertise among its membership in issues related to aging. ASHA formed its first committee addressing the communication needs of older adults in 1965 and more recently, created Special Interest Division 15, Gerontology, a group devoted to the study of communication behaviors and disorders in older individuals. ASHA has also published a number of technical and committee reports and position statements that further delineate the role of the speech-language pathologist working with the geriatric population.

A career in speech-language pathology requires a graduate degree, a passing score on the national exam, and completion of a 9-month postgraduate clinical fellowship. Many go on to achieve the Certificate of Clinical Competence (CCC) awarded by ASHA. This nationally recognized professional certification designates a level of excellence attained by meeting rigorous academic and professional standards. Certificate holders are expected to maintain their skills through regular continuing education and to abide by ASHA's Code of Ethics. In addition to the CCC, most states require licensure. At present, 47 states regulate the practice of speech-language pathology.

For more information about the field of speech-language pathology and career opportunities, contact the American Speech-Language-Hearing Association, 2200 Research Boulevard, Rockville, MD 20850-3289.

Phone: 800-638-8255
Web address: www.asha.org

THERAPEUTIC RECREATION

Nancy Richeson

The fastest growing segment of the U.S. population is the age group 65 years old and older. As Americans age, their health care needs also increase, and this will prove to be challenging for our society. The number of older people needing any type of long-term services is estimated to more than double from year 2000 (13 million needed services) to year 2050 (an estimated 27 million will need services).[18] One consequence of societal aging is that the demand for services to help in maintaining and/or improving the health of seniors will continue to grow.

According to Teague and MacNeil, one form of health service that has increasingly received attention for its preventive as well as therapeutic qualities is therapeutic recreation services.[19] Therapeutic recreation programs at facilities should be among the most important factors evaluated by consumers before selecting a long-term care facility. The Omnibus Budget Reconciliation Act (OBRA) of 1987 sets forth standards for long-term care facilities. Included in the law is the following provision: "The skilled nursing facility . . . must provide . . . an ongoing program, directed by a qualified professional, of activities designed to meet the interests and the physical, mental, and psychosocial well-being of each resident."

Currently, only 5% of the U.S. population age 65 and older live in long-term care facilities. This represents less than 2 million people. However, as more people live longer, the percentage of older people in long-term care is expected to rise to more than 20%. By 2040, 5.5 million people are likely to live in long-term care facilities.[20] Quality therapeutic recreation services are a necessity in long-term care.

The literature in therapeutic recreation describes the therapeutic approach as one intended to stimulate a change in behavior directed by one or more goals in different areas of functioning (e.g., physical, emotional, mental, social).[21] Therapeutic recreation specialists in long-term care use activities to accomplish the following objectives:

- Promote health
- Prevent impairment and dependence
- Maintain optimal functional capabilities
- Remediate disabilities

As stated by the American Therapeutic Recreation Association (ATRA), **therapeutic recreation specialists** (TRSs) are those professionals who have completed a degree in therapeutic recreation (or recreation with an emphasis in therapeutic recreation). National certification is available through the National Council for Therapeutic Recreation Certification (NCTRC). A few states regulate this profession through licensure, certification, or regulation of titles.

Therapeutic recreation specialists work as part of the initial health care team whose members gather pertinent information about long-term care residents through the administration of a standardized assessment, also referred to as the **minimum data set** (MDS). A completed MDS on each resident is required for long-term care facilities participating in Medicare and Medicaid programs. Therapeutic recreation specialists also collect information about leisure needs and interests from other sources such as medical records, medical staff, and family members. Based on the results of the assessments, the therapeutic recreation specialist writes an individual treatment plan. Activity programs are developed based on the residents' needs, abilities, and interests. Other documentation tasks the therapeutic recreation specialist must complete include writing progress notes, charting attendance records, developing a monthly calendar, and updating residents' records as required.

The therapeutic recreation specialist is responsible for the development of a comprehensive therapeutic recreation program. Often therapeutic recreation programs are provided on a continuum, with diversional activities provided simply to fill time in the resident's day on one end to treatment-oriented activities focusing on maintaining or improving functional abilities on the other. A balanced program provides treatment, education, and diversional opportunities to meet the residents' individual needs as determined by the therapeutic recreation assessment.[22]

An example of a therapeutic recreation treatment intervention in a long-term care facility is a sensory stimulation program designed to maintain or improve sensory functioning. This program is administered on a one-to-one basis or in a small group with other residents who have similar needs. Other therapeutic recreation treatment interventions include validation therapy, reminiscence/life review, animal-facilitated therapy, community outings, therapeutic activities, leisure education, physical activities, social opportunities, one-to-one treatment, and adult education opportunities. Additional responsibilities of the therapeutic recreation personnel might include coordinating volunteers, determining staffing needs, developing an operating manual, evaluating the program, and monitoring quality improvement measures.

Therapeutic recreation specialists are important members of the treatment team. Therapeutic recreation programs assist residents in increasing or maintaining their functional abilities and in developing their leisure skills. In addition, therapeutic recreation programs educate individuals about the value of leisure and provide recreational opportunities. The ultimate goal of any therapeutic recreation program is to help restore the individual to optimal health and well-being.

For further information on therapeutic recreation, contact the American Therapeutic Recreation Association (ATRA).

Phone: 601-264-3413
Web address: www.atra-tr.org

Or contact the National Therapeutic Recreation Society.

Phone: 703-858-2151
E-mail: NTRSNRPA@aol.com

SUMMARY

This chapter provides readers with valuable information related to the potential health team members working with older adults. The various health care providers do have certain traits in common: All seek to promote caring and respect for older people (as well as all their other clients). All the professions described are founded on a solid theoretical and/or knowledge base related to their specific scopes of practice and intend to provide ethical interventions at all times. All are bound by the Health Insurance Portability and Accountability Act (HIPAA), which protects the health information of those receiving health care services.[23]

Another commonality among these professionals is that they are generally obligated by law to report elder abuse. Although there is no federal standard, most states consider health care professionals to be "mandatory reporters," meaning they must report suspected abuse of older people. Abuse of older people consists not only of obvious physical abuse, but also health care fraud, sexual abuse, psychological or emotional abuse, financial exploitation, and neglect.[24] Any time a health care professional notes anything unusual that cannot be explained (e.g., odd behavior, documentation by others that does not fit what they observe, lack of cleanliness or sanitary surroundings), investigating and eventual reporting of the incident should be initiated. If your place of employment does not have a set protocol, the Elder Locator at 1-800-677-1116 can help.[24]

Also, the professionals discussed are generally guided by **evidence-based practice**, which relates to: those with the highest level of clinical expertise (i.e., those described earlier, among others) providing the most excellent, safe, and effective health care interventions based on the best research data available. The strongest evidence comes from large, randomized control studies, although these are relatively rare in the realm of rehabilitation and health care interventions. However, practice recommendations, guidelines, and options can also come from smaller research projects, which are easier to carry out in the realm of allied health care. In addition, an imperative for all providers is to consider the values and aspirations of the client and his or her family or other loved ones when designing and implementing interventions.[25] Indeed, building therapeutic rapport may be as important as, or even more important than, actual clinical skills in attaining positive outcomes in health care.[26] Health care professionals, by the very nature of their occupations, are obligated to engage in lifelong learning in their fields so that they can remain up-to-date on the most efficacious health care practices. In this way, they can provide the best health care possible for their older clients who need services.

Finally, most care providers offer health care intervention in the context of a health care team. The team concept predominates in health care today as a way to ensure efficacy and cost-effectiveness in health care delivery. By working together, collaborating, communicating clearly, pulling in team players who have the greatest expertise, and advocating for the most appropriate health care interventions possible, we can reach the ultimate goal of optimal health and best quality of life for the older people we serve.

Review Questions

1. HIPAA is best described as a law which:
   A. Regulates health care workers in long-term care
   B. Protects the health information of those receiving health care services
   C. Protects health care professionals from malpractice suits
   D. Regulates in-patient health care access

2. A health care team in which broad patient goals are shared by members of the team is called a(n):
   A. Interdisciplinary team
   B. Transdisciplinary team
   C. Multidisciplinary team
   D. Medical care team

3. EMS professionals do all of the following *except*
   A. Plan for the person's discharge from the hospital.
   B. Enter a person's home to begin treatment.
   C. Take note of the patient's surroundings.
   D. Evaluate vital signs and provide emergency medical care.

4. A health care professional who works on helping the patient adapt to a lower skill level through compensation and/or adaptation is called a(n)
   A. Gerontological nurse
   B. Nutritionist
   C. Radiologist
   D. Occupational therapist

5. One who develops specialized exercise techniques and programs is titled a(n)
   A. Occupational therapist
   B. Radiologist
   C. Physical therapist
   D. Social worker

6. Respiratory care practitioners perform all of the following tasks *except*
   A. Mechanical ventilation
   B. Monitoring life support systems
   C. Range of motion exercises
   D. Pulmonary function testing

7. The professional most likely to have the primary role of determining the plan for a person being discharged from the hospital is a(n):
   A. Social worker
   B. EMS professional
   C. Therapeutic recreation specialist
   D. Radiologist

8. If you notice your patient is having difficulty swallowing and coughs after every sip of water, the most appropriate referral for a consultation may be to a:
   A. Social worker
   B. Physical therapist
   C. Speech-language pathologist
   D. Dietician

Learning Activities

1. Sam, an older adult, has had a stroke (CVA) and has been admitted to a rehabilitation hospital. Who are likely to be members of his health care team and what roles are each of them likely to take?

2. How might the responsibilities of these team members change in the different kinds of health care teams: multidisciplinary, interdisciplinary, and transdisciplinary.

3. If you were going to start a commission with the purpose of improving health care specifically for older adults, whom would you invite to be participants (individual people *or* representatives of certain professions)? What major issues will they need to confront? Would you personally want to be a member of this commission? Why or why not?

REFERENCES

1. Prochaska, J, DiClemente, C. Stages and processes of self-change of smoking: toward an integrative model of change. *Journal of Consulting and Clinical Psychology*, 1983;51(3):390–395.

2. Velicer, WF, Prochaska, JO, Fava, JL, Norman, GJ, Redding, CA. Smoking Cessation and Stress Management: Applications of the Transtheoretical Model of Behavior Change. *Homeostasis*, 1998;38:216–233.

3. Case Management Society of America. What Is a Case Manager? Retrieved July 18, 2008, from http://www.cmsa.org/Home/CMSA/Whatisa CaseManager/tabid/224/Default.aspx

4. American Dietetic Association. American Dietetic Association Supports New Medicare Bill That Opens Doors to Medical Nutrition Therapy Expansion. Retrieved July 19, 2008, from http://www.eatright.org/cps/rde/xchg/ada/hs.xsl/media_17740_ENU_HTML.htm

5. Stanley, M, Beare, PG. *Gerontological Nursing: A Health Promotion-Protection Approach*. 2nd ed. Philadelphia: FA Davis; 1999.

6. Rempusheski, VF. Historical and Futuristic Perspectives in Aging and the Gerontological Nurse. In EM Baines (ed.), *Perspectives on Gerontological Nursing*. Newbury Park, CA: Sage; 1991.

7. Youngstrom, MJ. Introduction to the Occupational Therapy Practice Framework: Domain and Process, Continuing Education Article. *OT Practice*, September 2002, CE-1–CE-7.

8. Clark, F, Azen, SP, Zemke, R, Jackson, J, Carlson, M, Mandel, D, et al. Occupational Therapy for Independent-Living Older Adults: A Randomized Controlled Trial. *JAMA*, 1997;278:1321–1326.

9. Clark, F, Azen, SP, Carlson, M, Mandel, D, LaBree, L, Hay, J, et al. Embedding Health-Promoting Changes into the Daily Lives of Independent-Living Older Adults: Long-Term Follow-Up of Occupational Therapy Intervention. *Journal of Gerontology: Psychological Sciences*, 2001;56:60–63.

10. Guide to Physical Therapist Practice: Part 1: A Description of Patient/Client Management. Part 2: Preferred Practice Patterns. American Physical Therapy Association. *Physical Therapy*, 1997; 77(11):1160–1656.

11. Smith E, Serfass R. *Exercise and Aging: The Scientific Basis*. Hillside, NJ: Enslow Publishers; 1981.

12. McPherson, BD (ed.). *Sport and Aging: The 1984 Olympic Scientific Congress Proceedings*. Champaign, IL: Human Kinetics Publishers; 1986:5.

13. Hornbrook, MC, Stevens, VJ, Wingfield, DJ, Hollis, JF, Greenlick, MR, Ory, MG. Preventing Falls Among Community-Dwelling Older Persons: Results from a Randomized Trial. *The Gerontologist*, 1994;34(1):16–23.

14. Hausdorff, JM, Rios, DA, Edelber, HK. Gait Variability and Fall Risk in Community-Living Older Adults: A 1-Year Prospective Study. *Archives of Physical Medicine and Rehabilitation*, 2001;82(8):1050–1056.

15. Centers for Disease Control and Prevention, National Center for Injury Prevention and Control. Web-Based Injury Statistics Query and Reporting System (WISQARS) [online]. (2006) Retrieved January 15, from www.cdc.gov/ncipc/wisqars

16. Matteson, MA, McConnell, E. *Gerontological Nursing: Concepts and Practice*. Philadelphia: W. B. Saunders; 1988.

17. Barker, RL. *The Social Work Dictionary* (3rd ed.). Washington, DC: The National Association of Social Workers Press; 1995.

18. U.S. Department of Health and Human Services, and U.S. Department of Labor. *The Future Supply of Long-Term Care Workers in Relation to the Aging Baby Boom Generation: Report to Congress*. Washington, DC: Office of the Assistant Secretary for Planning and Evaluation; 2003. Retrieved August 4, 2008, from http://www.caregiver.org/caregiver/jsp/content_node.jsp?nodeid=440

19. Teaque, M, MacNeil, R. *Aging and Leisure: Vitality in Later Life*. 2nd ed. Madison, WI: Brown and Benchmark; 1992.

20. Cornman, J, Kingson, ER. Trends, Issues, Perspectives, and Values for the Aging of the Baby Boom Cohorts. *The Gerontologist*, 1996; 36(1):18.

21. Hawkins, B. *Therapeutic Activity Intervention with the Elderly: Foundations and Practices*. State College, PA: Venture Publishing; 1996.

22. Elliott, J, Sorg-Elliott, JA. *Recreation Programming and Activities*. State College, PA: Venture Publishing; 1991.

23. U.S. Department of Health and Human Services. Summary of the HIPAA Privacy Rule. 2003. Retrieved July 20, 2008, from http://www.hhs.gov/ocr/privacysummary.pdf

24. Jaffe-Gill, E, de Benedictis, T, Segal, J. Elder Abuse: Types, Signs, Symptoms, Risk Factors, and Prevention. 2008. Retrieved July 20, 2008, from http://www.helpguide.org/mental/elder_abuse_physical_emotional_sexual_neglect.htm

25. Institute of Medicine and the National Academy of Sciences. Chapter 6, Applying evidence to health care delivery. In *Crossing the Quality Chasm: A New Health System for the 21st Century*, pp.145–163. Retrieved July 20, 2008, from http://books.nap.edu/openbook.php?record_id=10027&page=145.

26. Graybeal, C. Evidence for the art of social work. *Journal of Contemporary Social Services*, 2007; 88(4):513–523.

Chapter 12

FUTURE CONCERNS IN AN AGING SOCIETY

PAUL D. EWALD, PhD

Anyone who gives you firm prognostications about what is going to happen is either a liar or a fool, because the uncertainties over trends in life expectancy, health and disability, and retirement age are quite high.
    —*Richard Suzman, Director of the National Institute on Aging's Office of Demography on Aging*

Chapter Outline

Behavioral Objectives

Upon completion of this chapter, the reader will be able to:

1. Identify three critical age-related issues facing the United States in the future.
2. Describe ways in which the future generations of older adults are different from the older adults of today.
3. Understand and describe the respective roles of the family, the public sector, and the private sector in caring for frail older adults.
4. Understand that populations around the world are aging at different rates and be able to explain some of the reasons for this and consequences of it.
5. Explain how societal responses to aging vary around the world because of differing rates of change as well as different social, political, and economic policies.

Key Terms

Age composition
Demographics
Fertility
Generational equity
Lifelong education
Migration
Mortality

Old-age dependency ratio
Private sector
Public sector
Volunteerism
Work life
Young-age dependency ratio

The aging of the U.S. population is not unlike a good news–bad news story. The good news is that more of us are living longer, often in better health, more independently, and with greater security. The bad news is that these advances carry considerable economic and social costs. The good news is that many of us have been, and will continue to be, the beneficiaries of technological and biomedical advances. The bad news is that we will be faced with increasingly difficult resource choices, ethical dilemmas, and political decisions. The good news is that there will be more opportunities for growth and personal enhancement in later life. The bad news is that there may be more years of dependency in later life.

Whether we attend to the good news or the bad news side of the story depends in large part on the social perceptions and attitudes we hold of old age, both individually and as a society. Do we think of it as a time of leisure, relaxation, reflection, and happiness? Or is it a time of greater dependency, illness, and loss? One can see elements of truth in both of these characterizations. Most of us hold dual stereotypes about the nature of old age because we can usually find validation for both the good and the bad in our day-to-day experiences: recalling our vibrant and wise grandparents one day; paying a visit to a nursing home the next.

As we come to terms with the realities of a society in which the number of older adults is increasing steadily, our perceptions and attitudes will undergo rapid change as well. Attitudes and perceptions, however, will not likely converge into a single way of understanding our elders. From the inception of gerontology as a field of study, researchers and observers have emphasized the diversity within the older population and the difficulty in drawing generalizations and conclusions. As the older population increases, it also is becoming more diverse, with multiple sources of variation.

Gerontologists have always been future-oriented. The engine that drives the enormous expansion of interest in the phenomenon of aging is **demographics**. Demographers have relentlessly drawn the attention of researchers, health care providers, and policymakers to the facts of a graying population. The basic facts are undisputed. The exact rates of growth and the consequences of this growth, however, are more speculative, and in some circles, hotly debated.

Demographers lay out their predictions of population growth and change on the basis of different assumptions. These assumptions most often concern fertility rates (adding new people into the population), mortality rates (subtracting people from the population), and migration (the addition and subtraction of people from the population). By examining trends over time, predictions about future growth and change can be made with a certain degree of confidence. But because the future can never be known with absolute certainty, demographers develop multiple series of projections based on assumptions of different rates. Which series to accept, of course, becomes critically important when faced with questions of health care planning or economic policy development. Beyond predicting basic rates of **fertility**, **mortality**, and **migration**, other factors quickly enter into discussions of the future of an aging population:

- Will health care costs continue to escalate at the present rates?
- How will family structures change as a result of divorce, separation, and an increasing number of never married?
- How secure is the Social Security system?
- Will older adults continue to retire at relatively early ages?
- Will Americans' savings rates improve?
- Will the U.S. economy continue to expand?
- Will young adult and middle-aged women continue to enter the full-time workforce at current rates?
- How will the demand for other federal expenditures change over the next 50 years?

The answers to these questions are often a great deal more speculative than fertility and mortality statistics, and yet, each will have a profound effect on the quality of the lives of older Americans in the next century—and consequently, the quality of American life. Thus, the task of prediction becomes precarious, and the careers of predictors often short. The seriousness of the concerns identified in this chapter rests on assumptions and, to a degree, on speculation. They will change as answers to some of the questions just posed change or become known. They are based on (usually conservative) demographic predictions and should be thought of in an if/then sense. *If* things develop as we suspect they will, *then* it is likely that . . . and so forth. You are encouraged to consider the issues identified in this chapter critically and with skepticism. Consider how the concerns may or may not materialize depending on how we come to view our elders; on how future generations of Americans come to understand issues of obligation, dependency, and entitlement; on how we behave toward different age groups; and on how we vote and behave politically. Shifts in our collective behavior will assuredly influence these concerns for better or for worse.

From among the many concerns in a rapidly aging population, this chapter focuses on three main categories of issues. First, some differences between today's older adults and the older adults of the future are identified. It is this future population with which we are mostly concerned, and they are unlike their predecessors in several important respects. Second, concerns over generational equity and distribution of resources have been raised since the 1980s and are likely to become more pressing as the expected population trends unfold. Third are concerns around how the burden of economic support, and social and medical care, will be distributed. This last concern is discussed from the perspectives of several different nations.

Populations around the world are aging at different rates, allowing us to look at different levels of societal response to the problems and challenges of aging. It will become clear that these are all very complex issues and the answers to many questions are not known. In many cases, the scope and dimensions of the problems and challenges are only partially understood. The goal in this chapter is to identify several of the major issues that have received the attention of planners, researchers, and the public and to try to provide some context for understanding and thinking about these issues. First, demographic shifts most important to an understanding of these concerns are reviewed.

SIGNIFICANT DEMOGRAPHIC SHIFTS

In 2006, there were 37 million Americans older than 65 years, and they constituted just over 12% of the population. This group is expected to grow to more than 71 million by 2030, representing about 20% of the U.S. population.[1] Within today's older population, the proportion that is older than age 85 numbers approximately 5.3 million. By 2050, the over-85 age group will number nearly 21 million. Much of our interest in, and concern over, our aging society is with this group that is older than 85, whose growth is outpacing all others. This is a heterogeneous and complex age group to study. They are often characterized as frail older adults. Indeed, the likelihood of hospitalization or nursing home placement rises considerably with advanced age. Dementias and cognitive impairments that many of us have come to associate with advanced age do in fact increase dramatically in rate to a point among surviving older adults. Mobility is reduced; chronic conditions multiply; impoverishment and social isolation are greater risks. There is reason for concern as we see the unprecedented expansion of this age group. And yet, there is evidence to suggest that for a substantial proportion of those who survive into their 80s, there is a sort of mortality grace period that is marked by vitality and relatively good health.[2] And as suggested in the following sections, today's population of individuals older than 85 may not be the best guide to understanding the future older adults.

Be cautious about generalizing circumstances found in the United States to other parts of the world. Societies throughout the world are aging at different rates as a result of different degrees of modernization, industrialization, and economic development. In general terms, developed nations have older populations. The countries of the developing world currently have relatively young populations, but over the next half century they will be experiencing population aging at a rate unprecedented in the developed nations. Countries like the United States have had the luxury, so to speak, of slower and steadier rates of aging throughout the 20th century and with considerable foreknowledge. The dual challenges of poorer countries will be to deal with the pace of aging and, concomitantly, the problems associated with economic development.

Another statistic of interest to demographers and gerontologists is referred to as the dependency ratio. This ratio refers to those people in the population who are usually thought of as economically dependent to those who are economically productive, and can be calculated and considered in several different ways. The **old-age dependency ratio** refers to the number of people in the population older than 65 as compared with those between the ages of 18 and 64. Although all of those older than 65 are not necessarily retired or nonworking, and all of those between ages 18 and 64 are not necessarily working and economically productive, this ratio serves as a general indicator of the economic burden confronting the working segment of the population at any given time. The old-age dependency ratio increased throughout the 20th century and will continue to increase gradually through about 2020. After this date, not long after the baby boom generation begins to retire, the ratio begins to increase dramatically. Today, in crude terms, 100 workers contribute to the health and economic welfare of approximately 21 or 22 older adults. In 2020, 100 workers will contribute to the well-being of 27 or 28 older adults and thus will carry a greater burden economically.

Another type of dependency ratio is the **young-age dependency ratio**, or the ratio of those younger than 18 years to those between the ages 18 and 64. Between 1970 and 1990, this ratio declined dramatically from about 61 young people to every 100 workers to 42. Since 1990, and well on into the middle of the 21st century, this ratio remains relatively constant with minor fluctuations.[3]

The young-age and old-age dependency ratios can be combined for a total dependency ratio (**Figure 12-1**). This statistic would show that in 1990, there were about 62 young and old people to every 100 workers. This number is expected to increase to 67 by the year 2020.[3] Note, however, that the share of the total dependency ratio accounted for by children is declining, while the share accounted for by older adults is increasing. Consider also that the care of the young in the United States is considered to be primarily a private family responsibility, whereas the care of older adults carries with it more of a public responsibility (primarily through the Social Security tax and other taxes imposed on the working population). This issue and the ratios of economic dependency to productivity become significant in the discussion, to follow, concerning generational transfers and questions of equitable distribution of economic resources. But first, we consider what is known about the older population of today and the older adults of the future.

OLDER ADULTS TODAY

Data from the 2000 U.S. Census provide a portrait of today's older adults and a basis for understanding and predicting some of the population characteristics of future older adults. The educational attainment of the over-65 population is significantly below that of the total adult population. For example, college degree completion rates for all U.S. adults

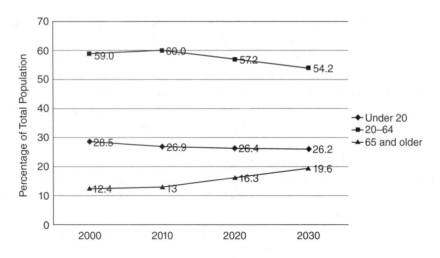

FIGURE 12-1   U.S. population, percent change by age.
Source: U.S. Census Bureau. U.S. Interim Projections by Age, Sex, Race, and Hispanic Origin. March 18, 2004. Retrieved February 17, 2009, from http://www.census.gov/population/www/projections/usinterimproj

are currently about 25%, whereas just 16% of adults over 65 have 4-year college degrees or higher. A more dramatic contrast can be seen in those with less than a high school diploma. Among the oldest-old, over age 85, nearly half did not complete high school. That figure for the total U.S. adult population over age 25 stands at about one-fifth.[1]

In 2000, 56% of older Americans were married, one-third were widowed, 7% were divorced, and 5% were never married. The number who are married declines with age. For example, two-thirds of those in the 65–74 age group were married compared to less than a third of the over-85 age group. This decline is explained largely by the difference in life expectancy for men and women, and the tendency for men to be slightly older than their wives. In 2000, there were 82.4 men for every 100 women in the 65–74 age group, and just 41 men to every 100 women in the over-85 age group.[1]

For the total over-65 population, in 2000, two-thirds lived in households with others, most often a spouse. Twenty-eight percent lived alone in a household. Women over 65 are about three times more likely to live alone than are men.[1]

For the over-65 age group, 18% of men and 10% of women are still in the workforce. The median earnings in 1999 for this age group were $31,556 for men and $22,511 for women. In households with at least one member over 65, 90% received Social Security in 1999. The poverty rate for older adults in 2000 continued at a rate lower than that of the total population (9.9% compared to 12.4%). Seventy-eight percent owned their own homes.[1]

The most common disabilities reported by older adults were physical in nature (27%), followed by difficulties with leaving the home (20%), and sensory difficulties such as blindness or hearing impairment (14%). All categories of disability increase significantly with age, with 47% of the over-85 population, for example, reporting difficulties leaving their homes.[1]

In sum, older Americans in 2000 had lower levels of educational attainment compared to the overall population; had high rates of home ownership and a modest level of financial security. Levels of disability, poor health, and living alone all rise with age, and women are more vulnerable than men because of their greater longevity. What is masked by this brief, stereotypical portrait is the considerable heterogeneity of the experience of aging and the variety of life circumstances found in late life. The future of aging in the United States is also changing as each successive cohort distinguishes itself from those that preceded them. The large baby boom generation begins entering late life in 2011 and will surely experience this period of life differently from how their parents and grandparents did.

FUTURE OLDER ADULTS

The older population of the future, the baby boomers, will be characteristically different from their older predecessors of today. Notably, they have many more years of formal education. Higher levels of educational attainment are associated with lower mortality, better health, reduced poverty, and higher probability of being married, and hence less likelihood of being alone.[4] Family size of the older population has already begun to change and will continue to shrink in the coming decades. Until 2005, family size of older adults was increasing, with 35% of older adults with four or more children, and 46% with two or three children. Since 2005, however, only 11% have four or more children, and 55% have two or three. Family size has important implications for social and economic support for older adults. Some estimates are that as much as 80% of care for older adults is provided by family members, often by adult children. As family size shifts downward, the availability of family care declines commensurately. The proportion of older adults requiring formal assisted care may then increase.

The gap in life expectancy for men and women is narrowing. During the 1980s, women gained about 0.2 years in life expectancy and men 0.6.[4] Under today's mortality conditions, older Americans reaching the age of 65 can expect to live an additional 18.7 years on average. For those who reach the age of 85, women can expect another 7.2 years of life and men an additional 6.1 years.[1] This trend results in higher rates of marriage among older adults compared to previous generations. Women do not lose their husbands as soon because of death and thus spend fewer years alone. Beneficial consequences of this will probably include reduced rates of isolation and subsequently lower rates of depression and suicide, interdependency of intact couples, and less dependency of single older adults on societal and familial aid. Also if the trends toward higher rates of divorce and separation among younger groups continue, combined with delayed childbirth and childrearing, available familial support is likely to decline even further than would be predicted by just the shrinking family size of older adults.

In the future, more women will retire from longer years of workforce participation. Participation in the workforce has increased among women over the last four decades. The largest increase has been among women ages 55–61, having gone from 44% working outside the home in 1963 to 64% in 2006.[1] For women older than 62, most of their increase in the workforce has occurred since the mid-1990s. This means that older women will be qualifying for their own pensions and Social Security benefits in larger numbers compared to years past.[4] This will have the effect of reducing poverty among older women and, combined with longer marriages, will increase the real income of older couples. Fewer are likely to need economic assistance. The paramount concern in this regard is how the Social Security system of revenue collection and benefits disbursement will be able to accommodate this larger cohort of beneficiaries with a reduced number of workers.

As the older population grows so too grows the number of voters who are old. Inasmuch as older people vote more than younger people, and are more politically active generally, older adults are likely to become a more vocal and potent political force. In 1990, approximately 30% of federal expenditures were directed to the older population. Were this level of expenditures to be maintained through 2030 they could conceivably reach 60% of the federal budget.[4] Age-related voting behaviors and budget expenditures are both nearly impossible to predict for the short term let alone over decades. If older adults vote in accordance with narrowly defined self-interests and maximize gains for older age groups, there will be fewer economic resources available for other purposes. If expenditures on defense and national security, for example, continue to increase as has been the case since 2001 to the present, pressure to reduce large federal budget items such as Social Security and other entitlements grows. There is little evidence, however, that older adults vote with one mind on age-related issues or any other issues for that matter. Still, age politics are likely to become more pronounced in the coming decades. This will be unavoidable if income transfers across generations become greater. Questions about the equity of shifting more resources to older adults are exacerbated by the downward trends in the welfare and quality of life for children in the United States. This issue is examined in greater detail in the section on generational equity later.

The difficulties in forecasting the future should be evident by now. Perhaps one of the greatest flaws in forecasting is in the assumption that today's notions about transitions from work to retirement will prevail in the future. The typical pattern of working from the completion of one's education in early adulthood to one's mid-60s, often for the same employer and in the same place, then abruptly leaving the workforce to pursue leisure and pleasure pursuits in retirement is not typical now—and for most Americans, never was. This is a pattern that fit middle- and upper-income white men for a relatively brief interval in our history. These are powerful stereotypes against which we must measure "the good life." The issues of generational equity and caring for frail older adults addressed in later sections are questions of resource availability and allocation. How we think about dependency, obligation, and the distribution of resources is influenced by whether we see others as needy, deserving, or a burden. In the United States, such determinations are made largely on the basis of what we believe one has earned through his or her own merit. Merit is awarded in our culture on the basis of education and training attained, work done, and contributions made. To what degree can we ascertain whether the future older adults will merit the benefits they reap? Are older adults cutting productive work lives unnecessarily short through early retirement? Could older adults stay on the productive side of the dependency ratio longer, thereby relieving some of the burden on younger generations?

WORK LIFE

Answers to these questions come from two very different directions that might be thought of as the supply and demand of work for older workers. As the absolute numbers of traditional-aged workers in the United States and other developed countries declines, employers are forced to rethink the attractiveness of older workers and modify work policies and practices. As life span, health, and opportunity extend, older Americans reconsider the balance of work, leisure, and social contribution in their lives.

Before the 1980s, retirement trends were quite clear. Women's participation in work outside the home stood at about half that of men. Most older workers retired as soon as they were able. The ability to retire was determined primarily on the basis of finances and health, factors working as incentives or disincentives depending on individual circumstances. By and large, the favorable balance of these two factors has provided great numbers of older male workers with sufficient incentive to take retirement at the earliest possible time. Labor force participation rates for older male workers declined steadily until the early 1980s. This decline was fueled by a reduction in the eligibility age for Social Security from 65 to 62 in the early 1960s. Older Americans had also accumulated greater amounts of lifetime wealth, allowing earlier retirement. Work participation for older workers leveled off in the mid-1980s for men. For men in the 65–69 age range, participation stood at 24% in 1985 but has shown a gradual rise to 34% in 2006. Most of the increase in labor force participation for women older than 62 began in the mid-1990s. These increases have been attributed to the elimination of the mandatory retirement age, changes in Social Security, and for women, significant cultural change and increased educational attainment.[1]

As the American economy and the labor market shifted in the 1980s and 1990s, downsizing and reduction in the workforce became familiar terms to American workers. Older workers were often targeted because of savings that would result from eliminating their higher salaries and the belief that their health insurance and benefits were more costly to employers. The Age Discrimination in Employment Act (ADEA) was introduced into law in 1967 to protect older workers from arbitrary and indiscriminate hiring and firing practices. The effect of downsizing is amply illustrated by the fact that between 1980 and 1987 one-fifth of all Fortune 500 companies' employees were eliminated.[5] In the early 1990s, an estimated 2 million people between the ages of 50 and 64 were able and wanting to return to work.[6] Workers in this age group often opt for "early retirement" after they have exhausted their work options. Those older than 65 years, generally in better health than previous generations, also show interest in continued employment, but more often in part-time or flexible employment opportunities.[6] These facts would suggest that the demand for work among older workers often exceeds the supply. Contrary to stereotypes, older workers have been found to be punctual, conscientious, sensitive to coworkers, and use fewer sick days for acute problems. They are also loyal to employers and experienced.[7]

It is questionable whether extending the **work life** of older workers beyond the gains already made over the last two decades is likely or realistic. There continue to be powerful incentives to leave the workforce among those whom employers would most like to retain. Foremost is the age of earliest eligibility for Social Security, which is 62 at the present time. Since the introduction of age 62 eligibility we have continued to see retirements spike at this age.[8] In addition, some portion of the over-62 population is not able to continue working because of ill health or disability.

There also appears to be a mismatch between the needs and desires of older workers and the economics of employing older workers. Older workers report consistently that full-time work is less attractive and that they prefer part-time or flexible work opportunities, which are often unavailable. Recent proposals put forward by the IRS may make phased retirement more feasible for older workers by reducing the extent of benefit coverage required by employers.[8,9]

Older workers tend to be the most expensive to employ. This can be balanced only by making them worth the cost to employers through, for example, ongoing educational, training, and professional development programs. Some industries, notably health care and higher education, have done well in this area by providing ongoing professional development, but by and large U.S. employers lag behind European and Japanese efforts in these areas.[10] In her comprehensive analysis, Munnell concludes that the only policy change likely to yield some significant extension of work life for older workers is to increase the earliest eligible retirement age from 62 to 64 or 65.[8] This is both politically challenging and would likely result in only marginal gains.

The pressure may come, however, from the other direction, that is, increased interest in and/or pressure to work among older adults themselves. People either work because they need to, they want to, or some combination of the two. The need to work, for some significant segment of the older population, may increase substantially, especially if the cost of living keeps rising at the current pace. Social Security in the future, for a variety of reasons, is not likely to cover as much of preretirement income as it now does. In 2006, the "average earner" who retired at age 65 received the equivalent of about 42% of previous earnings. After paying the automatically deducted Medicare premium, this drops to 38.7% of previous earnings. Current Social Security regulation is scheduled to reduce preretirement income replacement rates in the future through (1) the scheduled increases in the normal retirement age from 65 to 67, (2) increases in Medicare premiums, and (3) more taxation of Social Security resulting from exemption amounts not indexed to inflation.[8] Because Social Security provides the greatest source of aggregate income for older Americans, these changes are significant. In 2006, 37% of income for older Americans came from Social Security; 28% from earnings; 18% from pensions; and 15% from asset income.[8] Thus, the financial security of future older adults may be more tied to earnings than in the past. An AARP survey found two types of older workers, sustainers and providers, and estimated that about 61% of older workers do so at least in part out of financial need. This proportion may even increase in the future.[11] For this group, both income and health benefits are strong incentives to maintain employment.

For those who *want* to continue to work (estimated at 38% in the AARP survey) regardless of financial incentives, a number of powerful motives have been identified: maintenance of social networks, use of their knowledge, job autonomy, learning opportunities, involvement in decision making, supporting success in coworkers, job satisfaction, commitment to employers, a sense of responsibility, and making a contribution to society.[11] These motives are not far different from those identified by volunteers in a later section of this chapter.

In response to the displacement of older workers and the interests of retirees in extending their work life, a number of corporate and governmental initiatives have attempted to increase the supply side of work for older workers. For example, the Environmental Protection Agency has made deliberate efforts to recruit workers older than 55 for short-term projects. The Days Inn Corporation targeted workers older than 55 for recruitment and consequently reduced its absentee rate by 80%. Companies such as AT&T, NCR, Dow Jones, and the U.S. Postal Service have begun utilizing older workers for mentor programs. Gamse reports about a number of large-scale job fairs and job clubs designed to assist midlife and older workers who are changing careers or are unemployed.[7] These efforts constitute a mix of paid and unpaid work and affect workers in the 55- to 65-year-old age group as well as those past the traditional retirement age.

The future older adults will be considerably different from their predecessors with respect to interests in work, their work availability, and skills and talents. Gamse describes older workers of the future as a group with little loyalty to one employer or a single career path.[7] Their interests will be in finding work that, above all, gives them satisfaction. They will be better educated, more computer and technologically literate, and more comfortable with diversity. They will be in second and third careers relative to their earlier work histories and more interested in flexible work opportunities integrated with educational, leisure, and retirement activities. They also will be more likely to protest or litigate if treated unfairly.[7]

It is important to note that powerful determinants of work and retirement patterns are the lifelong expectations we hold of each. As family structures change, as women participate in the paid workforce longer, as maternity and paternity leaves become more commonplace, as education and retraining become more necessary, it is likely that older adults will become more accustomed to a mixed pattern of workforce entry, exit, and reentry. The expectation of a single sharp transition from work life to retirement will become less compelling. Combined with delayed benefit eligibility for Social Security, as well as general uncertainty about the stability of the Social Security system, specifically the economy in general, adults will plan differently for retirement and alter their expectations of what is typical. Work, education, volunteer service, and civic engagement are likely to become more integrated in the lives of older adults.

LIFELONG EDUCATION

The growth of secondary and postsecondary education in the United States since World War II has been dramatic and impressive. Although the GI Bill created opportunities for returning veterans to obtain college credentials and marked the beginning of an educational expansion that continues today, not all segments of the population (those slightly older or women, for example) benefited equally or at the same time in their lives. In 1965, just 24% of the older population had completed high school and only 5% had college degrees. In 2007, the number of high school graduates among older adults increased to 76%, and 19% had completed a 4-year college degree.[1] The rates of high school completion for older men and women in 2007 was about equal, but the rates of bachelor degree completion differed with 25% of men having completed but only 15% of women. Racial differences are more pronounced. In 2007, 81% of whites over age 65 had completed high school compared to 58% of African Americans and 42% of Hispanics. The respective bachelor's degree completion rates for whites, blacks, and Hispanics are currently 21%, 10%, and 9%.[1]

Later adult education takes many forms and, compared with the lock-step model of traditional early life education, is much more fluid and open-ended and can be considered **lifelong education**. Elderhostel has become a well-known national and international program offering thousands of short-term courses of study each year. Geared to the college level and cultural enrichment, Elderhostel does not offer college credit and tends to appeal to those who are already well educated. Also, at least one-quarter of community colleges target older adults for particular kinds of course offerings. Those most commonly enrolled tend to be in the areas of financial planning and management, health and cultural enrichment, and contemporary civic issues.[12]

Increased enrollments of older adults in college and university courses were a boon to institutions that had been bracing themselves for declining enrollments during the 1980s. At that time, there was a decline in the pool of graduating high school seniors on the order of 25%. Yet, college enrollments went from 12 million to 13.4 million during one year as a result of older learners returning to school.[13] Among the adult college population, there are now more women than men, whites dominate on the order of 90%, and 85% of older students work, mostly full-time. In order of frequency, the most common reasons given for returning to school are life transitions, learning as a satisfying activity, an opportunity to meet people, and a way to fill up free time. The kinds of life transitions precipitating a return to the classroom differ for older and younger adults. Those between 25 and 64 years cite career transitions. Those older than 65 more often cite leisure transitions and family transitions than do younger adults.[13]

It has been observed that adult education increases during periods of rapid social change. Changes in the economy, the age composition of society, technology, the family, and the roles of minorities and women all would appear to call for an increase in both traditional and less traditional forms of educational participation among older adults for some time to come.

VOLUNTEERISM

Wilson defines **volunteerism** as "engagement in proactive activities that involve commitment and whose benefits extend beyond the individual volunteers."[14] Similarly, Harootyan defines volunteering as "any activity intended to help others that is provided without obligation for which the volunteer does not receive pay or other material compensation."[15] Volunteering can be either formal or informal. According to the Current Population Survey of September 2005, 28.8% of the U.S. population engaged in formal volunteer work.[16] Older age groups participated somewhat less on average with about 1 in 4 persons over age 65 engaged as volunteers.[16] In a 2003 AARP study, the concept of volunteerism was broadened to include informal activity such as helping someone in the community. Among those older than age 70, 40% reported formal volunteer activity and another 40% reported informal assistance to someone in the community.[16]

Reasons given for volunteerism are multiple and include attaining higher levels of mastery, self-esteem, life satisfaction, and more energy[16]; to make a contribution to society, meet others[17]; to gain career-related experience, to enhance self-esteem, to reduce negative feelings, to strengthen social relationships, to learn more about the world, and to act on important values.[18]

Despite the significant contributions of older adults as volunteers, they are considered still to be an underutilized resource and one that is growing in size. In addition to those who volunteer there are a good many more who do not but say they would if asked.[19] Baby boomers who, relative to previous generations, are characterized by better health, higher levels of education, and greater financial security, report in high numbers (51%) that they intend to volunteer. Volunteer programs exist for most skill levels and interest areas. For example, the Older Volunteer Program of the ACTION Agency is an umbrella organization that includes the Retired Senior Volunteer Program (RSVP), Foster Grandparents, and Senior Companion Program. RSVP volunteers tend to be geared toward human services such as refugee services, literacy programs, long-term care, and youth counseling. Foster Grandparents and Senior Companions are targeted for low-income volunteers and provide small hourly stipends. RSVP allows for expense reimbursement. These programs are funded mostly with federal dollars, with some state and local contributions.[20,21]

AARP, formerly the American Association of Retired Persons, operates a Volunteer Talent Bank (VTB). The bank is set up for the purpose of matching volunteer interests and skills with agency and community needs. Set up originally to provide staffing for AARP volunteer needs, VTB now makes referrals to many outside agencies including the American Red Cross, the U.S. Fish and Wildlife Service, and the Peace Corps.[20]

The Service Corps of Retired Executives (SCORE) provides consulting and presents workshops for small business management assistance. By the early 1990s, SCORE had 13,000 volunteers providing voluntary assistance at 750 locations. Consulting services are free of charge to client businesses and managers, and a small fee is charged for workshops to cover expenses.[20]

The National Retiree Volunteer Center (NRVC) is underwritten by corporate sponsors and recruits from among corporate retirees. This program originated in the Minneapolis area and led to community initiatives ranging from food distribution centers, to board assignments with nonprofit institutions such as libraries and museums, to nutritional and childcare educational programs for young mothers. These initiatives are determined, staffed, and directed by senior volunteers with supporting corporate funding.[20]

In October 2006, the Older Americans Act (OAA) was reauthorized. The reauthorization included several steps to increase opportunities for volunteerism and civic engagement such as the availability of grants to organizations that engage older adults in services to meet community needs.[22] The OAA further asks area agencies on aging to participate in planning to support older Americans in civic engagement. Some proposals for policymakers include incorporating many of the structures of successful programs currently in place for younger age groups such as VISTA, the White House Fellows program, Troops to Teachers, and the Caro Fellows program. These proposals provide entry points, training, orientation, and structure to postcareer volunteer experiences.[22] Volunteerism is likely to play an enormous role in the lives of the future older adults.

THE QUESTION OF GENERATIONAL EQUITY

Substantial gains have been made among the older segment of the population in terms of income and living conditions. In 1959, older Americans had the highest rates of poverty of any age group, with 35% living below the federally defined poverty line. Children under 18 were the second most poverty-stricken group then, with 27% below the federally defined poverty level, followed by working-age groups at 17%. By 1993, the poverty rate for older adults had dropped to 12.4%. Children did not make comparable progress. Following significant gains in the 1960s, poverty rates among children climbed in the early 1980s and again in the early 1990s when it reached 22.7% in 1993,[1,23] making children the largest poverty-stricken age group in the United States.

Given children's dependency on the adults around them for survival and well-being, this fact is alarming and, some would argue, should be a source of national shame in a country as wealthy as the United States. These opposing trends have become the basis for the charge that older adults have become an overbenefited group at the expense of the young. There is concern that as the older population grows it will draw even more of our national resources away from an increasingly needy younger population. A way to remedy this circumstance and reverse the trend would be to recognize the importance of investing in young people, for example, by setting limits on expenditures and investments in the older population and redirecting those resources toward America's youth.

At first glance, this argument is a powerful one. It is indeed alarming to observe these opposing trends. It has been my experience that when even the most sympathetic students of gerontology become aware of these facts they quickly condemn the system that takes from children to benefit the old. The observation that the country's oldest adults seem to be enjoying an increasingly comfortable standard of living while the most dependent and vulnerable segment of the population is at greater risk carries with it images of selfishness, disregard for the future, and moral culpability. There are reasons to be cautious of these charges, however, and a need to examine the situation much more carefully. Researchers and gerontologists have argued that these impressions are misleading when taken out of context. Minkler summarized many of these contextual considerations and counterarguments at about the time when the disparity in age group poverty rates was reaching its peak.[24]

The way in which poverty is measured is sometimes different for the young and the old owing to estimated adjustments in living costs. Minkler argues that if the same definitions are used for the two groups, the poverty rate for older adults climbs about three percentage points. By any standard, income levels used to distinguish those in poverty from those not in poverty are artificial and set very low. When, for example, we consider 150% of poverty level as true poverty, sometimes described as poor and near poor, the poverty rate for older adults nearly doubles. In other words, although it is true that many of the old are no longer living below the poverty line as defined by the various government agencies, at least one-third of them are still living in extremely modest circumstances and would be considered by many to be poor. All of this is to suggest that poverty is more subjective and more complex than a magic cut-off number, and taken out of context these statistics can be misleading.[24]

More important is that the generational inequity argument strongly implies that monies are being taken away from the young and given to the old. In fact, the causes of childhood poverty and the causes of improved living standards for the old are quite independent and unrelated to one another. At the risk of oversimplification, the rise in poverty rates among children during the 1980s was attributable in large part to market forces. There was a decline in real wages among workers in the 1980s, an increase in substandard wage work, and loss of high-paying jobs in such areas as manufacturing, unfavorable employment trends for many, and an increase in single-parent, female-headed households. In other words, children are poor because young adults have declining opportunities in obtaining well-paying jobs and maintaining families. The declining poverty level among the old was primarily the result of changes in government policy in the 1970s. In 1972,

Social Security payments were increased 20% and tied to annual rises in the Consumer Price Index to protect against inflation. If Social Security were reduced to its pre-1972 levels, this would both increase real poverty among the old and do nothing to alter the changes in markets and family structure that affected the young during this time with such devastating consequences.[24]

Much of the cost burden of supporting an aging population is directly related to the costs of increased demand for medical care and health care resources. Those who argue for greater **generational equity** imply that the cost is inflated because of the demands for high-technology medical care among older adults. In fact, much of the crisis in health care is a result not of high technology but of the failure to control the costs of health care generally, costs that affect all ages. The costs of hospital care, for example, grew from $14 billion in 1965 to $167 billion in 1985. Health care costs increase at roughly twice that of the Consumer Price Index.[24]

Another flaw in the generational inequity argument is the suggestion that the distribution and redistribution of resources is a zero-sum game. This is not true of the political process generally, and there is no reason to believe that it should be true as the needs and demands of society change in a dynamic and fluid manner. The population is getting older. That calls for more resources of a particular kind. The Cold War ended almost two decades ago, reducing the need for economic resources for defense, and national security has consumed substantial resources since September 2001. As needs change and as the composition of society changes, so too, do the rules of resource acquisition and allocation change. This is evident in changes in tax laws, in retirement rules and benefits, in proposals for flextime for workers, and in uses of volunteer resources and energy. Corporate tax rates, for example, declined from 4.2% of the Gross National Product (GNP) in the early 1960s to 1.6% of GNP in the early 1980s. Although politically unpopular, perhaps we can no longer afford to forgo these sources of government revenues. Economic challenges, and the solutions identified to address them, must be understood as fluid and changeable.[24]

This section so far has considered inequities and imbalances between older adults and children. By the year 2000, the disparity in poverty levels between the young and old had narrowed to single digits, and by 2006 poverty rates stood at 9% and 17% for the old and for children under 18, respectively.[1] Today the debate is more often likely to focus on the equity of burden and benefit between the generations of working adults and retired adults. As the demographic shifts continue to move the United States toward an older age structure, and as grim economic forecasts predict insolvency in the Social Security system, age politics may take on a sharper edge. In 2006, Blackburn characterized the opposing camps in this debate on generational equity as the "generational accounting" supporters and the "generational solidarity" supporters.[25] The position held by the generational accountants, advanced in various forms since at least the late 1980s, is that taxing younger workers to finance the pensions of retirees is inherently unfair. This position amounts to a direct attack on the viability and equity of the Social Security program.

Such accounting calculates the total contributions and the total eventual benefits for a given generation and necessarily takes cohort or generational size into account. When combined with a portrayal of a bankrupt Social Security system, generational accountants advance an emotionally packed economic argument with clear generational winners (larger cohorts) and generational losers (smaller cohorts). Variations derived from this basic position include policies that advance health savings accounts, voluntary personal retirement accounts, and various Social Security privatization schemes.[26] When age cohorts vary substantially in size, questions of fairness, equity, and generational justice present formidable challenges.

Those who support a position of "generational solidarity" argue, no less emotionally, that there is a social bond between generations of parents and children that transcends precise accounting. Those who advance this position favor a pay-as-you-go system of generational transfers and consider claims of the imminent collapse of the Social Security system and the crisis of an aging population as alarmist propaganda. In contrast, generational accountants argue that each generation should pay its own way and that risk pooling within generations is preferable to risk pooling between them.[25]

Blackburn, in his review of these positions, favors the reasoning of generational solidarity supporters but suggests that it too is flawed. He points to the duties and obligations of each generation toward the other but maintains that these obligations are not without limit. The economic alarmism of the generational accountants, Blackburn maintains, is based on arbitrary assumptions and distant time horizons that, when combined, point to massive, and likely erroneous, shortfalls in the system.[25]

In contrast, generally accepted projections published annually by the trustees of the Social Security system and the Congressional Budget Office currently estimate that the system is solvent until 2041 by one methodology, or 2052 by another.[8,25] These projections have determined that an increase in Social Security payroll deductions of 1.92%, had it been implemented in 2006, would have restored solvency to the system through the 75-year time horizon used in the methodologies.[25] Delaying action until 2041 would call for an increased contribution on the order of 4.26%. Reading these same figures pushes the supporters of generational accounting and generational solidarity further into their respective corners.

As has been stated repeatedly, increasing the tax burden on a shrinking cohort of workers is not an attractive option for many. What alternatives does this leave if we are to retain a viable and equitable pension system for America's older adults? One approach that has been advanced in Sweden (discussed later), and that is under consideration in other developed countries indexes retiree public pension benefits to the actual size of the current working age cohort. Another approach altogether would be to focus reform efforts less on publicly funded pension support like Social Security and more on employer-sponsored defined benefit pensions. These private pensions were more the norm from post World War II until about the mid-1970s and resulted in considerably more retirement savings,[25,26] though at a higher cost to employers.

Related to the generational equity debate, and a large area of study in its own right, is whether age is being scapegoated when, in fact, there are sources of inequity within age groups that are greater than the inequities between age groups. It is important not to lose sight of the fact that older adults are certainly the most diverse age group in the population and that the aging experience varies enormously by race, sex, and class. To a lesser degree, this can be said of children as well. The likelihood of growing up in poverty, for example, is many times greater for an African American child in the United States than for a white child. The best predictor of poverty in old age is poverty throughout life. The study of aging from a life course perspective underscores the fact that economic resources and assets in old age result directly from continuous progressive employment throughout adulthood that has been the predominant traditional life pattern in U.S. society only for white males.[27]

PROVIDING FOR OLDER ADULTS

An analysis of the future of an aging society results in the recognition that the older population is growing at a rapid rate, and the segment of that population that is most frail and in need of greatest support (i.e., those 85 and older) is growing at an even faster rate than the rest. In response to that growing need, we can look to essentially three sources of resources and support. These include the family, the public government sector, and the private business sector. A brief review of the current system of resource provision and support in the United States follows. The U.S. system is then contrasted with the systems currently in place in Sweden and Japan.

Sweden is selected for two reasons. It has one of the oldest populations in the world and, in that sense, offers a glimpse of the future. It also has among the most elaborate public sector support systems for older adults in place anywhere. For that reason, it does not offer a probable glimpse of the future in the United States, inasmuch as few would suggest that the United States would or should adopt so extensive a social welfare arrangement.

Japan offers a startling demographic contrast to the United States. Compared to the 12.4% of the over-65 population in the United States, Japan today has an older population of more than 20%. Other contrasts exist in older labor force participation, cost and availability of health care, health care service utilization patterns, and societal attitudes toward older adults. Japan, because of the accelerated rate at which it achieved an older age structure, has had to consider and adopt many economic and health care policies the United States and other developed countries are just now considering.

Finally, general conditions in the developing world are described. These conditions differ enormously from those in the developed countries of western Europe and North America. Like Japan, though for very different reasons, these countries will experience a period of explosive old-age population growth in a relatively brief time.

Based on these sketches, we see several different scenarios for the future of the older population. The United States is in a state of flux right now, and the aging of its population is a political football. It is unlikely that younger generations can sustain substantially more of the burden of care for its elders both in terms of familial care and through tax support. Growth in the **private sector** is probable, but there is reason to be skeptical of the quality and sustainability of private sector options for the general older population. **Public sector** support involves a long-standing social contract that minimally must be sustained at near current levels and, some would argue, should be strengthened in certain areas.

In contrast, Sweden's system is impressive, but at a cost that would not be palatable to most Americans. In the future, the need will continue to expand in Sweden, although at a slower rate than in recent decades. As the need expands, it is unlikely that the Swedish public sector will expand any further. The difference is more likely to be made up by families and growth in the private sector.

Japan's greatest challenge is in the continued growth in its oldest population. The oldest-old is the fastest growing age group in the society and with increased disability and ambivalence about family care in younger age groups, providing high-quality care for this cohort will be challenging.

The developing world, by far, faces the greatest challenges. Most countries are ill equipped to cope with the growth in the older population. Governments in developing nations assume, out of necessity, that the traditional family structures will absorb the care of their older family members. Traditional family structures in the developing world, however, are undergoing significant changes as a result of urbanization and shifting labor markets, leaving families unable to provide the kind of support they might have in stable social systems or on the scale anticipated. In some countries the public sector recognizes this and is responding accordingly with the initiation of a variety of public economic programs. A more detailed picture is sketched later.

As described in Chapter 9, some of the care for the very old involves what is described as long-term care. This is a level of care usually needed for chronic and ongoing conditions that are more prevalent in the oldest-old. These chronic and ongoing conditions often limit mobility, functioning, and self-care. In many respects it is medically low-technology care, including social care and supervision. As disease conditions progress, the level of care intensifies and for some may require around-the-clock care and supervision as well as more intensive medical care. Long-term care may be provided in homes or in institutions, primarily nursing homes.

THE UNITED STATES

In the United States, funding for older Americans' health care comes from a combination of individual resources (or out-of-pocket payment), public health insurance, and a welfare approach. All Social Security recipients are eligible for basic Medicare coverage. Medicare is a public health insurance program for older adults and in 2004 covered 53% of the total health care costs for older Americans. Medicare beneficiaries have some allowances for long-term care but only on a short-term basis.

The major source of coverage for long-term care facilities is Medicaid, covering 48% of total costs in 2004, with out-of-pocket payment close behind at 45%.[1] Medicaid eligibility is income-based and provides payment for health care for those eligible, regardless of age, who do not have the private resources to pay for medical care. Medicaid was never intended to be the primary source of funding for long-term care for older adults, yet nearly half of nursing home revenues come from public funds, most of this from Medicaid.[1,3] Established in 1966 along with Medicare, Medicaid is jointly funded through state and federal funds, and by the 1980s it had become the biggest item in many state budgets, precipitating more stringent cost-containment measures.[28]

Because about 80% of nursing homes are privately owned and operated on a for-profit basis, the United States has the circumstance of having private sector nursing homes heavily subsidized with public funds. Critics have argued that this has created a two-tiered class system of care.[28] Because government funding sources are income-based and favor institutional care, institutions end up providing for an inordinate number of poor or impoverished older adults. Many of these individuals require more social than medical care but have neither the family nor other social support or financial resources to elect any other option other than nursing home care.

Olson argues that through the arrangement of publicly subsidized "private" homes, quality, access, and affordability have been compromised. Studies of nursing homes within the United States[28] as well as cross-national studies[29] paint a grim picture of conditions. Quoting Olson:[28]

> The vast majority of homes fail to provide for the basic health and safety needs of the occupants. Most are substandard facilities that do not comply with even minimum federal and state standards of care; many violations are serious and life-threatening, including lack of food, proper administration of drugs, and decent personal hygiene. Due to a scarcity of physicians, a significant percentage of patients do not receive needed lab tests or adequate medical attention. Many suffer from poor nutrition, insufficient nursing care, and generally squalid conditions.

Although this description may fit many nursing homes, if not a majority, there are also many high-quality, well-run nursing homes in the United States. Many of these better facilities, however, are expensive, may not accept Medicaid payments, and may have long waiting lists for admission. They may also not be equipped to meet the needs of the very sick or the very poor, thus reinforcing the two-class system.

Noninstitutional alternatives to nursing home care, which have increased in use in recent years, fall into either formal or informal service categories. *Informal care* refers to that which is provided by immediate family members or other relatives. In 2004, 16% of the total U.S. population provided care to someone over age 50. Among these care providers, about half provided care for 8 hours or less per week, while 17% provided 40 or more hours of care per week. Women make up 61% of care providers of people over age 50, are somewhat less likely than male providers to work full-time, and report more often that they had no choice in providing care. The combination of absence of choice and level of burden is the strongest predictor of physical and emotional strain and of experiencing financial burden. The average age of recipients of care is 75 years. Caregivers are most often taking care of a parent (44%) or a grandmother (11%). One-quarter of caregivers are assisting individuals with Alzheimer's disease, dementia, or other forms of mental confusion. Unpaid caregiving is estimated to provide services valued at about $257 billion per year.[30]

Formal support services pick up where family care leaves off or is unavailable. The availability and array of noninstitutional services vary considerably by community but may include in-home assistance with meals, homemaker services, home health aides, transportation, telephone monitoring, respite for family members, daycare, and legal services. These services have been designed largely to complement or aid family caregivers and less to replace them or sustain completely independent living conditions for older adults. Older people may first recognize the need for some form of long-term care during or after a hospitalization. Older people require hospitalization at about four times the rate of younger people. Approximately 20% of all older people use inpatient facilities in a given year.[3] What distinguishes the institutionalized from the noninstitutionalized older adults is often the availability of family help. Where family help is limited or unavailable, formal in-home and community services are intended to fill the gap and forestall institutional placement. Restricted availability, lack of awareness of and use of community services, fragmentation, and cost-containment measures, however, may all reduce the effectiveness of institutional alternatives. Findings from studies of demonstration projects comparing the costs of community care and institutional care have been mixed. They have not provided clear evidence that home-based care is more cost effective. There is considerable consensus, however, that it is preferred, more humane, and less dehumanizing.[31–34]

A longstanding criticism of formal in-home and community services has been the fragmented nature of the service delivery system. This fragmentation is largely a function of the financing mechanisms in place. Eligibility is usually income based, with the major funding sources being Medicare, Medicaid, Social Services (Title XX of the Social Security Act), Supplemental Security Income (Title XVI of the Social Security Act), the Administration on Aging, Veterans Administration, and Housing and Urban Development.[3] In addition to low-income requirements, many of the services are limited in volume per year or over the lifetime of the client. Other criticisms include limited access to services and a workforce providing care that is unskilled, untrained, underpaid, and overworked.[35]

In her review of care provision in the United States, Olson argues that the public sector falls short in providing for the eldest and neediest members of society.[28] Access to in-home and community-based services is limited and fragmented. With its emphasis on individualism and self-reliance, the United States places the primary financial obligation for care squarely on older adults themselves. When care providers are needed, family members take on the large majority of the responsibility. The public sector takes over when there are no resources or no family.

Since 1985 there has been a steady decrease in nursing home residence rates. The age-adjusted rate in 1985 was 54 people per 1,000 over the age of 65. This rate declined to 35 per 1,000 by 2004.[1] The sharpest declines were among the over-85 age groups. The decrease in rate of nursing home use is being replaced commensurately with more in-home alternatives and other forms of residential care and assisted living arrangements. Health care costs among residents of long-term care facilities averaged $52,958 annually in 2004, compared to $10,448 among community residents.[1] Even though there has been a decline in rate of use, the absolute number of occupied nursing home beds has increased as a result of the expansive growth of the older population.

The highest expenditures, naturally, occur among the oldest-old. Additional variability in health and health care costs, however, can be seen in demographic breakdowns of the population beyond age. For example, African Americans have higher costs than either whites or Hispanics. Low-income individuals and those with chronic conditions incur higher health care costs.[1]

The rising costs of prescription drugs have contributed significantly to the health care costs of older Americans. In 1992, prescription drugs constituted 8% of total health care costs for the older population. By 2004, they had reached 15%.[1] During this same period there were declines in both hospital stays and nursing home use that were offset by increases in outpatient hospital services and physician visits.[1]

In the aggregate, 53% of all health care services for older adults were covered by Medicare in 2004. Older Americans paid 19% of costs out of pocket, and another 19% was covered by other payers. Medicaid covered 9% of costs for all services.[1] The shift in the past decade to more community-based, noninstitutional care and services would seem to be a very positive one that adds to the quality of life for many older Americans. We have seen far less success in containing the costs of services and care, which continue to outpace nearly all other segments of the economy.

The coming decades will no doubt involve more political positioning and renegotiation of the social contract between society, older adults, and family support. Action has already been taken to prolong the work life, and thus reduce the dependency, of the next generations of older adults. Cutbacks in Social Security benefits are being discussed seriously. Shifts in the dependency ratio make it unlikely that any expansion in public sector financing and services will take place. More and more, one hears arguments for increasing family responsibility for care of older family members, but this ignores demographic trends that predict a reduction in the availability of care to the family, to say nothing of the economic, emotional, and psychological costs associated with prolonged caregiving. We are likely to see significant growth in the private sector. How well a free-market approach to elder care would meet the needs of older adults and the medical and human goals of an aging society remains to be seen.

JAPAN

Japan has the most rapidly aging population in history and consequently faces challenges unlike any other developed country. Japan's older population stood at 12% in 1990, and is approaching 22% today. By 2020, the over-65 population of Japan will constitute about 28% of the population. By contrast, the U.S. over-65 population is projected to reach 19.6% of the total population in 2030.[36] Most of the projected increase in Japan will be among the oldest-old. This growth in the older population will be accompanied by declines in the working-age population as well as the young age groups that would give birth to children. Fertility decline, however, is more linked to forgone and delayed marriage than absolute declines in birth-eligible women. Concomitant changes in attitudes toward child rearing, expectations to rely on one's children in old age, and toward older adults themselves are also evident in this rapidly changing society.[37]

Favorable post–World War II fertility and mortality conditions helped transform Japan into an economic superpower in the course of a few decades. These demographic conditions also contributed to relatively high savings rates. Both government and personal savings are expected to decline in the near term, which will in turn, of course, affect public pensions and health care funding.[37]

Population aging also slows labor force growth, a decline that has already begun. Participation in the labor force among older adults in Japan is actually considerably higher than it is in other developed nations; among men more than double that in the United States, for example. It is unlikely, therefore, that policies directed at lengthening life span workforce participation will yield further gains. Changes in marginal and social security tax rates could increase women's participation, though there is little evidence of movement in that direction.[37]

Japan has a publicly financed social insurance health care system. About 80% of health care in Japan is provided in the private sector, with costs heavily controlled by the government. The entire population is served through five main medical plans. Premiums amount to 8% of a worker's earnings equally divided by employers and employees. Premiums are not sufficient to cover total costs and the government has subsidized health care since 1972. Costs are paid directly to doctors and hospitals, with patients making copayments of between 10% and 30%. Health care costs for older adults rose from 14% of total health care costs in 1975 to 31% in 1995 and will reach 50% within the next decade. By international standards Japanese health care is relatively cheap at 7% of GDP, as compared to 14% in the United States. This is mostly because of cost containment and does not represent full actual costs. Among the disadvantages reported by MacKellar and Horlacher are unavailability of cost-effective treatments such as joint replacements and longer average hospital stays compared to other developed nations.[37]

Reforms in Japanese health care provision for older adults date to 1990 with the introduction of the "Golden Plan." This plan was directed toward increasing the number of nursing home beds and providing home-based services, short-term stay facilities, and elder daycare centers. These services are provided at low or no cost to older adults and their families, though there is some evidence that they have been underutilized. One explanation for this slow use rate has been provided by Asai and Kameoka, who invoke the cultural concept of *Sekentei*.[38] *Sekentei* translates as "social appearance" and is an important concept that reflects Japanese social values. The ideal of filial piety and care of one's elders commonly invoked in discussion of Asian cultures represents a set of social values that has undergone considerable change over the last several generations. The value of familial piety common to Confucian philosophy is considerably less relevant to younger generations of Japanese. Japanese scholars have challenged the concept for some time, arguing that older adults are no longer inordinately respected by family members or generally in Japanese society.[39,40] The suicide rate among older Japanese is the second highest in the world and is higher among older adults living with children than those living alone.[38] Other studies have found that Americans report higher levels of perceived parental care obligations compared to Japanese.[41,42] The concept of *Sekentei*, as used by Asai and Kameka, also translated as social pressure, results in a conflicted sense of shame in the use of nonfamily support services and thus may result in underutilization.

The Japanese pension system began as a fully funded arrangement but has gradually shifted to a pay-as-you-go system. It is a multitiered system consisting of a national flat beneficiary rate for all residents older than age 60, and a second tier employee pension that covers about 32 million private sector employees. There are also private corporation pension funds covering about 12 million workers. The beneficiary-to-worker ratio (or dependency ratio) within each of these systems is increasing markedly. Everyone between the ages of 20 and 59 contributes to the National Pension System. Pension reforms occurred in 1973, 1986, and 1994 and have variously increased pension levels, increased contribution rates, required mandatory coverage of employees' spouses, and imposed a minimum number of years of contribution for eligibility. Benefit formulas have been revised to discourage early retirement. The 1994 reforms raised the minimum eligibility age for the National Pension System from 60 to 65 to ensure that there would be sufficient reserves at the time of peak population aging.[37]

Additional reforms have been proposed and are under consideration including linking benefits to life expectancy, indexing pensions to real wages, linking the real incomes of beneficiaries to the real income of contributors (similar to Swedish proposals), and further raising eligibility to 67.

At the present time, pension payments account for about 70% of the income of older households, and about 50% of older Japanese rely exclusively on the public pension system. In the current arrangement younger Japanese (born after 1950), unlike their parents, will contribute more to the pension system than they will receive in benefits, likely adding additional pressure to reform efforts.[37]

SWEDEN

In many respects, it is not possible to fairly compare Sweden with the United States. With 8.5 million people and a land mass equivalent to a midsized U.S. state, Sweden offers a very different model of elder care based on very different social and political philosophies. Sweden, therefore, is being offered in contrast to the United States to present an alternative approach. Whether it is one that the United States can or should emulate is a question that goes beyond the purpose of this chapter. The other feature that makes Sweden a fascinating example is that, like Japan, it is ahead of the United States, as well as most of the rest of the world, in the aging of its population. Almost 18% of Sweden's population is older than 65, compared with about 12.4% in the United States. Four percent are older than age 80.

Sweden has one of the highest life expectancies in the world, and like other developed countries, its old-old population is the fastest growing segment. Much of Sweden's policy covering older adults is not age specific. In 1982, Sweden passed its Social Services Act, which provided municipal social services to all persons who needed them regardless of age. In the passage of this act, access to social services was established as a right of all Swedish citizens. The explicit goals of the act were to sustain self-determination and normalization by allowing for maximum choice and supporting the individual in remaining in his or her normal environment. The Health and Medical Services Act was passed in 1983 and provides health care and services to all members of society. Like social services, medical care and services are nearly all in the public sector. These publicly supported services available to all are supported through a tax system at the rate of about one-half of a working person's income. Approximately one-third of public expenditures goes to social insurance and social welfare programs. Of this expenditure, approximately 40% is used for various forms of old age support and care, mostly pensions and housing. There is widespread public opinion support for these policies in Sweden.[43]

Despite this generous public sector support directed toward independent living, Sweden does not differ from the United States in the proportion of its older adults who are institutionalized. It stands at about 5–6% of those older than 65 at any given time, with lifelong chances of being institutionalized being about 25–30%. The pattern of institutionalization for older adults, however, does differ somewhat. Generally, the older person is more likely to have a short-term stay in an institution and return home, possibly going back and forth several times. Trends are also for these stays to occur among the very old, near the end of life, and for shorter periods of time. The official policy goal is to keep people in their own homes to as great an extent as possible. The result has been that more are spending their final days in institutions but for a shorter time and at older ages. Also, as in the United States, Swedes' chances of spending time in an old-age home or nursing home are greater if they have no family.[43]

Sweden has one of the highest proportions of older adults who live independently. Estimates are that about 46% of Swedes older than 70 live alone. In Stockholm, 7 of 10 women older than 80 live alone. These rates are among the highest in the world. About 15% of older adults receives regular "Home Help" services. The trend in recent years has been toward more services being provided to fewer clients among the old-old. These services include cleaning, cooking, washing, and personal hygiene. The client pays a copayment of 5–10%, with the balance publicly subsidized.[41] The services are need-based, and the overall effect has been to reduce differences in use across classes. Studies have demonstrated that when health is controlled for, class differences in use disappear.[43]

Subsidized community-based services not subject to needs assessments include municipal transport services, food services, home-delivered meals, hairdressing, snow cleaning services, and district daycare centers. Most of these services are used by less than 10% of the elderly population.[43]

Studies of the Nordic countries generally find a ratio of formal caregivers to family caregivers of between 1:4 to 1:3. In Sweden, it is estimated that family and friends provide about two-thirds of all care.[43] Sweden's population is continuing to age and need will grow. It is unlikely that the public sector will expand any further. Sundstrom and Thorslund anticipate that the increased need will be met by a combination of increased family support and growth in private sector alternatives that, up until now, have not been common in Sweden.[43]

The Swedish pension system offers an intriguing model for other developed nations to consider. Pension contributions are made by the central government at a rate of 18.5% (in some cases based on pension credits awarded for such things as years spent on child care, national service, or studies), employers at a rate of 10.21%, and employees or the insured at a rate of 7%. Pension contributions are recorded on an ongoing basis in the bank books of the insured, but withdrawals are blocked until the age of retirement at 61. Savings accumulate with interest. Once retired, payment is reversed and disbursed to the insured for the remainder of their lives. Another feature of the system is that payment balances are affected by the survival rates of the cohort. That is, the pension balances of deceased members of the cohort, based on life expectancies, are added to the balances of surviving members of the cohort increasing payments. Pensions, therefore, are based on pension credits, accumulated interest, and these so-called inheritance gains. Annually, Swedish citizens receive a statement allowing them to track growth year to year.[44]

THE DEVELOPING WORLD

The expansion of the older population is a worldwide phenomenon, and the greatest increases by far will be in the developing world. The challenges this represents to societies in the developing world are compounded by the short time frame in which these changes will take place. For example, Guatemala, Singapore, Mexico, the Philippines, and Indonesia will all experience a tripling in the proportion of their older populations between the years 1985 and 2025. By comparison, growth in the United States in those years is estimated at 105%; in Canada, 135%; and in Sweden, only 21%.[44] In the next century,

China will age faster than any other country. Official policy in China has led to sharp reductions in birth rates, which, if continued into the next century, could result in a population that is 40% elderly.[45]

So, although the entire world is experiencing a shift in the **age composition** of its population, this is happening at very uneven rates. Currently, western Europe, North America, and developed countries in other parts of the world are the oldest countries with respect to age composition and will be aging at a relatively slow rate in the years to come. The developing world is very young in this sense, with Guatemala, for example, currently having fewer than one-fifth the proportion of older people in its population as Sweden. In addition to this rapid rate of increase, developing countries will face the challenges of aging while still dealing with all of the attendant problems of economic, social, and political development. The rapid aging apparent in these countries is, in fact, a result of past successes in the area of nutrition, vaccinations, and sanitation. Life expectancies in developing countries have increased from an average of about 40 years in the 1950s to almost 62 years in 1990.[46] The world population of persons older than 65 increases by 800,000 each month. Seventy percent of these older adults are in developing countries.[46]

It is not clear how the old will be provided for in many countries. Old-age pensions are not common in the developing world. In China, for example, only 10% of the workforce have pensions; in India, only 8%.[46] As economic development accelerates, traditional family patterns of care are likely to be disrupted. With urbanization, younger people move to the cities, often leaving older adults alone in villages and rural areas and without support.

In the developing world, health care provisions and expenditures are a fraction of those in the developed countries. According to World Bank figures, the U.S. per capita spending on health in 1990 was $2,763. By comparison, in Latin America, it averaged $105. In the world's poorest countries the average was $16.[46] As the populations of developing countries age, they will experience what demographers have referred to as the "epidemiologic transition" to the kinds of diseases and chronic conditions common to older age groups. This will occur while these countries are still grappling with infectious disease patterns common in younger age groups and developing countries. Hospitals, already available to only a fraction of the populations in these countries, may be overwhelmed with admissions, or demand for admissions, for cancers and cardiopulmonary diseases. Competition for resources could result in sharp class differences and age-based inequities.

Some of the wealthier countries in the developing world are initiating economic programs to reduce some of these problems. Taiwan, for example, has initiated a national health insurance system. Some Asian and Latin American countries have begun to look at mandatory pensions and savings plans.[46] But these sorts of reforms are still the exceptions rather than the rule. The more likely immediate solutions will be family and community based and emphasize low-tech, low-cost efforts to as great an extent as possible.

SUMMARY

Much has been said in this chapter about the way we might find the future as we grow older. Few of these claims are certainties. What is certain is that there will be many more older members of our society in the coming years, and the future cohorts of older adults will differ in significant ways from today's older adults. There are still gains to be made, although slight, in life expectancy, particularly among men. We can expect better overall health and greater independence. In the United States, the older adults of the future will be better educated as a group and, perhaps to an unprecedented extent, actively engaged in ongoing educational pursuits and community activities through both paid and unpaid work for longer periods of time. Despite this generally optimistic portrayal, the United States cannot afford to lose sight of the fact of heterogeneity in old age. This includes both a healthy diversity and a concern that aging is a very different experience for historically marginalized subgroups within the population. The aging population often magnifies the cumulative effects of inequality and inequity that have spanned lifetimes.

The major challenges facing our aging population in the future are the perennial concerns of today: care for those who cannot care for themselves, and the resources necessary for all persons to live their lives with dignity. These concerns will grow commensurate with the growth in the older population. To address these problems effectively, it is essential that they be reframed as shared national concerns, not as the problems of older adults. Younger generations, who must share the burden of growing costs and care, must be convinced that older adults merit their concern and their support and be assured that the same support systems and mechanisms will be there for them when they are old. This attitude toward the older adults of our society and confidence in the future are undermined by the divisive pitting of generations against one another in a falsely constructed zero-sum game. Such constructions must be rejected by an educated voting populace.

In terms of both age composition and ability to address the problems of aging, the United States finds itself on a middle ground relative to other nations of the world. Sweden was discussed as an example of an advanced and comprehensive system of care provision for one of the oldest populations in the world. Sweden's solutions, however, are not necessarily a good fit for the United States. Japan, as a result of the continuing rapid growth among older adults, is on a shorter timeline for solutions than is either Sweden or the United States. Issues of health care financing, pension reform, and public policy will continue to be acute in Japan for some time to come. In the upcoming years, the United States will be confronted with political and economic challenges in this arena that are unprecedented here. Effective policy formation and decision making will test our economic and political systems in unexpected ways. Solutions will call for creativity and probably the willingness to break with past patterns and expectations. Patterns of work, leisure, caregiving, and collective actions may all take forms not commonly practiced today. The uneven rates of change throughout the world will be one more strand in the complex web that draws us further into a global economy and worldwide network of associations. Just as the United Nations Children's Fund (UNICEF) was a global response to the needs of the world's children, there may also be the need for global responses to the concerns and problems of rapidly aging populations at a high risk for dependency.

Despite the uncertainties, the opportunity to live long, productive, and fully engaged lives in the United States is probably greater now than ever before. As aging becomes a more visible national phenomenon and more central to the national fabric, older adults will more often come to be seen as involved in all important aspects of public and private life. Attitudes among younger generations may well become more age-blind. We may become more adept at determining when and where age itself is or should be the significant criteria for sorting people into categories. What are age-related problems versus simply problems with living? When are age-based solutions called for versus need-based solutions? In what ways are the old and young alike rather than different? What do we share in common? These questions have not been prominent in the discussion thus far. They could mark a productive starting point for confronting some of the challenges that face us.

Review Questions

1. For future older Americans, family caregivers will
   A. Be more available to assist with care than they are today
   B. Be less available than they are today because of decreasing family size
   C. Be less available than they are today because of a declining willingness to help
   D. Be more inclined to provide financial support but not actual care

2. The number one reason older adults give for obtaining additional education is
   A. Boredom
   B. To socialize with younger people
   C. Life transitions
   D. Low cost

3. The most common reason older adults give for volunteering is
   A. To fill time
   B. To stay involved
   C. To meet new and interesting people
   D. Self-esteem

4. Recent trends suggest that older workers and retired persons are
   A. More interested in continued work than in the past
   B. Less interested in continued work than in the past
   C. More likely to be absent from work as a result of illness
   D. Less collegial and cooperative than younger workers

5. Childhood poverty in the United States
   A. Has been eliminated in the 1990s
   B. Has increased because of the growing older population
   C. Is restricted to rural areas
   D. Is caused primarily by market forces and the problems of young adults

6. In economic terms, older adults today are
   A. Better off than they were 30 years ago
   B. Much worse off than they were 30 years ago
   C. The same as 30 years ago
   D. All quite wealthy

7. The proportion of care for frail older adults that is provided by families is estimated to be about
   A. 10% of all care provided
   B. 25% of all care provided
   C. 50% of all care provided
   D. 80% of all care provided

8. According to Olson, the majority of nursing homes in the United States
   A. Are clean, safe, and well managed
   B. Are going to grow in number as the older population grows
   C. Do not meet the basic needs of older adults
   D. Are inexpensive and accessible

9. Worldwide, future growth in older populations is most dramatic in
   A. The United States and Canada
   B. Sweden and the Scandinavian countries
   C. The most industrialized countries
   D. The developing countries

10. Compared with the United States, care for older adults in Sweden has support from the public sector (government) to what extent?
    A. Greater
    B. Lesser
    C. About the same
    D. Almost none

Learning Activities

1. Discuss ways in which corporations could design work schedules to better serve their older employees. Discuss possible contributions older workers can offer their employers.
2. Describe potential models for work-to-retirement transition in the next century.

3. Develop a curriculum for an elder college. In addition to possible course offerings and student services, design a physical environment suitable for these older students.
4. Describe challenges faced by developing countries in caring for these growing older populations.
5. Discuss ways to achieve intergenerational harmony. What can the young offer the old and vice versa?
6. Interview three middle-aged individuals about what future concerns they have as they become older adults in an ever-aging society.

REFERENCES

1. Federal Interagency Forum on Aging–Related Statistics. *Older Americans 2008: Key Indicators of Well-Being. Federal Interagency Forum on Aging-Related Statistics.* Washington, DC: U.S. Government Printing Office; March 2008.
2. Perls, TT. The Oldest Old. *Scientific American,* 1995;10:70.
3. Kart, CS. *The Realities of Aging: An Introduction to Gerontology.* 5th ed. Boston: Allyn & Bacon; 1997:53.
4. Spencer, G. *What Are the Demographic Implications of an Aging US Population from 1990 to 2030?.* Washington, DC: American Association of Retired Persons and Resources for the Future; 1993:8.
5. Rupert, P. Contingent Work Options: Promise or Peril for Older Workers. In *Resourceful Aging: Today and Tomorrow, Conference Proceedings,* 1991;IV:51.
6. Patten, CW. Second Careers: New Challenges, New Opportunities. In *Resourceful Aging: Today and Tomorrow, Conference Proceedings,* 1991; IV:47.
7. Gamse, DN. Work and Second Careers: Executive Summary and Commentary. In *Resourceful Aging: Today and Tomorrow, Conference Proceedings,* 1991;IV:9.
8. Munnell, AH. *Policies to Promote Labor Force Participation in Older People.* Chestnut Hill, MA: Center for Retirement Research at Boston University; January 2006.
9. Munnell, AH, Sass, S. W*orking Longer: The Solution to the Retirement Income Challenge.* Washington, DC: Brookings Institute Press; 2008.
10. Taylor, P. Older Workers and the Labor Market: Lessons from Abroad. *Generations,* Spring 2007.
11. Roper, ASW. *Baby Boomers Envision Retirement II: Key Findings.* Washington, DC: AARP; 2004. Retrieved February 13, 2008, from http://assets. aarp.org/rgcenter/econ/boomers_envision_1.pdf
12. Feldman, NS. Lifelong Education: The Challenge of Change. In *Resourceful Aging: Today and Tomorrow, Conference Proceedings,* 1991;IV:17.
13. Aslanian, CB. Adult Learning and Life Transitions. In *Resourceful Aging: Today and Tomorrow, Conference Proceedings,* 1991;V:45.
14. Wilson, J. Volunteering. *Annual Review of Sociology,* 2000;26:215–240.
15. Harootyan, RA. Volunteer Activity by Older Adults. In JE Birren (ed.), *Encyclopedia of Gerontology: Age, Aging, and the Aged.* San Diego, CA: Academic Press; 2006: vol. 2, pp. 613–620.
16. Rozario, PA. Volunteering Among Current Cohorts of Older Adults and Baby Boomers. *Generations,* Winter 2006–2007.
17. Warburton, J, Terry, D, Rosenman, L, Shapira, M. Difference Between Older Volunteers and Non-Volunteers: Attitudinal, Normative, and Control Beliefs. *Research on Aging,* 2001;23: 586–605.
18. Clary, EG, Snyder, M. The Motivations to Volunteer: Theoretical and Practical Considerations. *Current Directions in Psychological Science,* 1999; 8:156–159.
19. Okun, MA, Schultz, A. Age and Motives for Volunteering: Testing Hypotheses Derived from Socioemotional Selectivity Theory. *Psychology and Aging,* 2003;18(2):231–239.

20. Costello, CB. Resourceful Aging: Mobilizing Older Citizens for Volunteer Service. In *Resourceful Aging: Today and Tomorrow, Conference Proceedings*, 1991;II:15.

21. Thompson, E, Wilson, L. The Potential of Older Volunteers in Long-Term Care. *Generations*, Spring 2001.

22. Gomperts, JS. Toward a Bold New Policy Agenda: Five Ideas to Advance Civic Engagement Opportunities for Older Americans. *Generations*, Winter 2006–2007.

23. Cornman, JM, Kingston, ER. Trends, Issues, Perspectives, and Values for the Aging of the Baby Boom Cohorts. *The Gerontologist*, 1996; 36:15.

24. Minkler, M. Generational Equity and the Public Policy Debate: Quagmire or Opportunity? In P Homer, M Holstein (eds.), *A Good Old Age*. New York: Simon and Schuster; 1990:222.

25. Blackburn, R. Age Shock: How Finance Is Failing Us. *Verso*, 2006;236–242.

26. Anrig, G. *The Conservatives Have No Clothes: Why Right-Wing Ideas Keep Failing*. New York: John Wiley and Sons; 2007:206–229.

27. Stoller, EP, Gibson, RC. Advantages of Using the Life Course Perspective. In EP Stoller, RC Gibson (eds.), *Worlds of Difference: Inequality in the Aging Experience*. Thousand Oaks, CA: Forge Press; 1994:3.

28. Olson, LK. Public Policy and Privatization: Long-Term Care in the United States. In LK Olson (ed.), *The Graying of the World: Who Will Care for the Frail Elderly?* New York: Haworth Press; 1994:25.

29. Kane, RL, Kane, R. *Long-Term Care in Six Countries: Implications for the United States*. Washington, DC: Department of Health, Education, and Welfare; 1976.

30. National Alliance for Caregiving and AARP. *Caregiving in the U.S.* New York: MetLife Foundation; April 2004.

31. Caro, FG. Relieving Informal Caregiver Burden Through Organized Services. In KA Pillemer, RS Wolf (eds.), *Elder Abuse: Conflicts in the Family*. Dover, MA: Auburn House Publishing; 1986:283.

32. Edelman, P, Hughs, S. The Impact of Community Care on Homebound Elderly Persons. *Gerontology*, 1990;2:570.

33. Pepper Commission, U.S. Bipartisan Commission on Comprehensive Health Care. *A Call for Action: Final Report*. Washington, DC: U.S. Government Printing Office; 1990.

34. Stephens, SA, Christian, TB. *Informal Care of the Elderly*. Lexington, MA: Lexington Books; 1986.

35. Cantor, MH. Family and Community: Changing Roles in an Aging Society. *The Gerontologist*, 1991;31:337.

36. U.S. Census Bureau. U.S. Interim Projection by Age, Sex, Race, and Hispanic Origin: 2000–2050. Washington, DC: Author; 2004.

37. MacKellar, L, Horlacher, D. Population Ageing in Japan: A Brief Survey. *Innovation*, 2000; 13(4):413–430.

38. Asai, MO, Kameoka, VA. The Influence of *Sekentei* on Family Caregiving and Underutilization of Social Services Among Japanese Caregivers. *Social Work*, 2005;50(2):111–118.

39. Hirayama, H. Public Policies and Services for the Aged in Japan. In R Dobrof (ed.), *Ethnicity and Gerontological Social Work*. New York: Haworth Press; 1987:39–51.

40. Kumagai, F. *Unmasking Japan Today: The Impact of Traditional Values on Modern Japanese Society*. Westport, CT: Praeger; 1996.

41. Maeda, D, Sussman, MB. Young Adults' Perceptions of the Elderly and Responsibility of Caring for the Aged Parents. *Shakai Ronen Gaku*, 1980;12:29–40.

42. Hashizume, Y. Salient Factors That Influence the Meaning of Family Caregiving for Frail Elderly Parents in Japan from a Historical Perspective. *Scholarly Inquiry for Nursing Practice: An International Journal*, 1995;12:123–134.

43. Sundstrom, G, Thorslund, M. Caring for the Frail Elderly in Sweden. In JK Olson (ed.), *The Graying of the World: Who Will Care for the Frail Elderly?* New York: Haworth Press; 1994:59.

44. Swedish Social Insurance Agency (SSIA). *Orange Report: Annual Report of the Swedish Pension System, 2006*. Stockholm: SSIA. 2006.

45. Cockerham, WC. *This Aging Society*. Englewood Cliffs, NJ: Prentice Hall; 1991:35.

46. Holden, C. New Populations of Old Add to Poor Nations' Burden. *Science*, 1996;273:46.

Chapter 13

THE LAST WORD: HEALTH LITERACY AND CLEAR HEALTH COMMUNICATION

TEACHING AND WRITING SO OLDER ADULTS UNDERSTAND

SUE STABLEFORD, MPH, MSB

Chapter Outline

Behavioral Objectives

Upon completion of this chapter, the reader will be able to:

1. Compare the reading level of health materials with the reading abilities of the majority of older adults, and discuss the mismatch or gap between them.
2. Define the terms *literacy* and *health literacy*.
3. Describe the health literacy skills of older adults according to their performance on the 2003 National Assessment of Adult Literacy as well as according to other research studies.
4. Describe the impact of older adults' limited health literacy skills on their health and on the health care delivery system.
5. List six plain language standards for verbal patient teaching.
6. List five to ten plain language standards for written information.
7. Discuss the impact that plain language and clear health communication could have if effectively implemented across health care delivery systems.

Key Terms

Chronic condition

Health literacy

Health Resources and Services
  Administration

The Joint Commission

Limited literacy skills

Literacy

Plain language

Plain language standards

Osteoarthritis

Reading levels

Sensory deficits

Shame-free environment

Teach-back

A PATIENT'S EXPERIENCE OF HEALTH COMMUNICATION

Meet Marjorie. She is 78 years old and lives independently in the same town as her daughter and grandchildren. She has **osteoarthritis**, which makes it a little hard for her to get around. At a recent medical visit, her doctor noticed that she was somewhat depressed and prescribed an antidepressant. When the office nurse called to see how she was doing, Marjorie was upset. Here is what she told the nurse.

> I don't know why the doctor thought I should take pills. I'm not crazy, you know. He asked me some questions about how I've been feeling and I told him. It's hard to get old and not be able to do all the things I used to be able to do. Sometimes I have trouble sleeping. And, I get lonely, especially when my daughter is too busy to come over and visit. The doctor said I'm depressed, but I don't understand how taking a pill will help. He gave me a pamphlet to read about it, but the print was so small and it was so complicated that I gave up.

PATIENT/CONSUMER COMMUNICATION: THE GAP BETWEEN HIGH LEVELS OF INFORMATION AND THE LIMITED LITERACY SKILLS OF AMERICAN ADULTS

Marjorie's experience is not unusual. Many, if not most, older adults have trouble understanding both verbal and written health communication. Sometimes this is because of **sensory deficits** in vision or hearing. Sometimes stress and anxiety are so high that it is impossible to listen or read with understanding. And sometimes communication fails because health professionals communicate at such high levels, both verbally and in writing—way beyond the abilities of most adults to understand.

Hundreds of research studies have documented the high **reading levels** of most health and medical information—typically high school and college level.[1] At the same time, researchers for the U.S. Department of Education have shown in two national adult **literacy** surveys (1992 and 2003) that most adults cannot read at these levels. On the most recent survey conducted in 2003, compared to other age groups, "Adults ages 65 and older had the lowest average prose, document, and quantitative literacy."[2]

On the **health literacy** section of that 2003 survey, older adults again scored the lowest of all age groups. About 60% had *below basic* or *basic* health literacy skills. Yet, one of the literacy tasks labeled as *intermediate* was this: "Determine what time a person can take a prescription medication, based on information on the prescription drug label that relates the timing of medication to eating."[3] Essentially, this means that a majority of older adults, lacking an intermediate level of health literacy skills, cannot read, understand, and use this type of medication label. Yet, this age group takes the most medications!

In this electronic age, you might think that "print is dead" and that the Internet is the major source of health information. For working-age adults, this can be true. According to Pew Internet surveys, about 75% of American adults go online and about 80% have searched for health information.[4] However, studies show that Web-based health information is usually at the same high reading level as print materials.[5] Studies also show that older adults are far less likely to go online or look for health information on the Web.

Finally, what happens when health care providers teach patients verbally? Patients again often struggle to understand, especially when time is rushed and much information is given quickly.

EXPANDING UNDERSTANDING: THE CONTEXT OF HEALTH LITERACY

Health literacy means using literacy skills—reading, writing, speaking, and computing (math)—in a health context. This context is, for many, like visiting a foreign country where they do not know the language or the customs.

Health literacy challenges include: (1) having the specialized vocabulary, knowledge, and skills to manage one's own health; (2) using multiple information formats in multiple locations to accomplish multiple tasks (e.g., reading food labels in the supermarket, medicine instructions at the pharmacy, safety regulations at work, consent forms in the hospital); (3) mastering the arcane American health insurance and health delivery systems; and simultaneously, (4) overcoming high levels of stress and anxiety associated with health decision making.

Viewed this way, it is likely that few adults have fully adequate health literacy skills. If an adult does not speak fluent English or does not know or accept the assumptions of Western medicine, understanding is further compromised. Health literacy challenges everyone, albeit in varying circumstances and to varying degrees. Older adults are an especially high-risk group.

LITERACY AND HEALTH LITERACY SKILLS: MAJOR KEYS TO GOOD HEALTH

Research studies conducted over the past 15 years have highlighted the huge impact of **limited literacy skills** on health and health outcomes.[1] One study of more than 3,000 older adults enrolled in a Medicare managed care plan (Prudential) provides rich data regarding the literacy skills of older adults and the relationship of limited literacy to health. In a series of publications, study collaborators shared these conclusions:

- Older adults with inadequate health literacy often misread simple prescription instructions, information about the results of blood sugar tests, and other vital health care information.
- Literacy and health literacy skills decline with age.
- Inadequate health literacy is independently associated with greater risk of hospital admission, lower use of preventive health services such as flu and pneumonia shots, poorer physical and mental health, and higher all-cause mortality.[6-11]

THE ROLE OF HEALTH LITERACY IN PATIENT SAFETY AND PATIENT-CENTERED CARE

Beyond the impact of literacy on individual patients is an overall impact on the health care system. Major national groups are speaking out about the problem.

The Joint Commission, which accredits hospitals around the country, points out in a report, "The typical informed consent form is unreadable for any level of reader." Further, it notes that communication failures are the underlying root cause of 65% of *sentinel events*—instances of serious patient harm. They urge hospitals to make effective communications a priority to protect patient safety.[12]

The American Medical Association has played a leading role in alerting physicians and other care providers about the health literacy problem and in supporting solutions. It is one of just a few health professions to publish a policy statement as well as reports and tools to address the issue.[13-15]

The federal government has also issued relevant policies—requiring linguistic access, culturally competent care, and public information written in **plain language**.* The **Health Resources and Services Administration** (HRSA) offers a freely accessible online training program titled *Addressing Health Literacy, Cultural Competency, and Limited English Proficiency*, linking these closely related issues.[16]

CLEAR HEALTH COMMUNICATION: AN OFTEN OVERLOOKED NECESSITY

Despite the research studies and policy pronouncements, which are just a few of many examples, public health and health care organizations often treat communication as an afterthought. Other issues command priority attention. Or it is assumed that adults working in health disciplines know how to speak, teach, and write well enough to get

---

* See www.PlainLanguage.gov for the plain language administrative order (first issued during the presidency of Bill Clinton and reaffirmed by the Bush administration) and www.omhrc.gov for Cultural and Linguistic Access standards.

their points across. As Marjorie's experience as well as research studies show, however, although clear communication is essential to good health outcomes, it does not happen automatically.

A large and only partially answered question is how to best communicate, both verbally and in writing, so that patients/consumers do understand critical health information. What are the best solutions? What works to increase the ability of patients/consumers to obtain, process, and use health and medical information?

Researchers have some partial answers, although much remains to be learned. One major national research review, completed in 2004, notes that we still have more questions than answers.[17] Research *has* shown that using specific patient teaching techniques such as "teach-back" and certain plain language writing techniques increases the likelihood that adults will understand and use health information.[18–20]

The organizations that have drawn national attention to this problem—The Joint Commission, the American Medical Association, the federal government, and others—have proposed similar solutions. The Joint Commission report contains 35 specific recommendations for improving communication in hospitals and across the continuum of care. Major emphasis includes teaching and writing in plain language.[12] Similarly, the AMA report, *Help Patients Understand*, states: "Providers should use clear communication skills, techniques and practices for interpersonal communication with *all* patients, not just those with limited literacy."[15] And the federal government devotes multiple websites to teaching employees and others how to communicate effectively in plain language.[21]

WHAT IS PLAIN LANGUAGE? HOW WILL I KNOW IT IF I *HEAR* IT?

Here are the six verbal communication tips that the AMA recommends that all physicians adopt to improve patient understanding.[22] (The author provides additional comments.)

1. *Slow down.* This is especially important to help older adults who may have hearing loss and who do not mentally process information as rapidly as when they were younger.
2. *Use plain, nonmedical language.* Another way to say this is to use everyday language or conversational language. Pretend you are talking with a relative or neighbor. Our usual spoken language is far simpler than formal communication.
3. *Show or draw pictures.* This is helpful in written materials as well. We know from research that pictures help older adults learn and remember information.[23]
4. *Limit the amount of information and repeat it.* This means prioritizing information to the 3–5 most important points. Most adults can remember only three things from a health care visit.
5. *Use the teach-back technique.* This means, have patients state what they understand they are to do. So, a provider might say something such as: "Ms. Smith, how will you explain this to your family when you get home?" This gives the provider a chance to learn what the patient understands and to fill in or repeat missing information.

6. *Create a **shame-free environment**: Encourage questions.* Some providers say: "*What* questions do you have" instead of the more common "*Do* you have any questions." By asking what questions, it is assumed that the adult has some and can feel safe asking them.

Two additional tips also help older adults learn more effectively from health care visits:

1. *Frame the conversation first.* This means, tell the adult what you will be talking about before launching into the discussion. This helps prepare him or her to listen and hear information with understanding.
2. *Encourage older adults to bring a friend or family member to the visit.* Another set of eyes and ears, or someone to actually take notes, can help the patient remember what to do at home.

If some of these techniques were used with Marjorie, how might the result have been different? If the doctor had used **teach-back**, he would have learned that Marjorie did not understand the diagnosis (depression) and did not agree with the treatment plan (medication). They could possibly have arranged an alternative plan that suited Marjorie better. If she had brought her daughter or a friend to the visit, they could have talked about it together later, and further understanding could have occurred.

WHAT IS PLAIN LANGUAGE? HOW WILL I KNOW IT IF I *SEE* IT?

The patient, Marjorie, also had trouble reading the information about depression that her doctor gave her. This is not surprising, given the high reading levels of most health and medical information. Although plain language is not a total solution to a complex problem, it is a great start at creating more accessible print and Web-based materials. Plain language principles also apply to designing information for other media, such as DVDs. Many groups publish **plain language standards**, including the National Institute on Aging. Their publication, *Making Your Printed Health Materials Senior Friendly*, is available online and in print.[24] Multiple expert groups agree that print and Web-based information should meet these minimum requirements.

- *Content*: Information is accurate, up-to-date, and limited. Focus is on behavior—what the reader needs to *do*. The average reader can use and remember no more than about five major points at one time. If a topic is complex, such as managing depression, break it up into smaller sections so that an adult can read small amounts at a time.
- *Structure/organization*: Structure and organize information from the user's perspective. This means putting the most important information first and creating small chunks with good headers or subtitles. Some readers read just the subtitles, so headings really need to convey key points. Health writers typically lead off with explanations about

anatomy or descriptions about how many people have a certain problem. Plain language reverses this and begins with clear action messages. The background information comes later because it is less critical.

- *Writing style*: As noted earlier, most adults best understand everyday language. These are typically short words (1 or 2 syllables) common in spoken language. When medical terms are used, such as the name of a condition, a pronunciation should be given and the term explained. Sentences should also be short, about 12–15 words on average. Use mostly active voice, a positive tone, and concrete examples. For example, instead of writing about regular exercise, write about walking most days of the week for at least one-half hour.

- *Appearance and appeal*: The first few seconds that an adult looks at a piece creates a lasting impression. So, we need to make sure our print materials and websites are attractive, inviting, and look easy to read. This almost always means plenty of white space, not a page crammed full of print. The size of the print needs to be large enough for reading ease (usually about 13- or 14-point typeface for older adults) and the print/paper contrast should be sharp with dark print and light paper. Limit the use of fancy typefaces, underlining, and other visual tricks. Use appropriate pictures to humanize materials and show adults how to do recommended action steps.

Many organizations publish plain language guides and checklists that are easy to access online. Try using them when you are creating easier-to-read information.[25–27] One of the best-kept secrets about plain language is that it takes practice to write simply and clearly. One key to success is planning what you want to write (or say) before you sit in front of the computer and start writing. You must know both your audience and your purpose well. Ask yourself over and over: Who will use this? What do they need to know to take the action I am recommending? How can I suggest this in a way that is appropriate and compelling to the intended audience?

Showing what you have written to prospective users before you make many copies of it is also important. Be brave and ask for feedback and ways to make your material more clear. You will be surprised at what your trial readers do not understand and the great ideas they will offer to improve your piece.

PLAIN LANGUAGE COMMUNICATIONS

Will using plain language and other clear health communication techniques ensure that older adults can read, understand, and use the information? There is no one solution to the complex problem of communicating effectively with diverse patients and audiences. We do know from research in the fields of health education, reading, social marketing, and psychology that well-planned and simply written information can make a big difference in understanding.

But simply knowing what to do is not the same thing as doing it, and many factors can interfere with adults taking actions beneficial to their health. Understanding, however, is almost always the first step, whether in getting preventive vaccines, managing a **chronic condition**, preparing for a medical test, or following discharge and medication instructions.

Health care providers have a challenge and an opportunity to enrich their practice and the lives of patients. Health professionals must take the lead in learning effective communication techniques for both verbal and written information. Good health and health care are too complex, important, and costly for us to continue bumbling along with materials that are too hard to read and verbal teaching that patients can not remember and use. You can use the online resources and training programs listed in the references and attend workshops to learn more.

Consider how Marjorie's life might have been enhanced if she had better understood her physician's concern for her mental well-being and they had been able to talk about how to improve her quality of life. Marjorie may have agreed to try medication, or perhaps she would have chosen other therapies first. She would have better understood that depression does not mean she is "crazy" and that it is not a normal part of aging. There are millions of Marjories managing chronic conditions who will benefit from the care we take with our communication.

Review Questions

1. Each of the following can negatively affect an older person's ability to understand our communication *except*
   A. Sensory decline in vision or hearing due to aging
   B. Professional use of medical terms
   C. Limited adult literacy skills
   D. Printed information written at the sixth grade level

2. Which statement about older adults' literacy skills is true?
   A. Those over 65 scored the highest on the 2003 National Assessment of Adult Literacy.
   B. Literacy skills tend to increase with age because of practice.
   C. Limited literacy skills are associated with greater health risks.
   D. Literacy skills are not related to hospital admission rates.

3. Which of these national groups issued an important report implicating communication failures as the cause of the majority of serious harmful patient events?
   A. American Association of Allied Health Professionals
   B. American Surgical Nurses Association
   C. The Joint Commission
   D. The American Medical Association

4. Which of the following statements about written plain language is *true?*
   A. Plain language is too boring to be helpful in increasing understanding.
   B. Plain language is conversational, meaning that it is clear and simple.
   C. Plain language does not include paying attention to any elements beyond words.
   D. Plain language dumbs down important health care information and may not be 100% accurate.

5. _____ have been shown to increase the likelihood that adults will use vital health care information.
   A. Written materials
   B. Verbal instructions
   C. Medically based instructions
   D. Teach-back techniques

6. Framing the conversation refers to
   A. Summarizing the conversation at the end
   B. Giving an overview of the information before you begin
   C. Asking repeated questions throughout the conversation
   D. Relating the four main points of the conversation

7. In printed material, content should meet of all of the following requirements *except*
   A. Content should be limited
   B. Content should contain headings
   C. Content should contain lots of detail
   D. Content should use direct and active language

Learning Activities

1. View the American Medical Association video *Low Health Literacy: You Can't Tell By Looking* and discuss. (The video is online at http://www.ama-assn.org. Using the search engine, type in *health literacy*, and click on videos.) This multimedia program is a great kick-off to start building knowledge about literacy facts and how limited literacy affects patients in medical situations.
2. Download the handouts from the *Ask Me Three* program (available at http://www.npsf.org/askme3). Discuss how the handouts might promote patient–provider interaction.
3. View Web-based health programs for older adults at http://www.NIHSeniorHealth.gov. Experiment with the various "buttons" on the site to see how users can change settings to suit individual needs. Consider how this site meets guidelines for plain language and accommodates possible sensory deficits in users.
4. Complete a health literacy "audit" of a local health care facility, preferably a hospital. Use the audit tool designed by Rima Rudd (available at http://www.hsph.harvard.edu/healthliteracy). Or, choose selected elements from the tool and create a mini-audit tool that can be completed more easily.

5. Use the checklist in the audit tool above or one noted in references 25–27 of this chapter to evaluate health and medical materials for plain language. How well do the materials meet plain language guidelines?
6. Read and evaluate a key national report about health literacy. The executive summary of the Institute of Medicine report *Health Literacy: A Prescription to End Confusion* can be found at http://www.nap.edu/catalog.php?record_id=10883.
7. Look for research articles that link health literacy and your health occupation. A search in major databases will reveal at least a few articles published in most health fields, including nursing, physical therapy, nutrition, pharmacy, and medicine.
8. Complete the online training program sponsored by the Health Services and Resource Administration (HRSA) (available at http://www.train.org). Look for the course titled "Unified Health Communication: Addressing Health Literacy, Cultural Competency, and Limited English Proficiency." You must register for the course (online), which is free, and you can complete one unit at a time and print out the course handouts.
9. Try writing a one-page, easy-to-read information piece related to a specific issue in your field. If you have a clinical practicum and access to patients, ask some of them for suggestions of what to include and for feedback about your first draft. Practice using your piece for patient teaching along with the teach-back method.
10. Look up the Cultural and Linguistic Access Standards (CLAS). You can find them at http://www.omhrc.gov/templates/browse.aspx?lvl=2&lvlID=15. Discuss how they pertain to health care organizations.

REFERENCES

1. Nielsen-Bohlman, L, Panzer, A, Kindig, D (eds.). *Health Literacy: A Prescription to End Confusion.* Washington DC: National Academies Press; 2004.
2. Kutner, M, Greenberg, E, Jin, Y, Boyle, B, Hsu, Y, Dunleavy, E. *Literacy in Everyday Life: Results from the 2003 National Assessment of Adult Literacy.* (NCES 2007-480). U.S. Department of Education. Washington, DC: National Center for Education Statistics; April 2007: 27.
3. Kutner, M, Greenberg, E, Jin, Y, Paulsen, C. *The Health Literacy of America's Adults: Results from the 2003 National Assessment of Adult Literacy* (NCES 2006-483). U.S. Department of Education. Washington, DC: National Center for Education Statistics; 2006: 6.
4. Maddow, M, Rajnic, L. *America's Online Pursuits: The Changing Picture of Who's Online and What They Do.* Washington, DC: Pew/Internet Reports; 2003.
5. Berland, GK, et al. Health Information on the Internet: Accessibility, Quality, and Readability in English and Spanish. *JAMA,* 2001;285(20): 2612–2621.
6. Gazmararian, J, et al. Health Literacy Among Medicare Enrollees in a Managed Care Organization. *JAMA,* 1999;281(6)545–551.
7. Baker, D, Gazmararian, J, Sudano, J, Patterson, M. The Association Between Age and Health Literacy Among Elderly Persons. *Journals of Gerontology Series B: Psychological Sciences and Social Sciences,* 2000;55B(6):S368–S374.

8. Baker, D, et al. Functional Health Literacy and the Risk of Hospital Admission Among Medicare Managed Care Enrollees. *American Journal of Public Health*, 2002;92(8):1278–1283.

9. Scott, T, Gazmararian, J, Williams, M, Baker, D. Health Literacy and Preventive Health Care Use Among Medicare Enrollees in a Managed Care Organization. *Medical Care*, 2002;40(5): 395–404.

10. Wolf, M, Gazmararian, J, Baker, D. Health Literacy and Functional Health Status Among Older Adults. *Archives of Internal Medicine*, 2005;165:1946–1952.

11. Baker, D, et al. Health Literacy and Mortality Among Elderly Persons. *Archives of Internal Medicine*, 2007;167(14):1503–1509.

12. Joint Commission. *"What Did the Doctor Say?" Improving Health Literacy to Protect Patient Safety.* 2007. Access here: http://www.jointcommission. org/NR/rdonlyres/D5248B2E-E7E6-4121-8874-99C7B4888301/0/improving_health_ literacy.pdf.

13. Ad Hoc Committee on Health Literacy for the Council on Scientific Affairs, American Medical Association. Health Literacy: Report of the Council on Scientific Affairs. *JAMA*, 1999; 281(6):552–557.

14. American Medical Association. *Improving Communication—Improving Care. An Ethical Force Program Consensus Report.* Chicago: AMA Press; 2006: 114.

15. AMA Foundation. *Health Literacy and Patient Safety: Help Patients Understand. Reducing the Risk by Designing a Safer, Shame-Free Health Care Environment.* Chicago: AMA Foundation; 2007: 13.

16. U.S. Department of Health and Human Services, Health Resources and Services Administration. United Health Communication 101: Addressing Health Literacy, Cultural Competency, and Limited English Proficiency. Retrieved February 17, 2009, from http://www.hrsa.gov/ healthliteracy/training.htm.

17. RTI International–University of North Carolina Evidence-Based Practice Center, Research Triangle Park. *Literacy and Health Outcomes: Evidence Report/Technology Assessment Number 87.* Rockville, MD: Agency for Healthcare Research and Quality, U.S. Department of Health and Human Services; January 2004.

18. Schillinger, D, et al. Closing the Loop: Physician Communication with Diabetic Patients Who Have Low Health Literacy. *Archives of Internal Medicine*, 2003;163:83–90.

19. Davis, T, et al. Intervention to Increase Mammography Utilization in a Public Hospital. *Journal of General Internal Medicine*, 1998;13: 230–233.

20. DeWalt, D, et al. A Heart Failure Self-Management Program for Patients of All Literacy Levels: A Randomized, Controlled Trial. *BMC Health Services Research*, 2006;6(30).

21. U.S. Department of Health and Human Services, Office of Disease Prevention and Health Promotion. Health Communication Activities. Retrieved February 17, 2009, from http://www. health.gov/communication/.

22. Weiss, B. *Health Literacy and Patient Safety: Help Patients Understand. Manual for Clinicians.* 2nd ed. Chicago: AMA Foundation; 2007: 29.

23. Houts, P, Doak, C, Doak, L, Loscalzo, M. The Role of Pictures in Improving Health Communication: A Review of Research on Attention, Comprehension, Recall, and Adherence. *Patient Education and Counseling*, 2006;61:173–190.

24. National Institute on Aging. Making Your Printed Health Materials Senior Friendly. Retrieved February 17, 2009, from http://www.nia. nih.gov/HealthInformation/Publications/ srfriendly.htm.

25. Maximus, CKF. National Program Office. *The Health Literacy Style Manual.* Covering Kids and Families. 2005. Retrieved February 17, 2009, from http://coveringkidsandfamilies.org/ resources/docs/stylemanual.pdf.

26. Centers for Disease Control and Prevention. *Scientific and Technical Information Simply Put.* Atlanta, GA: Centers for Disease Control and Prevention; April 1999. Retrieved February 17, 2009, from http://www.cdc.gov/od/oc/simpput. pdf.

27. Plain Language Association International. Website. Retrieved February 17, 2009, from http://www.plainlanguagenetwork.org/.

EPILOGUE

At the end we reflect. A decade has passed since the first edition of *Gerontology for the Health Care Professional* was published. How has the world changed for older people in the last 10 years? On average, we have gained a few more years of life expectancy and, our hope is that the additional years of life will be quality-filled with engagement in valued activities. The world has certainly grown in complexity with ever more information at our fingertips, and many more older adults are becoming cyber savvy. Also, although ageist stereotypes are still prevalent—rearing their ugly heads and causing harm to life

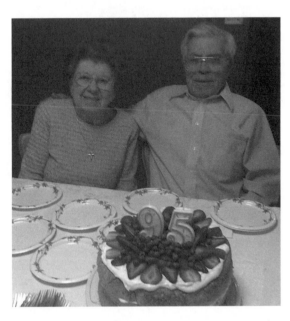

(Courtesy of Ann Altavilla and her grandparents)

quality in old age—perhaps, just perhaps and with optimistic anticipation, at least they are starting to be recognized for what they are—largely wrong.

Awareness is the first step toward eradication. It will be one fine day when we appreciate each life stage, perhaps especially those at the end of life. Once again, we hope that this book has done its share to dispel some of the myths of aging. Remember, resilience does *not* decrease with age. Time and again we are reminded of how such characteristics increase despite the multitudinous reasons (including age) we expect them to decline. Hold out hope for a better tomorrow and hope for "living life to its fullest" (as we say in occupational therapy).

Do not be surprised when the 95-year-old with multiple chronic conditions is eager to remain at or return to home. Someday this will no longer be the exception but the rule. Be sure to continue learning from these masters of life!

We enjoy hearing from our readers, so please let us know if you have any comments. Thank you for interest in gerontology and for taking the time to explore these issues of old age. This learning exercise will help you to become the very best health care practitioner you can be.

Regi Robnett, PhD, OTR/L, and Walter Chop, MS, RRT

ANSWERS TO REVIEW QUESTIONS

Chapter 1
1. B
2. E
3. B
4. C
5. D
6. B
7. C
8. C
9. B
10. D

Chapter 2
1. C
2. A
3. A
4. B
5. C
6. D
7. C
8. C
9. B
10. A
11. A
12. D
13. A
14. C

Chapter 3
1. C
2. C, B, F, A, H, E, D, G
3. A
4. C
5. D
6. E
7. B
8. B
9. B
10. B
11. E
12. D
13. B
14. A
15. B

Chapter 4
1. A
2. C
3. B
4. B
5. D
6. B
7. A
8. B
9. C
10. A
11. A
12. D

Chapter 5
1. B
2. D
3. C
4. A
5. C
6. C
7. C
8. D

Chapter 6
1. A
2. D
3. C
4. C
5. B
6. C
7. D
8. B
9. C
10. C

Chapter 7
1. C
2. C
3. C
4. A
5. A
6. D
7. B
8. B
9. D
10. B

Chapter 8
1. D
2. B
3. A
4. C
5. A
6. D
7. B
8. A
9. C
10. D
11. D
12. C

Chapter 9

1. C
2. A
3. A
4. D
5. B
6. B
7. C
8. C
9. C
10. A

Chapter 10

1. C
2. C
3. A
4. D
5. A
6. D
7. A
8. C
9. A
10. B
11. D
12. C

Chapter 11

1. B
2. A
3. A
4. D
5. C
6. C
7. A
8. C

Chapter 12

1. B
2. C
3. D
4. A
5. D
6. A
7. D
8. C
9. D
10. A

Chapter 13

1. D
2. C
3. C
4. B
5. D
6. B
7. C

GLOSSARY

A

Activities of daily living (ADLs): Normal everyday activities such as eating, sleeping, bathing, and toileting

Adaptation: Making accommodations to adjust to one's environment

Adherence: A therapeutic alliance or agreement between the patient and prescriber and the currently preferred term over the now outdated term *compliance*, which suggests the passive following of the prescriber's orders

Adult day services: Community-based group programs with specialized plans of care designed to meet the daytime needs of individuals with functional and/or cognitive impairments

Advance directives: In *advance* of something happening to the individual, he or she signs a written *directive* stating who should make decisions for him or her in the event of incapacity

Adverse drug reaction: An undesirable response associated with use of a drug that either compromises therapeutic efficacy, enhances toxicity, or both

Age cohort: Refers to a group or generation of elderly persons

Age-associated memory impairment (AAMI): The most common age-related cognitive decline that is associated with mild forgetfulness

Ageism: Based on stereotypes, myths about aging, and language that conjures up negative images of older adults

Agency on Aging: Community resource to assist older adults to connect with various services

Aging in place: The ability to continue to live in one's home safely, as independently as possible, and comfortably, regardless of age, income, or ability level. It means living in a familiar environment and being able to participate in family and other community activities

Agnosia: A decrease in perceptual skills, such as not understanding what common objects are used for

Alzheimer's disease (AD): A degenerative brain disease that is the most common form of dementia

Anemia: A decrease in hemoglobin level causing a lower than normal oxygen-carrying capacity of the blood

Aneurysm: Destruction of the inner layers of the artery wall that can cause a saclike enlargement that can weaken the arterial wall

Anhedonia: Difficulty experiencing pleasure doing formerly enjoyable activities

Anosmia: A complete loss of smell

Antacids: Drugs that reduce stomach acidity

Antidepressants: A class of drugs that combats depression

Anti-inflammatory: A class of drugs that decreases inflammation

Apraxia: The inability to carry out motor plans

Assisted living facility: Long-term residence option that provides resident-centered care in a residential setting. It is designed for those who need extra help in their day-to-day lives but who do not require 24-hour skilled nursing care

Atherosclerosis: The development of fatty plaques and the proliferation of connective tissue in the walls of arteries

Attention: Being able to focus or concentrate

Autoimmune disease: Diseases that are marked by the mistaken immunological destruction of the body's own cells. In such diseases, the body loses the ability to distinguish "self" from "non-self"

Average life expectancy: Mean length of life, usually differentiated by country

B

Baby boom generation: Those Americans born between 1946 and 1964

Beneficiary: The person to whom money or other value is distributed from a trust. The trust commonly names an immediate beneficiary and future beneficiaries

Benign prostatic hypertrophy (BPH): A benign enlargement of the prostate

Bereavement: A feeling of anguish at the death of a loved one

Biopsychosocial: Biological, psychological, and sociological factors associated with old age and aging

C

Carbohydrate: Carbohydrates are made up of one or more sugar molecules. They include bread, rice, grains, potatoes, sugar, and other like substances. Carbohydrates are classified as simple, which is made of fewer than three sugar molecules, and complex, which is made up of three or more sugar molecules

Caregiver: One who provides care for another. This usually involves caring for a family member

Cataract: An occurrence in which the eye becomes more opaque as its proteins become increasingly oxidized, glycosylated, and cross-linked

Cerebrovascular accident (CVA, or stroke): Infarction in the brain as a result of stenosis or occlusion of a blood vessel

Cholesterol: A waxy substance that is found in animal products and not in plant products. It is made by the human body and is necessary in making cell membranes, is a building block of some hormones, and is involved in the digestion of fats via bile

Chronic bronchitis: Common in older adults, especially in those with a long history of cigarette smoking. It is clinically defined as a chronic cough ("smoker's cough") productive of sputum, occurring on most days for at least 3 months' duration over at least 2 consecutive years

Chronic condition: A condition of long duration showing little or no improvement

Chronic obstructive pulmonary disease (COPD): Emphysema and/or chronic bronchitis

Cognition: Involves thinking, learning, and memory

Cognitive behavior therapy (CBT): A behavioral psychotherapy that emphasizes the importance of thinking about what we do and how we perceive ourselves

Cohousing: A type of collaborative housing in which residents actively participate in the design and operation of their own neighborhoods

Community spouse resource allowance (CSRA): An allowance of up to $104,400 for those who are receiving Medicaid in a nursing facility

Competency: A measure of an individual's mental processes

Congregate housing: Encompasses a multitude of different options, including independent living units, adult congregate living facilities, rental retirement housing, and senior retirement centers

Conservator: A person appointed to make financial, investment, and property decisions for another

Contracture: A condition generally caused by joint immobilization that results in decreased range of motion, stiffening and subsequent structural changes, and pain on movement at one or more joints

Crystallized intelligence: Intelligence that tends to remain strong in those who are aging typically, and includes skills such as language comprehension, educational qualifications, and life and occupational skills

D

Dementia: Progressive cognitive impairment that eventually interferes with daily functioning. The prevalence of dementia among 60-year-olds is only 1–2% but it becomes increasingly more common with advancing age

Demographics of aging: Study of vital statistics of the aging population including size, growth, density, and distribution

Depression: A mood disorder that is characterized by loss of interest in living. Symptoms that accompany depression can include sadness, hopelessness, loss of energy, tearfulness, loss of appetite, insomnia, and/or excessive sleep

Diabetes: A term used to describe any disorder characterized by excessive urine excretion. There are a number of different types of diabetes

Diabetes mellitus: A condition in which there is insufficient insulin. This can lead to elevated blood glucose levels

Dietary fiber: Nonnutrients that are considered important as a part of a healthy balanced diet because of their crucial role in health maintenance, disease management, and as a component of medical nutrition therapy

Discrimination: The act of exhibiting prejudicial behavior

Diuretics: A class of drugs used to promote fluid excretion

Diverticulosis: The development of small sacs where the large intestinal lining has herniated through the intestinal muscular wall

Durable financial power of attorney (DFPOA): Durable implies that the power of attorney document remains valid after the principal becomes incapacitated

Dysphagia: Difficulty swallowing

Dyspraxia: A decreased ability to plan and/or execute purposeful movements

E

Elderly, elders: Refers to older persons

Embolism: The blockage of an artery by a blood clot or other foreign material such as air or fat

Emphysema: A loss of functional elastic tissue in the lungs, resulting in the loss of alveolar wall surface area and the premature collapsing of small bronchioles during exhalation

Empowerment: Related to independence, or perhaps more aptly stated, freedom. It relates not only to people's ability, but also to the right to make choices affecting their own lives

Endurance: The ability to sustain involvement in a physical activity

Episodic memory: Memory oriented toward the past. This is what most people think of when they think of the global term *memory*. This type of declarative or conscious memory particularly involves remembering episodes or experiences in our lives (e.g., what we ate for lunch, our last birthday party)

Essential nutrients: The six classes of nutrients humans need to consume to be healthy: carbohydrates, proteins, fats, vitamins, minerals, and water

Exchanges for meal planning: A method that sorts foods into groups according to their carbohydrate, protein, fat, and calorie content

F

Failure to thrive: A condition in which a person fails to gain weight or in which the person loses weight

Fecal incontinence: The inability to voluntarily control defecation, largely because of the weakening of the external anal sphincter muscle

Fictive kin: When a niece or a nephew takes on the social role of a child, or a sibling takes on some of the traditional roles of a spouse

Fiduciary: A person who has legal authority and responsibility to make decisions for another

Fluid intelligence: Intelligence that involves the speed and accuracy of information processing, such as discrimination, comparison, and categorization. It has been deemed to be largely evolutionarily and genetically based

Free radicals: Molecules that contain at least one unpaired electron in their outer valence shells. Free radicals most notably form in the mitochondria of cells, the site of aerobic respiration

G

Gastritis: Inflammation of the stomach lining

Gastrointestinal: Refers to stomach, small intestine, and large intestine

Geriatric care managers (GCMs): Independently employed professionals who are commonly licensed as nurses or social workers

Geriatrics: A medical term for the study, diagnosis, and treatment of diseases and health problems specific to older adults

Gerontology: The scientific study of aging that examines the biological, psychological, and sociological factors (biopsychosocial) associated with old age and aging

Gerotranscendence: Associated with wisdom and a moving away from early and midlife materialism

Glucose tolerance: One's ability to maintain normal blood glucose

Grantor: The person who signs a trust document and establishes a trust

Guardian: A person (usually a family member) who is designated to make personal decisions for an incapacitated person, usually in the realm of medical, care, and residential issues

Guardian ad litem: A person appointed by the court to take legal action on behalf of one who cannot do this for him- or herself

H

Health literacy: The degree to which a person has the capacity to obtain, process, and understand basic health information and services needed to make appropriate health decisions

Healthy People 2010: A strategic plan set forth by the U.S. Department of Health and Human Services, the Healthy People Consortium, and other federal agencies to focus on preventable health threats (including disability and death) that affect citizens of all ages

Health Resources and Services Administration: A governmental organization that offers freely accessible online training in multiple areas, including health care literacy

Heat stroke: A condition caused by excessive exposure to heat in which the body temperature becomes dangerously elevated

Heterogeneous: Mixed, or consisting of dissimilar elements or parts

Home health care: Skilled health care provided to patients in the home

Hydrophilicity: Having a strong affinity for water molecules

Hyposmia: A decrease or diminished sense of smell

I

Incapacity: When illness and accidents leave a person unable to understand what is involved in a particular decision or unable to make and communicate his or her desires

Independent living: Maintaining living arrangements in one's lifetime home

Infantilizing: Negative portrayal of older adults that encourages dependency because it devalues the individual and does not foster independence. For example, referring to an unfamiliar older patient as "honey" or "dear"

Insomnia: The inability to fall asleep and/or abnormal wakefulness

J

Joint Commission: Organization that establishes standards of quality and performance as well as accreditation for health care organizations

L

Lactose intolerance: An inability to break down milk sugar, the carbohydrate (lactose) found in many dairy products

Learned helplessness: A condition that develops when living beings learn that their responses are independent of desired outcomes. Consequently, they learn to not respond to stimulation from their environments. For example, in experiments when dogs learn they cannot control the onset of electric shocks, they eventually give up and become helpless and apathetic

Lipid: A fat or fatlike substance, including fatty acids, neutral fats, waxes, and steroids

Lipofuscin: Fatty pigments found in aging cells

Lipophilicity: An affinity for fat

Long-term care: An array of long-term services and supports used by people who need assistance to function in their daily lives. It can include personal care, rehabilitation, social services, assistive technology, health care, home modifications, care coordination, assisted transportation, and more

Long-term care insurance (LTCI): Insurance that provides payment, or supplementary payment, for long-term care

Long-term care plan: A plan for the possible need for assisted living or nursing home care

Long-term memory: Permanent or long-term storage, for example, autobiographic information, early life experiences, or repetitive information

M

Malnutrition: A condition in which one suffers from a poorly balanced diet or has a deficiency in the digestive system

Maximum life span potential (MLP): The oldest age reached by an individual in a population

Maximum muscle strength: Muscular strength that tends to occur in early adulthood, whereas middle age is generally a time of only slight decline

Medicaid: A program jointly sponsored by the states and the federal government to provide health care for those who cannot finance their own medical expenses

Medicare: A federal program that provides health care for those age 65 and older and those with long-term disabilities

Medication-related problems: Events or circumstances involving a patient's drug treatment that actually, or potentially, interfere with the achievement of an optimal outcome

Mediterranean diet: A diet rich in fruits, vegetables, and healthy fats such as olive oil. It is thought to help reduce the risks of heart disease

Menopause: Refers to that time in life when menstruation ceases

Mild cognitive impairment (MCI): More serious cognitive losses that may portend the diagnosis of Alzheimer's disease (AD); those with MCI are at higher risk of developing AD

Monounsaturated fat: Fats, such as olive, peanut, and canola oils. They tend to be more liquid at room temperature

Motor coordination: Refers to fine and gross motor skills such as writing, self-feeding, and walking/running

Myocardial infarction: Blockage of the coronary arteries that can cause tissue death to part of the heart (a heart attack)

N

Naturally occurring retirement community (NORC): A neighborhood or building in which a large segment of the residents are older adults. In general, they are not purpose-built senior housing or retirement communities and were neither designed nor intended to meet the particular health and social services wants and needs of older adults

O

Obstructive sleep apnea (OSA): A cessation of breathing that, when the trachea is either totally or partially obstructed, causes the body's oxygen level to drop

Old-age dependency ratio: This refers to the number of people in the population older than 65 years as compared with those between the ages of 18 and 64 years

Old-old: Refers to those older than age 75 whose activities are often limited by functional disabilities

Older adult: A term used to describe people age 65 and older and the preferred term when speaking about aged individuals

Older Americans Act (OAA): Legislation passed in 1965 to specifically address the needs and rights of older adults. The OOA continues to be reauthorized and is expected to be reauthorized indefinitely. It is one piece of legislation that represents the United States' commitment to promoting the rights and welfare of older adults

Olfaction: Sense of smell

Orientation: Awareness of self, surroundings, and time

Osteoarthritis: A degenerative joint disease that is the second most common cause of disability in this country, affecting more than 27 million Americans

Osteoporosis: A disease in which bones become frail, making them more likely to fracture; disease is four times more common in women than in men

P

Peptic ulcer: An ulceration of the stomach, esophagus, or duodenum caused by gastric acid

Perception: The ability to make sense of incoming sensory information

Personality: Traits, behaviors, and qualities particular to an individual

Pharmacodynamics: The biological effects resulting from the interaction between a drug and its receptor site, and generally describes the relationship between plasma drug concentrations and an observed effect or response

Pharmacokinetics: The study of how drugs travel through the body over time. It deals with all aspects of drug disposition in the body, including *absorption* from the administration site, *distribution* into various body compartments, and *clearance* from the body

Plain language: Everyday or conversational language

Plain language standards: Standards of simple language for clients published by organizations such as the National Institute for Aging

Point size: Font size or typeface

Polypharmacy: Refers to the use of multiple medications in one individual

Polyunsaturated fat: Fats that are liquid at room temperature and that are found in plant products; examples are corn, safflower, and sunflower oils

Postural hypotension: A fall in systemic blood pressure upon rising from a supine to a standing position (usually too quickly)

Power of attorney (POA): The legal document setting out the legal authority of the agent to act for the principal

Power of attorney for health care (POAHC): Same as POA but specific to health care

Praxis: The ability to carry out purposeful motor actions

Presbycusis: The most common form of sensorineural hearing loss in adults

Presbyopia: A condition in which molecular changes render the lens less elastic and more rigid, which significantly impairs accommodation and thus the ability to focus on near objects

Primary memory: This type of memory has limited capacity and is used for information that is either used or generally forgotten in a matter of seconds

Procedural memory: Memory that is performance based, for example, remembering how to ride a bicycle or the motoric steps to completing a recipe or self-care task. Because these tasks are often overlearned and have become automatic, this type of memory is often maintained into old age

Prospective memory: This relates to remembering to do something in the future (e.g., appointments, medications, meetings, chores)

R

Range of motion: The ability of a joint to move through its natural pattern of movement

Rehabilitation: The process of helping someone regain his or her highest possible level of functioning after an injury or illness

Residential care facilities: Facilities that can have multiple labels, including adult residential facilities, adult group homes, domiciliary homes, personal care homes, family care, adult foster care, rest homes, board and care homes, and assisted living facilities

Restless leg syndrome (RLS): A neurological disorder including "creepy crawly feelings" or other unpleasant sensations in the legs usually while in bed

Retirement: That period of time after one retires from a work-related occupation

Reverse mortgage: A program that allows borrowers to use their home as collateral, and the bank sets up either an annuity or a line of credit to be used as needed until the home is sold or the loan repaid. This allows those with inadequate monthly income, but substantial home equity, to continue to reside in their own homes

Revocable living trust (RLT): A trust in which the grantor can be the initial trustee and the initial beneficiary

S

Sandwich generation: Adults caught between two caregiving roles, that of caring for older parents and caring for their own children

Saturated fat: Fats that are solid at room temperature and are primarily found in animal foods

Scotoma: An area of decreased vision (blind spots) surrounded by normal vision

Self-efficacy: The beliefs that each of us holds about the level of control we have over our future. Those who have strong self-efficacy, or internal locus of control, feel empowered to shape the future of their lives

Semantic memory: Involves a cumulative knowledge base about the world in general (e.g., language, including the meaning of words and the relationship of words, mathematical facts, symbols and formulas, vocational information learned during one's career, and recall of current events and worldly facts)

Senescence: Deleterious changes that occur as a result of the aging process

Sensory deficits: Common occurrence with aging that involves a diminishment or defect in one or more senses

Shame-free environment: Creating an environment that assures safety and encourages questions

Short-term memory: Involves remembering information for a short duration. An example of normal short-term memory is being able to recall a 7-digit number (for example, a telephone number) for a few minutes

Single-room occupancy (SRO) unit: Subsidized housing unit for individuals with very low incomes. These single-room units are usually found in cities and offer shared bathroom and kitchen facilities

Skilled care: A term used to describe services requiring a high level of skill that can only be provided by credentialed professionals to ensure safe and effective care

Sleep hygiene: Involves those activities and habits that are conducive to sleeping soundly

Sleep restriction: Refers to restricting one's time in bed

Social roles: Roles that define an individual's position in the community and dictate basic behaviors within social groups such as families, workplaces, and communities

Social Security: A major source of income for older adults in the United States. Ninety percent of older adults collected Social Security in 2004. The Social Security Act was signed into law by President Franklin D. Roosevelt in 1935

Stereotypes: A person, group, or event that is thought to conform, in a very formulaic manner, characteristic, belief, or pattern

Stimulus control: Refers to regulating the amount of time spent in bed, in this case, attempting to get to sleep or back to sleep

Stroke: Infarction in the brain that can occur as a result of occlusion or rupture of a cerebral artery

Suicide: The deliberate taking of one's life

Supplemental nutrition: Liquid nutrition products such as Ensure, Boost, and Glucerna that can help correct inadequacies in several areas

T

Teach-back: Refers to having the client state what he or she just heard and what he or she is supposed to do

Third-agers: French method of categorizing elderly persons 65 to 85 years of age

Thrombus: A stationary blood clot

Trust: The document that establishes the rules by which property will be managed for the benefit of another

Trustee: The person who administers the trust by following the rules in the trust

U

Uniform Health Care Decisions Act: A law that addresses the situation when a patient is incapacitated, unable to make or communicate a health care decision, and has no signed health care directive such as a power of attorney for health care or a court-appointed guardian

Universal design: The design of products and environments to be usable by all people, to the greatest extent possible, without the need for adaptation or specialized design

Urinary incontinence: The loss of voluntary control of micturition

V

Vision: The ability or act of seeing

Volunteerism: Proactive involvement in helping others without seeking payment or other forms of compensation

W

Working memory: Actively using or manipulating the information from this (short-term) storage base. For example, recalling the telephone number and actually dialing the number to make a call (one must retain the number while dialing)

X

Xerostomia: A condition in which dryness of the mouth occurs as a result of salivary gland dysfunction

Y

Young-age dependency ratio: The ratio of those younger than age 18 to those between the ages 18 and 64

Young-old: Denotes relatively healthy and financially independent older adults of any age, although usually referring to those between 55 and 74 years of age

INDEX